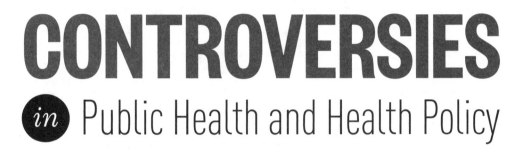

CONTROVERSIES

in Public Health and Health Policy

Jan K. Carney, MD, MPH

Associate Dean for Public Health
Professor of Medicine
University of Vermont College of Medicine
Burlington, VT

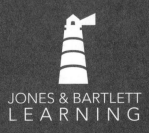

JONES & BARTLETT
LEARNING

World Headquarters
Jones & Bartlett Learning
5 Wall Street
Burlington, MA 01803
978-443-5000
info@jblearning.com
www.jblearning.com

Jones & Bartlett Learning books and products are available through most bookstores and online booksellers. To contact Jones & Bartlett Learning directly, call 800-832-0034, fax 978-443-8000, or visit our website, www.jblearning.com.

Substantial discounts on bulk quantities of Jones & Bartlett Learning publications are available to corporations, professional associations, and other qualified organizations. For details and specific discount information, contact the special sales department at Jones & Bartlett Learning via the above contact information or send an email to specialsales@jblearning.com.

Production Credits

VP, Executive Publisher: David D. Cella
Publisher: Michael Brown
Associate Editor: Nicholas Alakel
Associate Production Editor: Rebekah Linga
Senior Marketing Manager: Sophie Fleck Teague
Manufacturing and Inventory Control Supervisor:
  Amy Bacus

Composition: CAE Solutions Corp.
Cover Design: Kristin E. Parker
Rights and Media Manager: Joanna Lundeen
Media Development Editor: Shannon Sheehan
Rights and Media Research Coordinator: Mary Flatley
Printing and Binding: Edwards Brothers Malloy
Cover Printing: Edwards Brothers Malloy

Library of Congress Cataloging-in-Publication Data
Carney, Jan K., author.
  Controversies in public health and health policy / Jan K. Carney.
    p. ; cm.
  Includes bibliographical references and index.
  ISBN 978-1-284-04929-9 (paper)
  I. Title.
  [DNLM: 1. Health Policy--United States. 2. Public Health--United States. WA 540 AA1]
  RA393
  362.1--dc23
                                                            2015011869

6048

Printed in the United States of America
19 18 17 16 15   10 9 8 7 6 5 4 3 2 1

DEDICATION

To Mom—Margaret Emma Cline Carney—the smartest and most fun person I know—for always being there.

To Dad—Hallidae Kirk Carney, DDS—for your hard work, integrity, and . . . a sense of humor.

To Geoff—husband, dad, doctor, and chef extraordinaire.

To Ali—resolver of the arts and sciences.

To Sydney—sunshine and laughter—creative and strong.

To Geoffrey—science and arts, music and heart, swift and sure-footed.

To Nan—my only sister, whom I love and admire.

To Ham and Elmore—woof, woof, wag, wag—best dogs ever.

CONTENTS

PREFACE

Controversies in Public Health and Health Policy is designed to teach public health and health policy to a variety of audiences through the study of controversies.

Why study controversies? Public health issues don't often emerge in an orderly way. Sometimes they creep up on us and only then become obvious, such as the story of obesity in the United States. Other times, they have a dramatic entrance, as in examples of some antibiotic-resistant infections, or outbreaks of vaccine-preventable diseases. At other times, public health issues are enduring, such as ongoing challenges in improving mental health care or the social and economic factors determining our health.

Although this approach may seem like teaching and learning in reverse, many health issues only become obvious to the general public, public health and healthcare professionals, or policymakers as controversies. Controversies may be political or economic, or they may stem from scientific debate or not enough research, such as the history of firearm injuries.

Sometimes controversies help by raising awareness of immediate health crises. Other times they may hinder progress by sustaining inaction. In this book, controversies are *intentionally* presented in a way that highlights the breadth and resulting challenges, from myriad points of view.

Chapter topics reflect controversies in selected and significant public health and health policy topics. Many connect public health and health care, an important perspective given the Patient Protection and Affordable Care Act (ACA) and health system changes in the United States. Many health issues and their solutions are particularly challenging in different geographic areas, age groups, or among diverse social, economic, ethnic, and cultural groups, whether in the United States or on a global scale.

Some topics are recent and complex, such as health issues from climate change, E-cigarettes, or concussions in sports. Some health issues are so pervasive they risk becoming normalized in today's society—consider trends in adult obesity or binge drinking on college campuses.

Additionally, some public health issues require study over a longer time period to gain valuable insights. For example, it is difficult to examine current HIV prevention and treatment strategies apart from the history of HIV and AIDS. Similarly, the history of prescription drug abuse has deep roots in policy designed to alleviate pain and suffering. Today's controversies in health care for our nation's veterans are intertwined with their specific health needs and our changing healthcare system.

The textbook uses a structured format to examine each controversy and includes background, evidence base, discussion questions, and additional learning resources, challenging readers to consider public health and health policy by exploring these controversies and the issues behind them. For these public health and health policy issues, there is no simple answer. *Controversies* promotes self-learning, allowing readers to think for themselves and come to their own conclusions.

It is essential to remember why public health is so important, whether as a student, healthcare or public health professional, researcher, advocate, policymaker, or citizen. Public health uses a population approach and prevention strategies to protect and improve health, but public health's mission is improving the health and lives of *people*. Ultimately, if enough individuals use their combined public health knowledge, perhaps we *can* make progress on the far-too-challenging, complex, and controversial issues so important to the health of the public.

ABOUT THE AUTHOR

Dr. Jan K. Carney, MD, MPH is Associate Dean for Public Health and Professor of Medicine at the University of Vermont College of Medicine. She earned an AB from Middlebury College, an MD from the University of Cincinnati College of Medicine, and Master of Public Health (MPH) at the Harvard School of Public Health. Prior to her full-time faculty appointment at the University of Vermont College of Medicine, she served as Vermont's Commissioner of Health from 1989–2003, under three gubernatorial administrations, and participated in the design and implementation of a broad range of public health and health policy initiatives. At the University of Vermont College of Medicine, she is active in public health and health policy education; research, practice, and service; and also directs the University of Vermont's graduate programs in public health. She is also the author of *Public Health in Action: Practicing in the Real World*.

CHAPTER 1

Health vs. Health Care

LEARNING OBJECTIVES

- Compare health outcomes in the United States and their trends over time to 16 peer countries.
- Identify the "actual" causes of death in the United States.
- Describe all determinants of health and their proportional impact on the health of people in the United States.
- Compare, contrast, and critically assess public health models outlined by the Institute of Medicine.
- Discuss the role of socioeconomic factors on health, including the role of geographic location.
- Identify strategies to improve health outcomes in the United States.

THE CONTROVERSY

"U.S. health is *lousy* compared with peer nations," one newswriter says[1] reporting on a 2013 report from the U.S. National Research Council (NRC) and the Institute of Medicine (IOM), called *U.S. Health in International Perspective: Shorter Lives, Poorer Health.*[2] Another reporter asked, "What's ailing America?"[3] The committee chair overseeing the report's development summarized its findings simply as, "It's a tragedy."[3] The report's title describes the situation exactly, with the IOM president and NRC executive director writing, "The United States spends much more money on health care than any other county. Yet Americans die sooner and experience more illness than residents in many other countries."[2] An article in *The Atlantic* further lamented that, "Americans' health is even worse than we thought, ranking below 16 other developed nations."[4]

What is this report? What did it say? Why are Americans so unhealthy? This particular study was commissioned after another report issued earlier by the NRC in 2011[5] compared life expectancy in middle-aged Americans with 50 year olds in other high-income countries and found that U.S. life expectancy ranked behind other countries. The Office of Behavioral and Social Sciences Research (OBSSR) of the National Institutes of Health (NIH) asked the NRC and IOM—both prominent U.S. organizations—to join forces in order to study the factors behind health differences in high-income countries.[2]

A variety of health status measures were used to compare the United States to 16 other "peer" countries, focusing on the time period from the 1990s to 2008. In addition to shorter life expectancy, Americans had worse health outcomes in a variety of areas; these findings were seen even within higher socioeconomic groups in the United States compared to people in other peer countries.[2] One of the report's authors pondered whether our country's emphasis on individual freedom, characterized as "live free *and* die," might be contributing to these poor health findings.[4] Others called for immediate action, emphasizing that "mobilization of an unprecedented kind is now necessary in the United States."[6] *Shorter Lives, Poorer Health*[2] implicated factors beyond health care, such as behaviors, environmental conditions, and social and economic factors. However, one U.S. senator dismissed these, remarking that the Affordable Care Act "addresses many of these primary causes," while other members of Congress did not seem to notice the report at all.[4]

BACKGROUND AND SCOPE OF THE PUBLIC HEALTH AND HEALTH POLICY ISSUE

Health in the United States—Higher Costs and Worse Outcomes

Is it new news that the United State lags behind many other countries in our collective health? Not really. In 2000, the World Health Organization issued a 215-page report: *Health Systems: Improving Performance*,[7] which ranked the U.S. healthcare system 37th in the world.[8] In 2006, although the United States ranked number one in healthcare spending (per capita), it performed poorly on basic measures of health status, such as infant mortality (39th), adult female mortality (43rd), adult male mortality (42nd), and life expectancy (36th).[8] The authors asked, "Why do we spend so much to get so little?"[8] Not only was the U.S. ranking poor when compared to other countries, any improvements that were seen (e.g., mortality among males aged 15 to 60) happened more slowly than similar improvements in other countries.[8] Although lack of health insurance was part of the explanation, potentially preventable conditions also likely contribute, including smoking-related diseases, hypertension, obesity, physical inactivity, elevated blood glucose and blood lipids, all risks for chronic conditions, premature death, and increased healthcare costs.[8] Different populations within the United States as well as people living in different geographic regions had different rates of risk factors for chronic conditions.[8]

The 2013 publication by the IOM and NRC, *U.S. Health in International Perspective: Shorter Lives, Poorer Health,*[2] used extensive data and trends (from the 1990s to 2008) to highlight differences and illustrate the complexities of what determines the health of the U.S. population, something often oversimplified in a discussion of health insurance. Life expectancy in the United States is shorter than our peer (high-income) countries, and is also noted in different age groups.[2] Contrary to popular perception, differences in the health status of racial and ethnic minority populations or lower income individuals in the United States are not enough to explain these results; health differences between the United States and other peer countries are also seen in wealthier and more educated U.S. populations.[2]

Health status measures, also called health outcomes, were compared in 16 countries: Australia, Austria, Canada, Denmark, Finland, France, Germany, Italy, Japan, Norway, Portugal, Spain, Sweden, Switzerland, the Netherlands, and the United Kingdom.[2] In a commonly used measure of population health status, life expectancy at birth (in 2007) for men in the United States ranked 17th (of 17 countries), with an average length of life of 75.64 years, in contrast to men in Switzerland (ranked 1st) where men live an average of 79.33 years. For women in the United States, average length of life is 80.78 years, ranked 16th, in comparison to women in Japan, ranked 1st, who live an average of 85.98 years. Furthermore, the differences in life expectancy between the United States and other countries has become worse over the past 30 years[2] (see **Figures 1–1** and **1–2**).

The term "health disadvantage" describes the differences between the U.S. population and peer countries for all age groups (under age 75).[2] People in the United States who reach age 50 have worse health than their peers in other countries, and although lower socioeconomic populations experience a large share of poor outcomes, this "health disadvantage" is seen in all socioeconomic groups in the United States, including those with the highest levels of income and education.[2] Another interesting observation is that people who were born in the United States have worse health than people who have recently immigrated to this country, suggesting more complex and systemic reasons for observed health differences.[2] After age 75, people in the United States survive longer, have higher screening

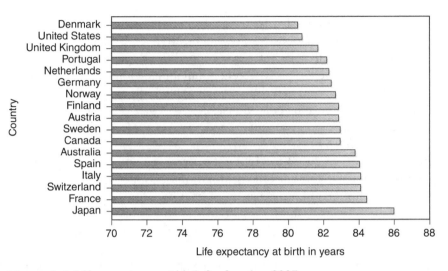

Figure 1–1 Life expectancy at birth for females, 2007.

Data from *U.S. Health in International Perspective: Shorter Lives, Poorer Health.*
The National Academies Press; 2013. Table 1–3; p.39. http://www.nap.edu/catalog.php?
record_id=13497

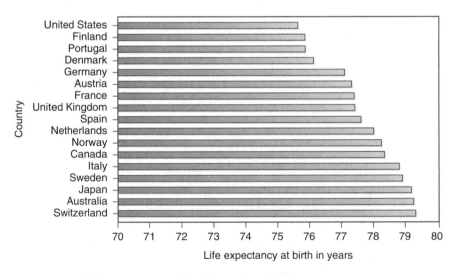

Figure 1–2 Life expectancy at birth for males, 2007.

Data from *U.S. Health in International Perspective: Shorter Lives, Poorer Health.*
The National Academies Press; 2013. Table 1–3; p.39. http://www.nap.edu/catalog.php?
record_id=13497

rates for some cancers, better control of cardiovascular risk factors (such as blood pressure and smoking), and access to life-saving care for some conditions.[2] Nine categories where U.S. health outcomes are worse than comparison countries include: infant mortality and low birth weight; injuries and homicides; teen pregnancy; HIV and AIDS; deaths from drug and alcohol abuse; obesity and diabetes; health disease; chronic lung disease; arthritis; and disability.[2]

Possible Explanations

Differences between the United States and other high-income countries could not likely be explained by a "single factor."[2] For example, lack of health insurance and financial access to primary and preventive care may contribute to some differences, but this alone is not enough to explain higher rates of injuries and homicides seen in the United States.[2] Smoking and obesity may also contribute, but higher rates of diseases (such as heart disease and diabetes) were seen in the United States, even in people without such risk factors.[2] On average, compared to peer countries, Americans eat more, have more firearms, don't wear seat belts, drink and drive, have higher rates of poverty (especially for children), are more likely uninsured, lack access to social services, or do not live in an environment that supports physical activity or access to nutritious food, all compared to other peer countries.[2] Unfortunately, there is no "quick fix" for these problems, and the authors of this report called for a systemic understanding of social, education, transportation, health care and other policies that can together promote better health in the United States.[2] A national campaign to educate the public, greater use of existing health objectives, and evidence-based approaches were all recommended, with the worry that health differences between the United States and peer countries will continue to worsen in future years, unless immediate actions are taken.[2]

What Really Kills Us?

In the United States, the Centers for Disease Control and Prevention (CDC), through its National Center for Health Statistics (NCHS) and Web-Based Injury Statistics Query and Reporting System (WISQARS) publishes annual summaries of leading causes of death and injury, including statistics by age group. For 2011, NCHS reported the leading causes of death

Rank	<1	1–4	5–9	10–14	15–24	25–34	35–44	45–54	55–64	65+	Total
					Age Groups						
1	Congenital Anomalies 5,013	Unintentional Injury 1,337	Unintentional Injury 761	Unintentional Injury 874	Unintentional Injury 12,330	Unintentional Injury 15,518	Unintentional Injury 15,230	Malignant Neoplasms 48,897	Malignant Neoplasms 112,572	Heart Disease 475,097	Heart Disease 596,577
2	Short Gestation 4,106	Congenital Anomalies 493	Malignant Neoplasms 441	Malignant Neoplasms 419	Suicide 4,822	Suicide 6,100	Malignant Neoplasms 11,717	Heart Disease 36,100	Heart Disease 69,742	Malignant Neoplasms 397,106	Malignant Neoplasms 576,691
3	SIDS 1,910	Homicide 412	Congenital Anomalies 182	Suicide 282	Homicide 4,554	Homicide 4,185	Heart Disease 10,635	Unintentional Injury 20,749	Unintentional Injury 15,158	Chronic Low. Respiratory Disease 121,869	Chronic Low. Respiratory Disease 142,943
4	Maternal Pregnancy Comp. 1,591	Malignant Neoplasms 353	Homicide 129	Congenital Anomalies 176	Malignant Neoplasms 1,611	Malignant Neoplasms 3,499	Suicide 6,599	Liver Disease 8,864	Chronic Low. Respiratory Disease 15,044	Cerebro-vascular 109,323	Cerebro-vascular 128,932
5	Unintentional Injury 1,163	Heart Disease 165	Heart Disease 92	Homicide 154	Heart Disease 998	Heart Disease 3,301	Homicide 2,519	Suicide 8,858	Diabetes Mellitus 12,688	Alzheimer's Disease 84,032	Unintentional Injury 126,438
6	Placenta Cord. Membranes 1,004	Influenza & Pneumonia 112	Chronic Low. Respiratory Disease 64	Heart Disease 111	Congenital Anomalies 432	Diabetes Mellitus 686	Liver Disease 2,449	Diabetes Mellitus 6,012	Cerebro-vascular 11,205	Diabetes Mellitus 52,402	Alzheimer's Disease 84,974
7	Bacterial Sepsis 526	Septicemia 61	Influenza & Pneumonia 63	Chronic Low Respiratory Disease 72	Influenza & Pneumonia 220	HIV 666	Diabetes Mellitus 1,842	Cerebro-vascular 5,705	Liver Disease 10,749	Influenza & Pneumonia 45,386	Diabetes Mellitus 73,831
8	Respiratory Distress 513	Chronic Low Respiratory Disease 53	Benign Neoplasms 40	Influenza & Pneumonia 55	Cerebro-vascular 186	Cerebro-vascular 530	Cerebro-vascular 1,718	Chronic Low. Respiratory Disease 4,634	Suicide 6,521	Unintentional Injury 43,258	Influenza & Pneumonia 53,826
9	Circulatory System Disease 500	Benign Neoplasms 45	Cerebro-vascular 40	Cerebro-vascular 47	Complicated Pregnancy 172	Influenza & Pneumonia 515	HIV 1,619	HIV 2,781	Septicemia 4,953	Nephritis 37,796	Nephritis 45,591
10	Neonatal Hemorrhage 456	Cerebro-vascular 42	Septicemia 38	Septicemia 31	Chronic Low. Respiratory Disease 170	Liver Disease 505	Influenza & Pneumonia 859	Septicemia 2,461	Nephritis 4,754	Septicemia 26,746	Suicide 39,518

Figure 1–3 Ten leading causes of death by age group, United States – 2011.

Reproduced from Centers for Disease Control and Prevention: Injury Prevention and Control: Data & Statistics: Ten Leading Causes of Death and Injury, 2011. Available at http://www.cdc.gov/injury/wisqars/LeadingCauses_images.html http://www.cdc.gov/injury/wisqars/leadingcauses.html

as: heart disease (596,577 deaths); cancer (576,691 deaths); chronic lower respiratory diseases (lung disease; 142,943 deaths); stroke (cerebrovascular disease; 128,932 deaths); accidents (unintentional injuries; 126,438 deaths); Alzheimer's disease (84,974 deaths); diabetes (73,881 deaths); nephritis, nephrotic syndrome, and nephrosis (kidney diseases; 45,591 deaths); influenza and pneumonia (53,826 deaths); suicide (39,518 deaths)[9,10] (see **Figure 1–3**).

The top 10 leading causes of death in the United States, for all ages, reflect summaries of deaths collected in vital records and reported from all states in the United States.[10] This type of data has many practical uses, such as determining the magnitude of different causes of death and their trends over time, whether in response to new diseases and conditions, medical improvements, or demographic changes in the overall population. In 1993, in a very novel approach, McGinnis and Foege published a paper called *Actual Causes of Death in the United States*.[11] Instead of using the disease and medical conditions causing deaths, they quantified the impact of underlying risk factors for these deaths by searching for and using high-quality published studies to calculate estimates of "actual" causes of death.[11] In 1990, the leading contributors to death in the United States were tobacco (estimated 400,000 deaths), diet and activity (300,000 deaths), alcohol (100,000), microbial agents (90,000), toxic agents (60,000), firearms (35,000), sexual behavior (30,000), motor vehicle deaths (25,000), and illegal drug use (20,000).[11] In total, these factors, which all represent potentially preventable conditions, contributed to about half of all deaths in the United States in 1990.[11] The impact of social and economic factors could not be determined in this study, but quantifying the "actual causes of death" highlighted the missed opportunities and enormous potential for prevention in the United States each year.[11]

This study, using similar methods, was repeated 10 years later, for all deaths in the United States in the year 2000.[12] In a 10-year period, tobacco was still the leading actual cause of death, causing 18.1% of the total U.S. deaths (435,000), poor diet and physical inactivity (sedentary behaviors) were next, causing 15.2% of United States deaths (365,000), and alcohol consumption caused 3.5% of U.S. deaths (85,000).[12] The growing contribution of poor diet and physical inactivity to deaths in the United States reflect the worsening obesity epidemic, and the authors argue that in the face of rising healthcare costs, disease prevention is desperately needed in the United States.[12]

What Determines Health?

Public perception and media focus support the notion that health care is the primary determinant of health. Much scientific literature argues against this belief, recognizing that while access to quality health care is an essential determinant of our collective health, it is certainly not the only one, nor the most influential, despite how much the United States spends on health care per capita.[13] Determinants of health include our genetic predisposition to disease, our habits and behaviors (such as tobacco and alcohol use, the quality of our diet, and how active we are), access to health care, environmental factors (including the quality of the air we breathe and water we drink, as well as whether our environment hinders or promotes our health, such as in neighborhood designs), as well as social circumstances (where we live, our income and education).[13] In fact, estimates of the relative contributions to premature death in the United States emphasize the important contribution of behavioral patterns (contributing 40%), followed by our genetic predisposition (30%), social circumstances (15%), health care (10%), and environmental exposures (5%).[13] In a famous Shattuck lecture, Dr. Steven Schroeder explained, "First, the pathways to better health do not generally depend on health care, and second, even in those instances in which health care is important, too many Americans do not receive it, receive it too late, or receive poor-quality care."[14]

Experts generally agree that directly impacting our genetic make-up is difficult, if not impossible, however, we can sometimes limit genetic risks through our behavior, our environment, or access to health care.[14] Preventing tobacco use, obesity, and alcohol excess, all require behavior changes. Recent successful approaches to reducing smoking in the United States are cited as a potential model to help with other analogous but different health challenges, such as preventing obesity.[14] Successful tobacco reduction in the United States required a collective and sustained approach that included programs to help smokers quit, laws and policies to limit access to environmental tobacco smoke, educational initiatives to prevent children from using tobacco products, and price increases to reduce consumption, especially in young people.[14] However, many authors note tobacco's ongoing public health impact,[11,12] especially in less educated and lower income individuals, and as a major contributor to the premature death of people with mental illness in the United States.[14]

Changing demographics in the U.S. population also have public health implications. Since 1950, the U.S. population is more than twice as large (from 152.3 million to 308.7 million people).[15] As a whole, the population is getting older, with an increasing number of people aged 65 and older. This is significant because of the increased prevalence with age of many chronic conditions. As a consequence of population aging, ensuring that adequate numbers of healthcare professionals are available to care for the growing population of older individuals becomes a priority.[15] In addition, the racial and ethnic composition of the U.S. population is changing, becoming more diverse.[15] CDC highlights public health concerns in people living in mostly minority communities; they may experience higher risks for illness, have more challenges getting health care, and often have lower socioeconomic statuses.[16] Difference in deaths, illness, risk factors, and access to care have been widely documented. For example, risk for premature death from cardiovascular disease is higher in non-Hispanic black individuals than in whites; infant mortality in non-Hispanic black women is more than twice as high as in non-Hispanic white women; homicide rates are 665% higher in non-Hispanic black individuals when compared to non-Hispanic white individuals.[16] CDC regularly issues findings and recommendations for national public health strategies related to these changing demographic factors, such as *The State of Aging and Health in America 2013*[17] and the *CDC Health Disparities and Inequalities Report— United States, 2013.*[16]

Social and economic factors, and their influence on U.S. health, are both the most complex and controversial health determinants to study and influence. Americans with limited incomes in the United States often have higher rates of habits and behaviors associated with premature illness and death, but these alone are not sufficient to explain differences in health outcomes within the United States or compared with health status indicators in peer countries.[2,16] Using the National Heart, Lung, and Blood Institute's Atherosclerosis Risk in Communities Study, a study in four U.S. communities in North Carolina, Mississippi, Minneapolis, and Maryland, investigators studied characteristics of neighborhoods, including such factors as income, education, and occupation, and the subsequent risk of developing coronary heart disease.[18] For each neighborhood they studied, they developed a summary measure of the socioeconomic environment. After a period of 9 years, they found that people who lived in disadvantaged neighborhoods, even after adjusting for individual factors of income level, education, and occupations, and known risk factors for coronary heart disease, had higher risks for developing heart disease.[18] In other words, the socioeconomic characteristics of communities, in addition to individual risk factors, contributed to health differences.[18]

Other authors note substantial health variations within the United States. For example, white men in the 10 healthiest U.S. counties live an average of 76.4 years, compared to a life expectancy for black men in the least healthy U.S. counties, who have life expectancies of 61 years (Philadelphia), 60 years (Baltimore and New York), and 58 years (District of Columbia).[19] Using international comparisons, people with low income in the United States (despite the fact their incomes exceed those in many countries) may have poorer health status and shorter lives than people living in some poor countries internationally.[19] The Whitehall studies of British civil servants showed that deaths from both heart disease and all causes were inversely related to the social grade of employment.[19]

An elegant study of disease and social and economic factors in the United States and England tried to sort out some of the factors contributing to health differences between the United States and other countries.[20] This study focused on people aged 55 to 64 from the United States and England, using national surveys from each country that measured comparable indicators, and limited the study to non-Hispanic whites in both locations. The researchers measured rates of chronic conditions such as diabetes and heart disease, based on people's own reports, and also used actual biological measures (blood tests) for inflammation and cholesterol levels to ensure their findings were not due to differences in the two counties in how people perceived or defined their own illness.[20] The investigators found that when compared to the population in England, middle-aged people in the United States have higher rates of diabetes, high blood pressure, heart disease, myocardial infarction, stroke, lung disease, and cancer.[20] Furthermore, the differences in health between the two countries was not simply due to differences in rates of known risk factors for chronic diseases (i.e., smoking, obesity, alcohol). In both the United States and England, self-reported disease rates were highest in people with lowest income and education, and this relationship followed a "gradient" of socioeconomic factors.[20] The findings were still seen when the biological measures were used, and the authors concluded that, at every socioeconomic level, people in the United States were not as healthy as people in England.[20] Another study compared health outcomes for six chronic diseases in 10 European countries, with the results analyzed according to categories of income.[21] At all levels of income, people in the United States reported worse health than people in Europe, and differences were even worse among people in the United States with the lowest incomes.[21]

What Is Public Health? Who Is Responsible for Public Health?

"Public health is what we, as a society, do collectively to assure the conditions in which people can be healthy."[22] In 1988, the IOM published *The Future of Public Health* in response to a growing national concern that public health was not well understood, "in disarray," and not-at-all prepared to deal with current, emerging, and complex public health issues.[22] These findings presented a sharp contrast to improvements seen in many other areas due to public health measures, such as infectious diseases, safe drinking water, childhood immunizations, and others. The role of governmental public health agencies was carefully scrutinized, and despite the importance and role of private agencies, individuals, nonprofit organizations, and others in public health, this report concluded that "the governmental public health agency has a unique function: to see to it that vital elements are in place and that the mission is adequately addressed."[22] The core functions of public health agencies were defined as "assessment, policy development, and assurance,"[22] terms that remain resonant today in public health practice.

The role of government public health agencies continued to change, as public health issues evolved and future study committees expressed their findings. In 2003, the Institute of Medicine, in *The Future of the Public's Health in the 21st Century*,[23] reported that the role of government was no longer enough to ensure the public's health. Although the committee acknowledged that governmental agencies have the responsibility to "promote and protect" the health of the public, they could not do this alone. Public resources were shrinking, improving health required other sectors, and collaborative relationships were critical to improving health.[23] Their promotion of a new "intersectoral" public health system was designed to enhance the ability of governmental public health agencies to protect and improve health—still their designated responsibility. In this model, the governmental public health infrastructure, communities, academia, healthcare providers, employers, and businesses all shared responsibility for health.[23] Extensive recommendation were outlined in each of these areas. Some sectors continued to be natural partners, such as the ongoing connections of governmental public health agencies with health care, communities, and academia, whereas collaboration with others, such as business and the media, required new approaches.[24,25]

However, there are both tensions and opportunities in relationships between public health agencies and businesses. For example, the relationship between public health agencies and the tobacco and alcohol industries is often adversarial.[24] In addition, public health has many regulatory responsibilities that may prevent even preliminary discussion of partnerships with employers and businesses.[24] Furthermore, some authors cite challenges of communicating with diverse stakeholders, including the public, about public health. These authors argue that the first "language" of the United States is built on individualism and personal responsibility, and they emphasize the importance of developing and strengthening a "second language" in the United States, that better describes connections between the factors contributing to poor health and the strategies needed for current and pervasive public health issues.[26]

Centers for Disease Control and Prevention: Public Health Achievements and Threats

CDC has highlighted 10 great public health achievements from 1900 to 1999, which collectively added 25 years to the life expectancy of Americans.[27] These include immunizations, motor-vehicle safety, workplace safety, infectious disease prevention and control, reductions in deaths from heart disease and stroke, food safety, maternal and child health, family planning, water fluoridation, and decline in tobacco use.[27] For 2013, CDC cites achievements in public health related to a national media campaign that resulted in 200,000 Americans quitting smoking, advanced laboratory methods of detecting listeria, a cause of death from foodborne illness, public health role in the Million Hearts campaign, improved national tracking of healthcare-related infections, and international efforts to prevent HIV/AIDs, called the U.S. President's Emergency Plan for AIDS Relief (PEPFAR).[28] But also in 2013, they cite leading imminent health threats: antibiotic-resistant infections, prescription drug abuse, global health security, HPV and the need for vaccination, and polio.[28]

Community, state, national, and global collaboration and sustained and evidence-based public health efforts are both required as approaches for new threats and for public health successes. Although funding has been under repeated challenge,[29] many share optimism about new resources for public health through the Prevention and Public Health Fund created by the Patient Protection and Affordable Care Act (ACA)[30] and the National Prevention Strategy advanced by the National Prevention Council, also created by the ACA.[31]

EVIDENCE BASE FOR PREVENTION AND PRACTICE

Measuring Health Outcomes: *Healthy People 2020*

In 1990, the U.S. Public Health Service announced *Healthy People 2000*, measurable goals and objectives for the nation to improve the health of the public in many areas, such as immunizations, smoking rates, cancer screening, and many others, building on the first such initiative a decade prior.[32] Some authors noted that improvements in the delivery of clinical services were easier to achieve than changes in risky behaviors, such as tobacco and alcohol use, because changing behaviors required broader engagement of a variety of stakeholders and often controversial policy changes.[32] Evidence-based strategies are familiar for clinical preventive services,[33] but are less well known for community preventive services,[34] both of which use scientific evidence to make recommendations for individuals and populations respectively.

Decades after it was first used, *Healthy People 2020* continues as a national public health strategy to improve health through the use of measurable health outcomes, collaborative strategies, and policies.[35] Topics and objectives range from access to health services to oral health, nutrition, and health of older adults. Some *Healthy People 2020* areas emphasize clinical objectives (e.g., diabetes), whereas others (e.g., physical activity) require clinical and community prevention. There are a total of 42 topic areas and about 600 measurable objectives. Priority health areas, called *leading health indicators*, are measured and reported on a regular basis, and include such areas as maternal, infant, and child health; injuries and violence; social health determinants; and measures of nutrition, physical activity, and obesity,[35] all areas where the United States fares measurably worse than peer countries.[2] This approach, using measurable outcomes, is flexible, allowing states and communities to choose priority indicators that are the most important in their geographic areas. It is also strategic, promoting focus on the most pressing issues and setting priorities. In addition, the use of measurable health objectives (health outcomes) reflects collective actions, and supports the approaches described in the newest models of public health as well as approaches needed to best influence current public health issues.

DISCUSSION QUESTIONS: TEMPLATE FOR DISCUSSION

1. Significance of this public health issue:
   a. Why is this health issue important?
   b. How many people does it impact?
   c. How serious is it?
   d. Is it preventable?
2. What is the evidence base for prevention?
3. What specific strategies should be used to achieve progress on this health issue?
   a. What evidence-based approach would you use?
   b. Where would you start if you are an individual citizen; public health professional; healthcare professional; community, state, or federal policymaker?
4. Specific questions for this topic:
   a. How does health differ from health care?
   b. What approaches might be used to educate the public about determinants of health?
   c. How might the 2013 report *U.S. Health in International Perspective* be used as a catalyst for health improvements in the United States?

5. What is the controversy?
   a. Define the controversy.
   b. Is controversy a good or bad thing? (Does it help or hinder progress?)
6. *Why* is this health issue controversial?
   a. What specific factors are involved?
   b. Do economics, government, scientific uncertainty, or politics play a role?
   c. What is the role of the media?
7. How would you respond to the controversy?

PERSPECTIVES TO CONSIDER

The fundamental question is: Why isn't the IOM and NRC's *Shorter Lives, Poorer Health* report causing a national stir? Why aren't people talking about this in schools, communities, college campuses, state legislatures, in congress, and over coffee? Their question "Why do we spend so much and get so little?" remains unanswered.[8] Health is not the same as health care. Research comparing the United States to other similar countries, and especially to England,[20] is very revealing, and highlights the facts that health is dependent on health care and much, much more. Genetics and biology, habits and behaviors, our environment (whether effective in worsening or promoting good health), social and economic factors (education, income, housing, transportation and others), as well as access to health care (especially primary and preventive care) all determine our collective health.[13]

Improvements in all areas are desperately needed if we want better *health* in the United States. Why is this so difficult to accomplish? Some note that the language of public health explaining connections between education, services, programs, and policies relevant to health determinants is complicated, compared to talking about habits and behaviors or health care.[26] Others worry about the public health system itself, and the perpetual challenge for sufficient resources, a well-educated workforce, and the increasing dependence on accountability for health outcomes by organizations whose primary mission is not related to health. The authors of the *Shorter Lives, Poorer Health* report[2] note the need to evaluate policies, both health and social, the need for a national conversation about *health,* and a more systematic use of currently available national health metrics.

Continually challenged by needed improvements in critical health-related behaviors that require methods, models, programs, and policies external to health care, we need a **wide-angle lens**. Public and population health may be viewed through the lens of health care, rather than one that recognizes root causes of poor health and the need to partner with individuals, groups, and organizations that share the potential to change it. Focusing the public's attention on *health*, while we reform health care, and expand the use of population-based models of care, makes great sense. The use of measurable outcomes, such as *Healthy People 2020*,[35] on a national, regional, and local level, along with the systematic use of evidence-based public health and clinical prevention, might begin the collective shift in decades of worsening health in the United States. **The tested, but underutilized *Healthy People* model, uses evidence-based, measurable objectives to improve population health, linking prevention in individuals and populations. In addition, much of the data are readily available through CDC or health departments.**

Achieving 10-year outcomes requires partnerships in defined geographic or population settings, an approach easily applied to the geographic differences in health seen in many areas of the United States, with available tools such as health impact assessments (HIA).[36] Objectives for chronic disease management, clinical prevention, and habits and behaviors (40% of preventable mortality[13]), could easily be tied to data measures for healthcare quality. If we can embrace a broadened view of population health, we can achieve better health for patients and populations—all needed to improve our "dead last"[4] ranking.

FOR ADDITIONAL STUDY

Banks J, Marmot M, Oldfield Z, Smith JP. Disease and disadvantage in the United States and in England. *JAMA*. 2006;295(17):2037–2045.

REFERENCES

1. Brown E. U.S. health is lousy compared with peer nations, report says. *Los Angeles Times.* 2013. http://articles.latimes.com/2013/jan/09/news/la-heb-us-health-lags-peers-20130109. Accessed January 30, 2014.
2. *U.S. Health in International Perspective: Shorter Lives, Poorer Health.* Washington, DC: The National Academies Press; 2013.
3. Paramaguru K. What's ailing America? New report finds U.S. falls behind international peers in health and life expectancy. *Time.com.* 2013. http://newsfeed.time.com/2013/01/11/whats-ailing-america-new-report-finds-u-s-falls-behind-international-peers-in-health-and-life-expectancy/. Accessed January 29, 2014.
4. Rubenstein G. New health rankings: Of 17 nations, U.S. is dead last. *The Atlantic.* 2013. http://www.theatlantic.com/health/archive/2013/01/new-health-rankings-of-17-nations-us-is-dead-last/267045/. Accessed January 29, 2014.

5. *Explaining Divergent Levels of Longevity in High-Income Countries.* Washington, DC: The National Academies Press; 2011.

6. Bayer R, Fairchild AL, Hopper K, Nathanson CA. Public health: Confronting the sorry state of U.S. health. *Science.* 2013;341(6149):962–963.

7. WHO. The world health report 2000. 2000. http://www.who.int/whr/2000/en/whr00_en.pdf?ua=1. Accessed January 30, 2014.

8. Murray CJ, Frenk J. Ranking 37th—measuring the performance of the U.S. health care system. *N Engl J Med.* 2010;362(2):98–99.

9. CDC. FastStats: Leading causes of death. 2013. http://www.cdc.gov/nchs/fastats/lcod.htm. Accessed January 31, 2014.

10. CDC. Ten leading causes of death and injury. 2012. http://www.cdc.gov/injury/wisqars/LeadingCauses.html. Accessed January 31, 2014.

11. McGinnis JM, Foege WH. Actual causes of death in the United States. *JAMA.* 1993;270(18):2207–2212.

12. Mokdad AH, Marks JS, Stroup DF, Gerberding JL. Actual causes of death in the United States, 2000. *JAMA.* 2004;291(10):1238–1245.

13. McGinnis JM, Williams-Russo P, Knickman JR. The case for more active policy attention to health promotion. *Health Aff (Millwood).* 2002;21(2):78–93.

14. Schroeder SA. Shattuck Lecture. We can do better—improving the health of the American people. *N Engl J Med.* 2007;357(12):1221–1228.

15. Shrestha LB, Heisler EJ. The changing demographic profile of the United States: Congressional Research Service Report. 2011. http://fas.org/sgp/crs/misc/RL32701.pdf. Accessed August 14, 2014.

16. Frieden TR, CDC. CDC health disparities and inequalities report—United States, 2013. [Foreword]. *Morbidity and mortality weekly report. Surveillance summaries.* 2013;62(Suppl 3):1–2.

17. CDC. The state of aging and health in America 2013. 2013. http://www.cdc.gov/features/agingandhealth/state_of_aging_and_health_in_america_2013.pdf. Accessed August 14, 2014.

18. Diez Roux AV, Merkin SS, Arnett D, et al. Neighborhood of residence and incidence of coronary heart disease. *N Engl J Med.* 2001;345(2):99–106.

19. Marmot M. Inequalities in health. *N Engl J Med.* 2001;345(2):134–136.

20. Banks J, Marmot M, Oldfield Z, Smith JP. Disease and disadvantage in the United States and in England. *JAMA.* 2006;295(17):2037–2045.

21. Avendano M, Glymour MM, Banks J, Mackenbach JP. Health disadvantage in US adults aged 50 to 74 years: A comparison of the health of rich and poor Americans with that of Europeans. *Am J Public Health.* 2009;99(3):540–548.

22. *The Future of Public Health.* Washington, DC: The National Academies Press; 1988.

23. *The Future of the Public's Health in the 21st Century.* Washington, DC: The National Academies Press; 2003.

24. Simon PA, Fielding JE. Public health and business: A partnership that makes cents. *Health Aff (Millwood).* 2006;25(4):1029–1039.

25. Majestic E. Public health's inconvenient truth: The need to create partnerships with the business sector. *Prev Chronic Dis.* 2009;6(2):A39.

26. Wallack L, Lawrence R. Talking about public health: Developing America's "second language". *Am J Public Health.* 2005;95(4):567–570.

27. CDC. Ten great public health achievements in the 20th Century. 2013. http://www.cdc.gov/about/history/tengpha.htm. Accessed January 31, 2014.

28. CDC. CDC's top ten: 5 health achievements in 2013 and 5 health threats in 2014. 2014. http://blogs.cdc.gov/cdcworksforyou24-7/2013/12/cdc%e2%80%99s-top-ten-5-health-achievements-in-2013-and-5-health-threats-in-2014/. Accessed January 29, 2014.

29. Kliff S. The incredible shrinking prevention fund. *The Washington Post WONKBLOG.* 2013. http://www.washingtonpost.com/blogs/wonkblog/wp/2013/04/19/the-incredible-shrinking-prevention-fund/. Accessed January 31, 2014

30. Benjamin G. Public health investments critical in 2014 omnibus spending bill. 2014. http://www.apha.org/about/news/pressreleases/2014/omnibusspendingbill.htm. Accessed January 31, 2014.

31. U.S. Department of Health and Human Services. National prevention strategy. 2011. http://www.surgeongeneral.gov/initiatives/prevention/strategy/. Accessed September 6, 2013.

32. McGinnis JM. Health in America—the sum of its parts. *JAMA.* 2002;287(20):2711–2712.

33. U.S. Preventive Services Task Force 2014. http://www.uspreventiveservicestaskforce.org/. Accessed January 31, 2014.

34. The Community Guide: What works to promote health. 2014. http://www.thecommunityguide.org/index.html. Accessed January 31, 2014.

35. *Healthy People 2020.* http://www.healthypeople.gov/2020. Accessed January 30, 2014.

36. CDC. Healthy places: Health impact assessment. 2009. http://www.cdc.gov/healthyplaces/hia.htm. Accessed January 31, 2014.

CHAPTER 2

Improving Health Literacy: Finding High-Quality, Web-Based Information

LEARNING OBJECTIVES

- Describe the attributes of websites providing "higher quality" information on health topics.
- Identify factors contributing to consumers' finding and using poor quality or inaccurate Web-based health information.
- Design practical strategies to improve the quality of health information that consumers find when searching the Web.

THE CONTROVERSY

Thirty-four Texas high school students participated in a well-designed experiment to see how well they could determine the accuracy of scientific information about vaccine safety and vaccine danger from Internet searches.[1] Results of their Google searches, their subsequent opinions about the accuracy of their search results, and answers to written questions asking about the strength of evidence were all evaluated by study investigators.[1]

Although more than half the sites that students found were inaccurate, nearly 60% of the students thought they were indeed accurate, and in their written assessments of the accuracy of the information, more than half the students had erroneous factual knowledge about vaccine safety and danger.[1] For example, based on their Web search, student participants thought the evidence to support the statement that "vaccines prevent epidemics" was "mixed," but after later viewing an evidence-based video on vaccines, rated the evidence as "strong to very strong," a statistically significant difference.[1] Similarly, after their Internet search, they noted the evidence was "mixed to strong" that "vaccines do not cause autism," but later rated

19

this significantly higher, as "strong to very strong" after viewing the evidence-based video.[1]

Although the number of high school students in this study was small, and it is not known whether similar results might happen in any high school in the United States, among these 17- and 18-year-old study participants, a Google search of a controversial scientific topic resulted in students gathering much erroneous knowledge, largely because their searches produced many credible-appearing but inaccurate sites.[1]

BACKGROUND AND SCOPE OF THE PUBLIC HEALTH AND HEALTH POLICY ISSUE

Have you ever tried to quickly find accurate and high-quality information about health on the Internet? If you Google a topic, you may find a list of sites that may or may not be what you are really looking for. Health information is everywhere, but much of the information may be misleading, inaccurate, and not of the highest quality, depending how and where you search.

Contributing Factors—Internet Use Climbs

Nearly three-quarters of U.S. adults use the Internet and more than 60% have conducted searches for health or medical information; nearly half of Internet users have searched for websites that provide information about a specific health condition.[2] The National Center for Health Statistics published estimates from the 2009 National Health Interview Survey, a national health survey of the U.S. population conducted with in-person interviews and using data collected from more than 7,000 adults from the first 6 months of the year. From this survey, they found that 51% of adults had searched for health information on the Internet in the past year, with women (58%) searching more frequently than men (43.4%)[2] (see **Figure 2–1**). In another report, it was estimated that 4.5% of Internet searches globally are for health information.[3]

More recently, in a 2012 nationwide telephone survey of more than 3,000 U.S. adults, the Pew Research Center's Internet and American Life Project found that 81% of U.S. adults used the Internet.[4] In their report, they also noted that of people who use the Internet, 72% reported searching for health information on the Internet in the previous year, a percentage that translates to 59% of all U.S. adults.[4] Additionally, nearly one-third of all cell phone users in the United States used their phone to search for health information,

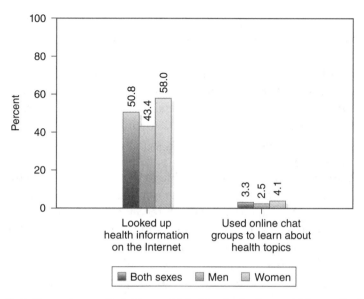

Figure 2–1 Percentages of adults aged 18–64 who in the past 12 months looked up health information on the Internet.

Reproduced from Cohen RA, Ph.D., and Stussman B, B.A., Division of Health Interview Statistics, Health Information Technology Use Among Men and Women Aged 18–64: Early Release of Estimates From the National Health Interview Survey, January-June 2009. National Center for Health Statistics. Available from http://www.cdc.gov/nchs/data/hestat/healthinfo2009/healthinfo2009.htm

with adults under 50, African Americans, Latinos, and those with college education most often conducting phone searches for health information.[4]

How Do People Search for Health Information?

A qualitative study conducted in Germany provides many clues about how consumers find and evaluate the quality of health information.[5] Investigators in this study held focus groups, conducted interviews, and directly observed participants as they searched for health information in response to specific questions. Questions to the study participants included such topics as, for example, the need for malaria prophylaxis for travel to specific geographic locations, or the definition of being overweight.[5] Twenty-one participants in focus groups noted that characteristics of high-quality sites included the organization's expertise, a professional appearance, and referencing scientific materials, as well as being able to easily understand the site's material.[5]

However, when the researchers directly observed how 17 of the study participants actually performed the search, they found some different results. Participants did not begin their searches in government or academic sites, but instead used search engines such as Google and Yahoo, and most used a single search term, even for complicated questions.[5] In addition, when searching, study participants usually chose links appearing on the first search page. By measuring "clicks" the investigators determined that 71.3% used one of the first five links, and 97.2% used a link from the first 10 on the page.[5]

In this study, people were usually able to find the information they were looking for quickly: the average time to find answers to the questions was less than 6 minutes, and ranged from 38 seconds to 20 minutes.[5] However, during their searches, study participants did not use available information to verify the credentials of the authors of the Web-based information they used, and nearly 80% of the time they couldn't remember whether the information was from a government, academic, or commercial source when they had completed their search.[5]

In the Pew Internet and American Life Project report, *Health Online 2013*, the vast majority (77%) of Internet users looking for online health information reported using a search engine, for example, Google, Bing, or Yahoo. More specific health or medical information sites (e.g., WebMD) were only used by an additional small percentage (13%).[4]

What Determines Which Internet Sites Appear First?

Several factors may determine what appears on the first search page, such as consumer-driven searching strategies,[6] website "optimization" at the level of the webmaster,[7] or commercial ads and "pay for placement" strategies.[3] Searching strategies taught in most colleges and universities and also available in public libraries can help people use accurate search terms and improve searching strategies. One example of this, using the word "AND" to narrow a search, is called using Boolean logic and connectors (also called Boolean "operators"), such as AND, OR, or NOT.[8] There are existing guides for businesses and people who develop websites to help them influence how often their site is prominently located during Web searches. Google publishes a *Search Engine Optimization Starter Guide* to instruct users in how to improve website structure, content, and pages, which may "optimize" what is found when people search for topics.[7] Advice is plentiful for business owners about strategies to best use ads on their websites, sometimes making it more challenging for consumers.[9] Studies suggest that many searchers use just the first page, or frequently, they just use the first few links to find and act on health information.[5] The important perspective for people searching online for health information is to realize that a number of influences determine what links might appear first after searching, at the top of the list and on the first page, and these sites may or may not be the most high-quality or evidence-based websites, unless specific searching strategies are used.

What Health Information Are People Searching For?

People most often search for information on specific health or medical conditions. In the 2012 Pew Internet and American Life Project report, 35% of all U.S. adults have searched online for specific health information related to a specific medical condition.[4] Stated differently, the survey noted that of all the Internet users in the United States who have searched for health information, more than 72% have searched for information related to a specific medical condition.[4] Previous studies found that people may search for information for either themselves, a family member, or a friend.[3,10] Women, adults under 50, and people with some college education and higher incomes were more likely to conduct online searches for specific medical information. Men, older adults, and people with lower incomes also queried health topics online, but not as often.[4]

Another multivariate analysis of the Pew surveys found that women; people employed less than full time; frequent Internet users; or individuals with ongoing medical problems, new medical diagnoses, or those receiving a new medical treatment were all associated with frequent online searching for health information.[11] Frequent health topics of interest (in addition to information about specific diseases or medical conditions) included specific medical treatments, losing or controlling weight, health insurance information, food or drug safety, or information about an advertised pharmaceutical[4] (see **Figure 2–2**). When comparing white, African American, or Latino Internet users, the frequency of searching online for different topics differed only in searches about weight control (higher in African American and Latino individuals), pregnancy and childbirth (highest in Latino individuals), advertised pharmaceuticals (highest in African Americans), and whether the search was done for a specific condition (highest in white Internet users).[4]

Limited published information is available about differences in online health searching by country. For example, about one-quarter of individuals

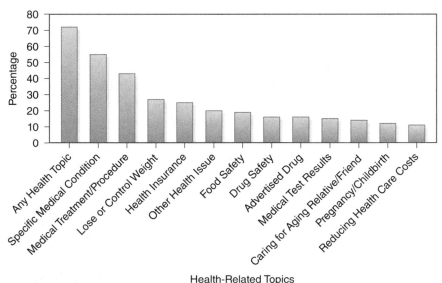

Figure 2–2 Adult Internet users–topics for recent health-related searches 2012.

Data from Fox S, Duggan M. Health Online 2013. *Pew Internet & American Life Project.* Page 10. January 15, 2013. http://www.pewinternet.org/Reports/2013/Health-online.aspx

from the United States and Germany and 19% of individuals from France searched for specific health information frequently, and the percentage was much lower (6%) in people living in Japan. Furthermore, in Japan, more than one-third of those looking for any health information on the Internet do not look for specific medical information.[3,12]

The Pew Internet and American Life Project also looked at social aspects of Internet users who were searching for health information, using the term "e-patient" to describe this group.[13] In this report, more than half of searches (52%) were for someone else. There were many instances where online health searchers were looking for additional healthcare information about a health or medical condition. For example, about one-quarter searched for rankings or reviews of health professionals or hospitals, and 41% read blogs or commentaries about the illness.[13] Use of social networking sites, like Facebook or Twitter, is less common, with only 12% of e-patients using Twitter for information about specific medical conditions, although people aged 18 to 49 are the highest users.[13] About 60% of e-patients report that their health information search affected their own health decisions, or decisions related to someone else, most often for less serious situations.[13] In addition, from 2002 to 2009, several topics have increased in popularity for online searches, such as information about exercise, weight loss, specific medical conditions and treatments (including medications), mental health conditions, alternative medicine, health professionals and hospitals, and health insurance.[13]

Do People Trust the Health Information They Find on the Internet?

Web surfers looking for health information don't *always* trust what they find. A 2002 Pew study showed reasons why people may reject certain websites, with nearly half of people looking for health information reluctant to use the information because the site was "too commercial."[10] However, in the same report, nearly three-quarters (72%) of people searching for online health information felt they could "believe all or most of the health information online."[10]

Another important perspective is how people actually use the health information they find, especially if the health condition is more complex or serious. In the *Health Online 2013* survey, when people were asked who they consulted for help when they had a "serious health issue," 70% relied on a physician or other health professional and 60% relied on family and friends.[4] In addition, following their Internet searching, more than half the people subsequently talked with a medical professional about the information.[4] But in another study of more than 6,000 U.S. adults from the Health Information National Trends Survey, investigators compared respondents' preferred and actual behavior when looking for health information.[14] What they found was that although nearly two-thirds of respondents trusted physicians, and nearly half wanted to ask his or her physician first for specific health information, in terms of their actual behavior, only 10.9% went to their physician first and nearly 50% went online first.[14]

EVIDENCE BASE FOR PREVENTION AND PRACTICE

Do We Need Quality Measures for Websites?

For well over a decade, health professionals from large national organizations, such as the American Medical Association (AMA) have warned patients about the potential for inaccurate or misleading health information from Internet searches. The AMA has advocated for quality standards that include authors and credentials, references, disclosure of website ownership, and publication dates to ensure information is current.[15] Other authors agree that health professionals should advocate for quality standards for health information, recommend specific websites to patients, and teach consumers how to search and critically appraise the credibility and quality of what they find.[3]

Berland and colleagues studied the quality of health information in specific health topics, in both English and Spanish.[16] Using ten search engines in English and four in Spanish, they systematically evaluated the quality and reading level of health information in response to hypothetical patient questions about breast cancer, depression, obesity, and childhood asthma. When combining all health information topics, the authors found that for English-language searching, 34% of the links on the first page were relevant, but ultimately only 20% of the links identified on the first page resulted in content directly relevant to the initial search question.[16] In Spanish-language search engines, the percentages were even lower: only 18% of the links found on the first page were relevant, and only 12% of the links identified on the first page ultimately produced relevant content.[16] They also found substantial variation in the extent and accuracy of coverage of these four clinical topics, worse for the Spanish-language sites. They further observed that the general literacy level required to navigate health information on these topics was high, requiring the equivalent of some college-level education to navigate the English-language sites, and high-school level education to understand the Spanish-language sites.[16]

In a review of 1,512 abstracts and 186 published papers, Crocco and colleagues specifically looked for evidence of harm from using online health information.[17] They reported cases in which consumer Internet searches resulted in emotional distress from the inability to find relevant health information or that medical decision making was based on entering different keywords; they found one instance in which dogs were poisoned because of inaccurate information found online and one patient who had an adverse reaction to alternative cancer treatment found on the Internet. Whether the reporting of harm from searching for and using Internet health information was rare or if the risk of harm was actually low could not be determined from this study.[17]

Efforts to Promote Quality of Online Health Information

Numerous organizations have attempted to educate health information consumers about ways to find high-quality and accurate information.

"Codes of conduct" contain criteria to help consumers determine the quality of websites.[18] One example of an organization promoting quality of health information is the Health on the Net Foundation (HON), created in 1995 as a nonprofit and nongovernmental organization.[19] The organization publishes (on the Internet) a voluntary certification system, search function for certified websites, a list of tools and special topics available to individuals, health professionals, and Web publishers. HON principles include: authority, complementarity, confidentiality, attribution, justifiability, transparency, financial disclosure, and advertising.[19] Entering the search term "cancer" in the search box results in a first page with lists of large educational organizations, nonprofit organizations, or healthcare institutions.[19]

Another example of efforts to promote quality includes the AMA[20] principles for websites that was designed for their own materials, but may be useful to other organizations. These include principles for content, advertising and sponsorship, privacy and confidentiality, and principles for e-commerce.[20] There are other examples of organizations such as Health Internet for member states of the European Union[18] and the e-Health Code of Ethics of the iHealth Coalition, from an "e-Health Ethics Summit" hosted by the World Health Organization/Pan American Health Organization in 2000.[21] Quality labels, filtering tools, systems to help Internet users, and third-party labels have also been described.[22]

In a large systematic review of all the methods different investigators have used to assess quality of online health information (both published and unpublished reports in any language), 79 studies were included that reviewed nearly 6,000 health websites and more than 1,000 Web pages.[23] These investigators noted a wide variety of criteria used to measure quality, but often included such attributes as accuracy, readability, disclosures, and presence of references. In 70% of the studies included in this review, authors were concerned about the quality of information, but there was much variation in the approaches taken by the different studies included, making comparisons challenging.[23] Gagliardi and Jadad found that of 98 published methods to evaluate the quality of health-related websites, many were no longer being used only 5 years later.[24] In addition, there were over 50 new methods reported in their study, but most of these could not be verified as effective.[24] Other authors are skeptical of efforts to measure the quality of Internet health information.[25] All of these articles emphasize the challenges of finding effective, sustainable, and practical strategies to educate the public about how to find high-quality health information on the Internet.

Strategies to Find Higher-Quality Health Information Online

Despite the proliferation of codes of conduct and other strategies, the literature suggests most consumers searching for health information use available and popular search engines, like Google.[3,5] At the same time, they do often consult with their physician or other healthcare professional to confirm the accuracy of the information they have found and especially seek medical consultation for serious health conditions.[4] Despite the challenges of defining and measuring the quality of health information, there are some especially helpful resources for Internet users, in addition to the HON and AMA principles already discussed.

The Medical Library Association (MLA) has published (online) a user's guide called "Find and Evaluate Health Information on the Web."[26] In their approach, they both help people using search engines, by suggesting ways to improve search quality, and also direct people to respected health information sites such as MedlinePlus,[27] or Healthfinder,[28] or their "Top 10" list.[26] In addition, the MLA has guidelines to evaluate the quality of the website and information found, including identifying sponsorship of the site, how frequently it is updated, clarity and referencing of the information, and the target audience.[26] The "MedlinePlus Guide to Healthy Web Surfing" emphasizes teaching consumers the principles and strategies for finding high-quality online health information.[29] This site emphasizes the need to find the primary source of the information, and encourage searchers to be a "cyber skeptic." In addition to recommending that consumers look at health information with a critical eye, they advise consumers to consult with their own healthcare professional. In addition, there is a user-friendly tutorial available on their site[29] (see **Figure 2–3**).

What Are the Public Health Benefits of Finding High-Quality Health Information Online?

For 2 months in 2003, during the SARS global outbreak, SARS was the most searched-for topic at Yahoo.[3] More recently, in addition to searching for information about specific health or medical conditions, many adults have also looked for health information about public health topics: 27% of adults who had searched for health information online during the past year looked for information about losing or controlling weight, and 19%

Who or what is the source of the information?

Is the information current?

Are there links and references to the actual research (primary sources)?

Is the information clear and easy to read?

Who are the intended audiences for the information?

What is the source of funding for the site?

Is there bias in how information is presented?

Have you considered discussing the information with your health professional?

Figure 2–3 Searching for health information online–questions to ask.

Data from Medical Library Association. Find and Evaluate Heatlh Information on the Web. 2014 http://www.mlanet.org/resources/userguide.html NS MedlinePlus Guide to Healthy Web Surfing. 2013; http://www.nlm.nih.gov/medlineplus/healthywebsurfing.html

looked for information about food safety, both important and relevant public health topics.[4] These examples highlight the potential benefits of having the general public skilled in health-related Internet searching for the prevention of chronic conditions, or in times of epidemics, natural disasters, or public health emergencies, to help with preparedness. In addition, benefits of becoming more health literate might have implications for health care, facilitating patients' active participation in maintaining their own health. With our changing population demographics, increasingly complex health conditions and treatments, and the availability of new public health information on a daily basis, the challenges of reaching people of different ages, genders, cultures, and education and literacy levels are daunting, but potential benefits are huge.

DISCUSSION QUESTIONS: TEMPLATE FOR DISCUSSION

1. Significance of this public health issue:
   a. Why is this health issue important?
   b. How many people does it impact?
   c. How serious is it?
   d. Is it preventable?

2. What is the evidence base for prevention?
3. What specific strategies should be used to achieve progress on this health issue?
   a. What evidence-based approach would you use?
   b. Where would you start if you are an individual citizen; public health professional; healthcare professional; community, state, or federal policymaker?
4. Specific questions for this topic:
   a. What are the characteristics of "higher quality" websites containing health information?
   b. What are the characteristics of websites containing health information that are *not* as "high quality"?
   c. Can you find specific examples of websites containing health information that are "higher quality" and not as "high quality"?
   d. Can you compare and contrast the sites that you found?
5. What is the controversy?
   a. Define the controversy.
   b. Is controversy a good or bad thing? (Does it help or hinder progress?)
6. *Why* is this health issue controversial?
   a. What specific factors are involved?
   b. Do economics, government, scientific uncertainty, or politics play a role?
   c. What is the role of the media?
7. How would you respond to the controversy?

PERSPECTIVES TO CONSIDER

The ability to quickly find "higher-quality" Web-based information about health is a great skill, but the increased use of the Internet can also potentially result in finding and using misleading or inaccurate information. Conversely, finding high-quality information on reputable sites may improve health literacy, enhance shared decision making between patients and health professionals, and contribute to improvements in public health. The challenge is: how can we best teach the public to find high-quality, Web-based resources about health in a way that improves both individual and population health? Do we give patients a list of example websites or teach them how to be critical of what they find? Probably both are needed. Teaching adolescents how to search for and critically appraise health-related information could, if systematically taught in educational settings, increase the health literacy of young adults. Giving patients lists of credible and reputable sites and encouraging conversations might contribute to improved healthcare communication and decision making. Additional educational efforts by public health professionals could reinforce the importance of Internet health literacy in areas of clinical medicine and public health issues.

What was notable from currently published studies was how few studies, with the exception of the extensive Pew Internet and American Life Project,[4] have been conducted recently. The most frequent online searchers tend to be more highly educated, and some studies raise questions about literacy levels required to best use available higher-quality health information.[16] Gaps are prevalent in our detailed knowledge of how Internet searching influences health decisions in different geographic locations, different racial and ethnic populations, and especially in those with less income and education. But from the available literature, despite a lack of extensive documentation of harm, it seems obvious that there is the potential for risk. People acting on health-related information from websites that are not evidence-based or from reputable sources, and who don't discuss the findings with healthcare professionals, may not be using the best possible information for these important decisions.

Based on growing Internet use, how people actually search for health information, and Web optimization strategies that place certain sites strategically on the first page, it is possible that many people find and use health-related information from sites of lower quality. Conversely, what was intriguing, were potential possibilities to improve the health of individuals and entire populations, if patient searches could more frequently be connected to credible health information, including public health sources and integrated into actual conversations in healthcare settings. Both public health and healthcare professionals have critical roles in educating individual patients and the general public about how to find high-quality health information online.

FOR ADDITIONAL STUDY

Morahan-Martin JM. How Internet users find, evaluate, and use online health information: a cross-cultural review. *Cyberpsychol Behav.* 2004;7(5):497–510.

Fox S, Duggan M. Health Online 2013. *Pew Internet and American Life Project.* 2013. [complete report.] Available at http://www.pewInternet.org/Reports/2013/Health-online.aspx

REFERENCES

1. Kortum P, Edwards C, Richards-Kortum R. The impact of inaccurate Internet health information in a secondary school learning environment. *J Med Internet Res.* 2008;10(2):e17.

2. Cohen R, Stussman, B. Health information technology use among men and women aged 18–64. *NCHS Health E-Stats.* 2010. http://www.cdc.gov/nchs/data/hestat/healthinfo2009/healthinfo2009.pdf. Accessed September 18, 2013.

3. Morahan-Martin JM. How Internet users find, evaluate, and use online health information: A cross-cultural review. *Cyberpsychol Behav.* 2004;7(5):497–510.

4. Fox S, Duggan M. *Health Online 2013.* Pew Internet and American Life Project. 2013. http://www.pewInternet.org/Reports/2013/Health-online.aspx. Accessed September 18, 2013.

5. Eysenbach G, Kohler C. How do consumers search for and appraise health information on the world wide web? Qualitative study using focus groups, usability tests, and in-depth interviews. *BMJ.* 2002;324(7337):573–577.

6. Searching Databases Effectively. 2013. http://www2.smumn.edu/deptpages/tclibrary/tutorials/finding/search.pdf. Accessed September 20, 2013.

7. *Search Engine Optimization Starter Guide 2010.* http://static.googleusercontent.com/external_content/untrusted_dlcp/www.google.com/en/us/webmasters/docs/search-engine-optimization-starter-guide.pdf. Accessed September 18, 2013.

8. *Database Search Strategies: Boolean Operators.* 2010. http://libguides.uwb.edu/content.php?pid=82016&sid=608681. Accessed September 20, 2013.

9. Dahl D. Real-life lessons in using Google AdWords. *The New York Times.* 2009. http://www.nytimes.com/2009/10/15/business/smallbusiness/15adwords.html?pagewanted=all&_r=1&. Accessed September 20, 2013.

10. Fox S, Rainie, L. Vital decisions: How internet users decide what information to trust when they or their loved ones are sick. Pew Internet and American Life Project. 2002. http://www.pewinternet.org/files/old-media//Files/Reports/2002/PIP_Vital_Decisions_May2002.pdf.pdf Accessed September 18, 2013.

11. Rice RE. Influences, usage, and outcomes of Internet health information searching: Multivariate results from the Pew surveys. *Int J Med Inf.* 2006;75(1):8–28.

12. Taylor H, Leitman R. Four-nation survey shows widespread but different levels of internet use for health purposes. *Health Care News.* 2002. http://www.ehealthstrategies.com/files/hi_v2_11.pdf. Accessed September 18, 2013.

13. Fox S, Jones S. The social life of health information. 2009. http://www.pewInternet.org/2009/06/11/the-social-life-of-health-information/. Accessed August 25, 2014.

14. Hesse BW, Nelson DE, Kreps GL, et al. Trust and sources of health information: The impact of the Internet and its implications for health care providers: findings from the first Health Information National Trends Survey. *Arch Intern Med.* 2005;165(22):2618–2624.

15. Silberg WM, Lundberg GD, Musacchio RA. Assessing, controlling, and assuring the quality of medical information on the Internet: Caveant lector et viewor—Let the reader and viewer beware. *JAMA.* 1997;277(15):1244–1245.

16. Berland GK, Elliott MN, Morales LS, et al. Health information on the Internet: Accessibility, quality, and readability in English and Spanish. *JAMA.* 2001;285(20):2612–2621.

17. Crocco AG, Villasis-Keever M, Jadad AR. Analysis of cases of harm associated with use of health information on the Internet. *JAMA.* 2002;287(21):2869–2871.
18. Wilson P. How to find the good and avoid the bad or ugly: A short guide to tools for rating quality of health information on the Internet. *BMJ.* 2002;324(7337):598–602.
19. HON: Health on the Net Foundation. 2013. http://www.hon.ch/. Accessed September 18, 2013.
20. Winker MA, Flanagin A, Chi-Lum B, et al. Guidelines for medical and health information sites on the internet: Principles governing AMA web sites. *JAMA.* 2000;283(12):1600–1606.
21. Rippen H, Risk A. e-Health Code of Ethics (May 24). *J Med Internet Res.* 2000;2(2):e9.
22. Brock D, Abu-Rish E, Chiu CR, et al. Interprofessional education in team communication: Working together to improve patient safety. *BMJ Qual Saf.* 2013; 22(5):414–423.
23. Eysenbach G, Powell J, Kuss O, Sa ER. Empirical studies assessing the quality of health information for consumers on the world wide web: A systematic review. *JAMA.* 2002;287(20):2691–2700.
24. Gagliardi A, Jadad AR. Examination of instruments used to rate quality of health information on the internet: Chronicle of a voyage with an unclear destination. *BMJ.* 2002;324(7337):569–573.
25. Deshpande A, Jadad AR. Trying to measure the quality of health information on the internet: Is it time to move on? *J Rheumatol.* 2009;36(1):1–3.
26. Medical Library Association. Find and evaluate health information on the Web. 2014. http://www.mlanet.org/resources/userguide.html. Accessed September 18, 2013.
27. MedlinePlus: Trusted health information for you. 2013. http://www.nlm.nih.gov/medlineplus/. Accessed September 18, 2013.
28. Healthfinder.gov. 2013. http://healthfinder.gov/. Accessed September 18, 2013.
29. *MedlinePlus Guide to Healthy Web Surfing.* 2013. http://www.nlm.nih.gov/medlineplus/healthywebsurfing.html. Accessed September 18, 2013.

CHAPTER 3

Obesity—Is Fat the New Normal?

LEARNING OBJECTIVES

- Describe data and trends in obesity in children, adolescents, and adults in the United States.
- Discuss variation in obesity according to demographic factors and geographic regions in the United States.
- Evaluate the overall public health impact of obesity in the United States.
- Summarize evidence-based approaches for clinical and community prevention.
- Identify future predictions for obesity and implications for public health.

THE CONTROVERSY

In 2005, the Institute of Medicine reported "[W]e begin the 21st century with a startling setback—an epidemic of childhood obesity. The epidemic is occurring in boys and girls in all 50 states, in younger children as well as adolescents, across all socioeconomic strata, and among all ethnic groups."[1] A Huffington Post blog[2] reported that by 2030, if all continues, we might expect half the U.S. population to be obese, referencing a July 2011 survey of 1,000 Americans conducted by Russell Research for Pollock Communications.[3] The survey showed that slightly more than half of respondents believed they were overweight or obese, in stark contrast to national surveys showing 67% as the actual percentage. Men and younger individuals were even less likely to believe they were overweight than women or middle-aged people. A registered dietician quoted in the news release noted, "With numerous environmental changes, from stretchy fabrics to larger car and movie theater seats, many American feel they are a normal weight despite actually being overweight. Overweight is the new normal weight in the United States."[3] Another 2011 survey found a significant decline in just a year's time in the percentage of people changing their diet, increasing physical activity, trying to lose weight, or even considering themselves overweight.[4] Taken together, these findings suggest that Americans may be getting a bit too comfortable with a society in which so many people are now overweight or obese, a perception that might be even worse in the future, as today's young people are the least likely to think they are overweight.[3]

BACKGROUND AND SCOPE OF THE PUBLIC HEALTH AND HEALTH POLICY ISSUE

The World Health Organization (WHO) defines overweight and obesity as "abnormal or excessive fat accumulation that may impair health."[5] *Body mass index* (BMI) is defined as weight in kilograms divided by the square of height in meters (kg/m^2), classifying overweight as BMI greater than or equal to 25 and obesity as a BMI greater to or equal to 30.[5] (This can also be calculated in adults by dividing weight in pounds by height squared then multiplying 703.[6]) The National Heart, Lung, and Blood Institute adds a category of extreme obesity, a BMI greater than or equal to 40, but adds measurement of waist circumference to BMI when screening adults.[7]

Obesity is potentially preventable. WHO statistics define one-third of the world's population as overweight (1.4 billion adults as of 2008) with more than 40 million overweight children under age 5. Since 1980, overall obesity rates have nearly doubled across the globe and more than 10% of the entire adult population meets the definition for obesity.[5] A 2014 report summarizing the Global Burden of Disease Study concurred with the global severity of obesity in children and adults.[8] In the United States, from 1990 to 2000, obesity was the fastest growing "actual cause of death,"[9,10] with poor diet and physical inactivity estimated to contribute to 400,000 annual deaths in the United States. The concern for the future was, based on current trends, obesity could overtake tobacco as the leading preventable cause of death in the United States.[9,10]

Data and Trends

A variety of national surveys are used to collect information about health risks, including obesity. The National Health and Nutrition Examination Survey (NHANES) began in the 1960s and is designed to gather information about the health of children and adults in the United States. It includes both an interview and direct measurements and laboratory tests of a sample of 5,000 people each year. It is a program of the National Center for Health Statistics (NCHS), which is part of the U.S. Centers for Disease Control and Prevention (CDC), and helps in the research of a wide variety of health conditions and risk factors.[11]

Another source of data is the Behavioral Risk Factor Surveillance System (BRFSS), the largest national phone survey, collecting monthly data in all 50 states, the District of Columbia, Puerto Rico, the U.S. Virgin Islands, Guam, American Samoa, and Palau.[12] The survey, now 30 years old, uses regularly asked core questions and rotating groups of questions on a variety of health topics and risk behaviors, allowing comparisons of risk behaviors over time and state-by-state comparisons.[12] There is also a Youth Risk Behavior Surveillance System (YRBSS) that collects similar data about adolescents.[13] The National Health Interview Survey (NHIS), established in 1957, uses personal interviews to collect data on a wide range of health indicators.[14]

To account for children's growth during childhood and adolescence and differences between boys and girls, age and sex-specific percentiles for BMI (CDC growth charts) are used for children and adolescents ages 2 to 19, rather than the simple calculated BMI that is used for adults.[15] Using these growth charts, overweight is defined as BMI between 85th and 95th percentile and obesity as BMI at or above the 95th percentile.[15] Using NHANES data, the NCHS estimates 16.9% of children and adolescents were obese in 2009–2010, with 18.6% of boys and 15.0% of girls meeting this definition.[16] Overall trends from 1971–1974 to 2009–2010 show an increase from 5.1% to 16.9%[16] (see **Figure 3–1**).

In adults, using NHANES data, the NCHS estimated obesity rates for U.S. adults from 2009–2010: 33% of adults aged 20 and older were overweight, 35.7% were obese, and 6.3% extremely obese.[17] When analyzing trends in U.S. adults since 1960, obesity has more than doubled since 1976–1980, although rates of overweight have remained at about the same level[17] (see **Figure 3–2**).

In addition, there are both racial and ethnic similarities and differences. For example, in children, there were increasing obesity trends seen in non-Hispanic white, non-Hispanic black, and Mexican-American adolescent boys and girls (ages 12–19) when comparing 1988–1994 and 2009–2010. However, during 2009–2010, non-Hispanic black adolescent girls were statistically significantly more likely than non-Hispanic white adolescent girls to be obese (24.8% vs. 14.7%).[16]

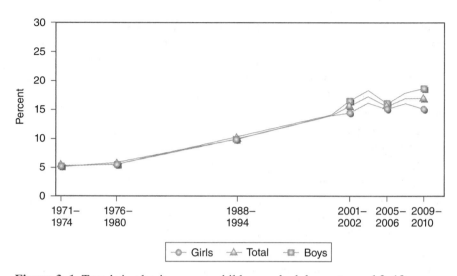

Figure 3–1 Trends in obesity among children and adolescents aged 2–19 years.

Reproduced from Fryar CD, M.S.P.H.; Carroll MD, M.S.P.H.; and Ogden CL, Ph.D., PPrevalence of Obesity Among Children and Adolescents: United States, Trends 1963–1965 Through 2009–2010. National Center for Health Statistics. Available from http://www.cdc.gov/nchs/data/hestat/obesity_child_09_10/obesity_child_09_10.htm

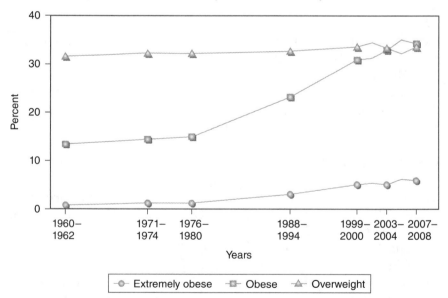

Figure 3–2 Trends in overweight, obesity, and extreme obesity among adults aged 20–74 years.

Reproduced from Fryar CD, M.S.P.H.; Carroll MD, M.S.P.H.; and Ogden CL, Ph.D., Prevalence of Overweight, Obesity, and Extreme Obesity Among Adults: United States, Trends 1960–1962 Through 2009–2010. National Center for Health Statistics. Available from http://www.cdc.gov/nchs/data/hestat/obesity_adult_09_10/obesity_adult_09_10.htm

What Are the Health Risks?

Adults who are overweight or obese have an increased risk for chronic health conditions such as coronary heart disease and stroke, type 2 diabetes, hypertension, lipid abnormalities, some types of cancer (endometrial, breast, colon), and osteoarthritis.[18] In the Nurses' Health Study (115,195 U.S. women who were followed for 16 years), there was a significant relationship between weight and mortality.[19] Women with higher BMIs were more likely to die from any cause, compared to women with a BMI of less than 19, and this risk increased as BMI increased. For example, in this study, women with a BMI between 27.0 and 28.9 were 60% more likely to die and women with BMI between 29.0 and 31.9 were more than twice as likely to die as women with BMI less than 19 during the study period.[19]

In the Coronary Artery Risk Development in Young Adults (CARDIA) study, a study of white and African American men, weight gain over a 15-year period was related to changes in risk factors for cardiovascular disease.[20] In another 20-year study of more than 7,000 British men, risk of cardiovascular disease and diabetes were higher in men with higher BMI; risks were also increased in men who gained weight during a 15-year period.[21]

For children and adolescents, according to CDC, obese children have greater risks for hypertension, type 2 diabetes, asthma, musculoskeletal problems, and low self-esteem.[15] These children may also experience one of the greatest risks, the risk of becoming overweight adults, with increased risks for many chronic health conditions later in their lives.[15] Other researchers also note that preventing childhood obesity is critically important because of the impact it may have years later, because of the biology of chronic conditions.[22] As the prevalence of obesity has risen dramatically, type 2 diabetes mellitus, previously seen infrequently in children, has also risen.[23]

The American Heart Association, in a scientific statement, noted that both individual treatment and population-level prevention is needed.[22] In the National Heart, Lung, and Blood Institute Growth and Health Study, a study of 1,166 Caucasian and 1,213 African American girls, found that obesity during childhood increased subsequent risk for adult obesity by as much as 30 times. Furthermore, overweight girls as young as age 9 were more likely to experience a range of cardiovascular disease risk factors, including high blood pressure and blood lipid levels.[24] In a study of more than 300 children followed for 8 to 12 years, children (both boys and girls) with a BMI between the 75th and 85th percentiles were as much as 20 times more likely to become overweight as young adults; the increased risk began to increase at BMIs greater than the 50th percentile. In addition, in boys, increased BMI during childhood was associated with an increased risk of hypertension in young adulthood.[25]

Psychosocial issues are also common in obese children. In a study of 197 young children and parents, being overweight was associated with lower self-esteem in children as young as 5 years old.[26] Overweight adolescents are more often subjected to teasing about their appearance than their normal-weight peers, potentially resulting in social isolation, loneliness, and poorer self-image,[27] all of which may hinder efforts to achieve normal weight and activity levels.

Using the National Health Interview Survey (1984–2000) and U.S. Census Bureau data, Narayan and colleagues estimated that for children born in the year 2000, the lifetime risk for developing diabetes was more than 30% for boys and nearly 40% for girls, and was even higher in Hispanic populations; these risks are also associated with a shortened life expectancy.[28] In 2005, it was predicted that if we do not stop current obesity trends, children born today would not live as long as their parents.[1,29]

What Causes Obesity?

At a basic level, imbalance from energy taken in (from foods and beverages) and energy out, in the form of physical activity, contributes to rising obesity rates.[30] Environmental factors can promote or hinder good nutrition and physical activity. Availability of sugar-sweetened beverages, pervasive food marketing, and uneven access to healthier and affordable foods in all communities, are cited as contributing factors.[31] High quality and daily physical activity is not universally available in all schools, television and computer screen time is rampant, and in many communities there are insufficient safe places for children to be active, making daily physical activity challenging.[30] CDC cites a role for behavioral, environmental, genetic, and socioeconomic factors as contributing to obesity.[18] According to the Surgeon General's Call to Action in 2001, behavior and the environment have the greatest potential role in prevention.[32]

Place Matters

Epidemiologists describe populations and public health issues in terms of person, time, or place, looking at characteristics of individuals, trends over time, or different geographic locations. Looking at data in this descriptive way helps provide hints or generate hypotheses as to why this is happening, and helps set priorities for action. For example, a map of overall adult obesity across the United States shows states or regions that are higher or lower than other places. Looking at such maps and how they change over time, as CDC shows in obesity prevalence maps on its website,[6] gives a different picture; not only can you see variation in different states (place), but when compared to earlier years it is readily apparent that obesity is getting worse over time. Looking at public health issues in these ways may help our understanding of the issue itself and how we might potentially prioritize our interventions, whether direct services, policies, programs, or educational messages.

As an example, using results from the Behavioral Risk Factor Surveillance System there is variation in the prevalence of self-reported obesity in U.S. adults in different states, with lowest rates of obesity reported in Colorado (21.3%) and Hawaii (21.8%) and highest rates in West Virginia (35.1%) and Mississippi (35.1%) in 2013; on a regional basis, the highest percentages are generally reported in the Midwest and South[33] (see **Figure 3–3**).

In addition, in adults, when self-reported obesity rates are compared in non-Hispanic white, non-Hispanic black, and Hispanic populations, geographic differences appear striking.[34] When looking only at non-Hispanic white adults, no state in the United States had a self-reported obesity prevalence of 35% or higher. However, when looking only at Hispanic adults, 5 states had an obesity prevalence of 35% or higher.

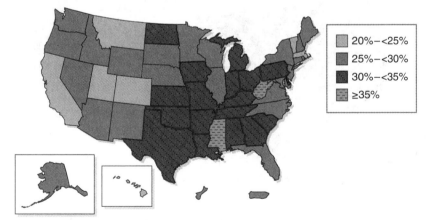

Figure 3–3 Prevalence of self-reported obesity among U.S. adults by state and territory, BRFSS, 2013.

Reproduced from Centers for Disease Control and Prevention (CDC). Behavioral Risk Factor Surveillance System Survey Questionnaire. Atlanta, Georgia: U.S. Department of Health and Human Services, Centers for Disease Control and Prevention 2013 http://www.cdc.gov/obesity/data/prevalence-maps.html

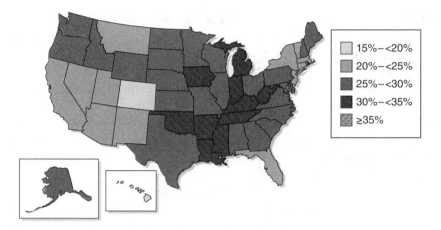

Figure 3–4 Prevalence of self-reported obesity among non-Hispanic white adults by state, BRFSS, 2011–2013.

Reproduced from Centers for Disease Control and Prevention (CDC). Behavioral Risk Factor Surveillance System Survey Questionnaire. Atlanta, Georgia: U.S. Department of Health and Human Services, Centers for Disease Control and Prevention 2011–2013 http://www.cdc.gov/obesity/data/table-non-hispanic.html

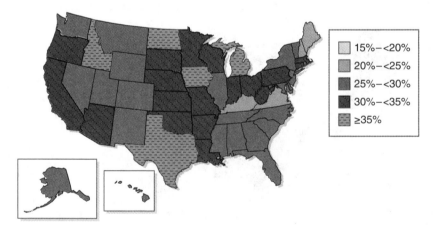

Figure 3–5 Prevalence of self-reported obesity among Hispanic adults by state, BRFSS, 2011–2013.

Reproduced from Centers for Disease Control and Prevention (CDC). Behavioral Risk Factor Surveillance System Survey Questionnaire. Atlanta, Georgia: U.S. Department of Health and Human Services, Centers for Disease Control and Prevention 2011–2013 http://www.cdc.gov/obesity/data/table-hispanics.html

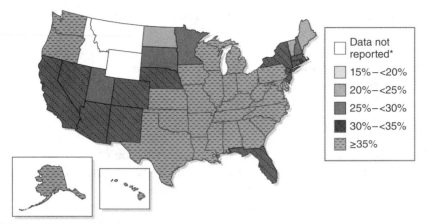

*Sample size <50 or the relative standard error (dividing the standard error by the prevalence) ≥ 30%

Figure 3–6 Prevalence of self-reported obesity among non-Hispanic black adults by state, BRFSS, 2011–2013.

Reproduced from Centers for Disease Control and Prevention (CDC). Behavioral Risk Factor Surveillance System Survey Questionnaire. Atlanta, Georgia: U.S. Department of Health and Human Services, Centers for Disease Control and Prevention 2011–2013 http://www.cdc.gov/obesity/data/table-non-hispanic-black.html

In non-Hispanic black adults, 28 states in the United States as well as the District of Columbia had an obesity prevalence of 35% or higher[34] (see **Figures 3–4, 3–5** and **3–6**).

Environmental Influences

Patterns of eating away from the home, physical inactivity, increased portion sizes, television advertising, and food pricing all contribute to observed increases in obesity.[35] Much attention is also focused on the built environment and evidence from an urban planning perspective suggests that how cities are designed and transportation systems developed may be important factors in strategies to improve walking and bicycling on a population level.[36] A study by Young and Nestle of trends in portion sizes of food servings showed a dramatic increase in the 1980s, far exceeding federal standard portion sizes. The study also demonstrated that portion size increases were accompanied by population increases in rates of overweight and obesity.[37]

Much research has been published about fast food consumption and risk for weight gain or developing type 2 diabetes. French and colleagues studied the impact of fast food consumption on energy intake and weight studied in 891 women aged 20 to 45 who filled out dietary question-naires, had weight and height measured, and were followed over a 3-year period. Results showed that more frequent fast food restaurant eating was associated with increased body weight and also with decreased physical activity.[38] In the CARDIA study, a study of more than 3,000 black and white adults, results showed that consuming fast food more often was associated with weight increases in all populations studied.[39] In a study in New Orleans, where researchers mapped the location of fast food restau-rants, investigators found differences in the density of fast food restau-rants in neighborhoods with mostly white or black residents.[40] There were 1.5 fast food restaurants per square mile in predominantly white neigh-borhoods, whereas there were 2.4 fast food restaurants per square mile in mostly black neighborhoods.[40]

The Nurses' Health Study II, a study of more than 91,000 women for 8 years, found that women drinking one or more sugar-sweetened soft drink per day had an increased risk of developing type 2 diabetes (relative risk of 1.83) when compared to women who drank less than one sugar-sweetened beverage per month.[41] Women in this study who increased the number of sugar-sweetened beverages they drank from 1 or less per week to 1 or more per day, showed the most weight gain over 4 years of the study.[41]

EVIDENCE BASE FOR PREVENTION AND PRACTICE

Upstream vs. Downstream

The discussion of population-based approaches to obesity prevention commonly invokes a call for more emphasis on "upstream" rather than "downstream" approaches, meaning the use of policy or environmental approaches, rather than just treating clinical conditions.[7] The analogy of people falling into a river is commonly used to illustrate this point.[7] Imagine a river flowing and you are standing on the bank and see someone in the river who is drowning, then another, then another, etc. The downstream approach, as the analogy goes, would require more and more clinicians to save the drowning people in the river.[7] If you hiked up the bank (walking upstream), to look for reasons why people were falling in the river, you might, for example, find that the bridge was out. An upstream or public health approach might involve fixing the bridge or at worst, creating a tem-porary detour until bridge repair could be accomplished, in order to stop the growing number of people falling into the river, while still rescuing downstream those who have already fallen in.[7] Likewise, in preventing obesity, prevention efforts aimed at the population level would aim to reduce the number of obese individuals while at the same time, clinical care, screening, and treatment continued.[7] Some authors note that stronger upstream strategies, such as policy and environmental approaches, may be especially needed and helpful in populations with lower incomes[7] and in some ethnic and cultural settings.[42]

Government Strategies and Solutions

Environmental changes in homes, schools, communities, and child care settings—places where children spend time—to promote better nutrition and more physical activity are effective strategies.[30] CDC makes recommendation for states, communities, healthcare providers, and parents about ways to improve nutrition and increase physical activity.[43] The U.S. Department of Agriculture (USDA)'s Center for Nutrition Policy and Promotion (CNPP)[44] "was established in 1994 to improve the nutrition and well-being of Americans." CNPP's activities include such priorities as establishing Dietary Guidelines for Americans, implementing USDA food guidance, such as MyPlate,[45] based on the 2010 Dietary Guidelines for Americans[46] and previous food pyramids. MyPlate is a visual representation of dietary recommendations, along with educational materials, which also reinforces physical activity, in collaboration with *Let's Move*, launched by First Lady Michelle Obama on February 9, 2010.[47]

Evidence-Based Prevention—Community Prevention

The Community Preventive Services Task Force systematically reviews community-based intervention to determine "what works" in the area of community prevention.[48] In their review of obesity prevention and control, the task force recommends interventions to reduce screen time (TV, video games, or computers) with evidence of reduced screen time and sedentary behavior, and improvement in weight-related outcomes and nutrition, in children and adolescents. Skills building, goal setting, and parent or family support were effective in supporting screen time reductions.[49] Likewise, in the area of increasing physical activity, the task force recommended strategies to change individual behavior, educational campaigns, and environmental policy approaches.[50] Based on the evidence, they recommended strategies to increase physical activity using behavior change programs aimed at individuals, social support, improved school physical education (where more children are more active for longer times), and improved community design to make places for physical activity more available and accessible.[50]

Evidence-Based Prevention—Clinical Prevention

The U.S. Preventive Services Task Force (USPSTF), an independent panel of nongovernment experts in prevention and evidence-based medicine, systematically reviews scientific evidence for clinical prevention and develops recommendations for healthcare professionals using a grading system in which an "A" or "B" grade provides an evidence-based service recommended for clinical practice.[51] USPSTF recommends health professionals screen children for obesity, starting at age 6, and refer them to further interventions as needed to improve weight status.[52] They also recommend screening all adults for obesity in clinical settings and referring patients with a BMI of 30 kg/m^2 or higher to further interventions.[53] Some authors argue that families and schools are the best vehicles for prevention and health professionals caring for children can provide "anticipatory guidance" related to television viewing to further support parents' efforts.[54]

Environmental Strategies and the Built Environment

There is evidence that local food environments are important in obesity prevention. Investigators studied food stores in Mississippi, North Carolina, Maryland, and Minnesota and compared them to rates of obesity and overweight, in over 10,000 individuals participating in the Atherosclerosis Risk in Communities (ARIC) study.[55] They specifically looked at whether the availability of larger supermarkets, smaller grocery stores, or even smaller convenience stores was related to the percentage of people with obesity in that geographic location. Researchers found that percentages of obesity and overweight were lowest in areas with only larger supermarkets and highest in places that had only convenience stores and smaller grocery stores. They suggested that what types of food stores (and food products) are available in a given location may be important in the development of strategies to prevent overweight and obesity.[55]

In considering how neighborhoods might also differ in ways other than the types, size, and numbers of food stores, Morland and colleagues compared food stores, housing values, and whether neighborhoods had mostly white or black residents, in Mississippi, North Carolina, Maryland, and Minnesota to estimate how social, economic, and cultural factors might play a role. In their study, more supermarkets were found in wealthier neighborhoods and in predominantly white neighborhoods.[56] Another study of 1,295 adults in some Mississippi and North Carolina neighborhoods showed an association between large chain supermarkets, smaller grocery and convenience stores, fast food restaurants and the percentage of obesity in the population.[57] The presence of at least one large supermarket was associated with a lower prevalence of obesity. Areas with at least one smaller grocery store, at least one convenience store with a gas station, or more than one fast food restaurant were associated with higher population percentages of obesity.[57]

A cross sectional study in Atlanta, GA, looked at weight, time spent in a car, and demographic information through a survey of more than 10,000 individuals, also measuring land use and density of residential areas in areas where participants lived.[58] Of all factors studied, land-use mix had the strongest relationship with obesity, as did increased time spent in a car, while walking was associated with lowered risk of obesity. The authors concluded that land-use and strategies to increase walking and reduce car use could have positive public health benefits.[58]

Changing Dietary Behavior

There are also published studies about interventions to decrease the amount of sugar-sweetened beverages that children consume. A randomized controlled pilot study in adolescents, using home deliveries of noncaloric beverages in the intervention group showed a reduced consumption of sugar-sweetened beverages and reduction in BMI among the heaviest participants.[59] An educational trial in England in children aged 7 to 11 to reduce consumption of sugar-sweetened drinks resulted in fewer drinks consumed and fewer overweight and obese children.[60] Recent studies discuss the potential of "traffic-light" labels promoting healthy food choices. In a study in a large hospital cafeteria, foods were labeled like a traffic light—green, yellow, or red, to reflect healthier to less healthy choices, and records were kept of cafeteria sales.[61] Over a 2-year period, the sale of red (unhealthy) food choices decreased and green (healthy) food choices increased, both statistically significant changes. Similar significant changes were also seen with labeled beverages.[61]

Systematic Reviews

A review of interventions to prevent childhood obesity in Sweden included 24 studies that involved more than 25,000 children.[62] Authors found 41% of the studies reviewed had positive effects from school-based interventions that included both physical activity and promotion of healthy diets.[62] Systematic reviews of childhood interventions to prevent obesity highlighted the importance of school environments,[63] but also demonstrated the challenges of finding specific programs and best practices, and the need for more and ongoing research.[7,63,64]

Some authors simply call for a more systematic approach to improving the built environment to enhance physical activity, including improved education in training public health professionals, research, and creating an infrastructure to promote physical activity.[65]

What Might the Future Hold?

The Robert Wood Johnson Foundation and Trust for America's Health have projected what we might expect in the United Stated in 2030 under two different set of assumptions, one in which current obesity trends continue and another that assumes a 5% reduction in average BMI.[66] If obesity rates continue on the present course, the authors projected more than half of adult Americans would be obese in 39 states by 2030; type 2 diabetes, coronary heart disease and stroke, hypertension, and arthritis would "increase 10 times between 2010 and 2020 and double again by 2030;"[66] and healthcare costs could rise by as much as $66 billion per year.[66] Under a projection in which BMI is decreased by 5% among the U.S. population, over half of adult Americans would be obese in 24 states, fewer Americans would develop chronic conditions, and healthcare cost savings could be as high as $81.7 billion in some states.[66] Recommendations in this report included such priorities as protecting needed prevention and public health funding, and investing in effective prevention programs.[66]

The 2012 report titled "F as in Fat: How Obesity Threatens America's Future," captured wide public and media attention, with such controversial headlines such as "Most U.S. residents will be obese within next 2 decades,"[67] "Fat and getting fatter: U.S. obesity rates to soar by 2030,"[68] and called attention to the present by projecting consequences for the future. Meanwhile, Elizabeth Kolbert, in *The New Yorker*, reminds us that the impact of obesity can be subtly integrated, without our really noticing, into daily life: "Hospitals have had to buy special wheelchairs and operating tables to accommodate the obese, and revolving doors have had to be widened."[69]

Why are such attempts to project obesity rates and the related health risks and healthcare costs so important? Because when there is a slow, steady rise in the prevalence of a risk factor or chronic condition, unless continued attention is paid, the risk is that is it not very noticeable until there is a dramatic change. This is most easily seen on the CDC website[6] where their use of color maps gives a vivid picture of the geographic variation and worsening of adult obesity throughout the United States over the last 25 years. Other types of epidemics, such as those caused by infectious diseases may be much more apparent in a short time period. In contrast, the insidious but continued worsening of the obesity epidemic becomes obvious only when it becomes substantially worse, potentially hindering public attention and progress in the interim.

However, there is encouraging news. Using data from NHANES to study trends in abdominal obesity (high waist circumference) in more than 16,000 U.S. children and adolescents from 2003 to 2012, rates of abdominal obesity were stable in most age groups, and decreased significantly in young children, aged 2 to 5.[70] In August 2013, CDC reported in its publication *Vital Signs*[71] that there is demonstrable progress in childhood obesity in some states in the United States. Small decreases in obesity rates in low-income, preschool-aged children were reported in 19 of 43 states included as a part of this report.[71] Although there was worsening in 3 states, and no difference in 21 states and territories, this was a welcome change after many years of increases and the grim statistic that about 1 in 8 preschoolers are obese.[71] To build on this progress, CDC recommends changes in communities to ensure access to healthy and affordable foods, encouraging availability of places for physical activity for children, and supporting healthcare professionals in counseling children and families about nutrition and physical activity.[71]

DISCUSSION QUESTIONS: TEMPLATE FOR DISCUSSION

1. Significance of this public health issue:
   a. Why is this health issue important?
   b. How many people does it impact?
   c. How serious is it?
   d. Is it preventable?

2. What is the evidence base for prevention?
3. What specific strategies should be used to achieve progress on this health issue?
   a. What evidence-based approach would you use?
   b. Where would you start if you are an individual citizen; public health professional; healthcare professional; community, state, or federal policymaker?
4. Specific questions for this topic:
   a. What is the evidence that environmental and behavioral factors contribute to obesity? What specific factors play a role?
   b. What is the evidence that a combination of individual and population-based approaches will reduce the health consequences of obesity in both children and adults?
   c. Is there a role (or not) for the beverage industry in creating solutions?
5. What is the controversy?
   a. Define the controversy.
   b. Is controversy a good or bad thing? (Does it help or hinder progress?)
6. *Why* is this health issue controversial?
   a. What specific factors are involved?
   b. Do economics, government, scientific uncertainty, or politics play a role?
   c. What is the role of the media?
7. How would you respond to the controversy?

PERSPECTIVES TO CONSIDER

Scientific evidence supporting obesity as a risk for a variety of health conditions—and death—is not a new finding. Systematic reviews of evidence-based prevention strategies highlight commonalities in approaches and solutions, but also highlight challenges and research gaps, and lack of a clear cookie-cutter approach to successful interventions.[7,62–64] This is not surprising given what we know about how place, demographics, and environmental factors play a role, with obesity rates dramatically higher in some populations and in some geographic locations.[33,34] There is intriguing research about social networks and the interconnectedness of how we live, work, and socialize that can provide additional hints for new approaches.[72] Policy leverage to prevent obesity is supported by many authors, but is also controversial. It is important to think about policy in the broadest sense, from implementing the National Prevention Strategy[73] and ensuring full funding for the Prevention and Public Health Fund established by the Patient Protection and Affordable Care Act;[74] to local initiatives, such as school policies, price increases or decreases, or funding strategies concerned with improving the built environment.

Obesity is complicated. The good news is that there are hints of progress and research continues at a rapid pace. Recent studies regarding the benefits of low-carbohydrate diets in weight loss and improving risk factors for cardiovascular disease[75,76] have sparked debate, once again, as to what dietary recommendations we should be following. The role of controversies in obesity is also complex. Consider the use of language—fat vs. overweight. Does this help or hinder the conversation? Academic debate and statistical sparring about obesity and the risk of death[77–79] are essential for the clearest research on this complex topic, but may also confuse the public; such controversies[80,81] advance our knowledge, but nuances must also be clearly communicated.

Is obesity the "new normal"[3] in our society? Have we really gotten used to obesity as an expected health condition? Prevention messages are challenging to create and sustain, and one risk from becoming too accustomed to a health issue is a risk of complacency. However, at least at the present time, with regards to obesity, there is certainly no shortage of controversy.

FOR ADDITIONAL STUDY

Kumanyika SK, Obarzanek E, Stettler N, et al. Population-based prevention of obesity: The need for comprehensive promotion of healthful eating, physical activity, and energy balance: A scientific statement from American Heart Association Council on Epidemiology and Prevention, Interdisciplinary Committee for Prevention (Formerly the Expert Panel on Population and Prevention Science). *Circulation.* 2008;118(4):428–464.

Ng M, Fleming T, Robinson M, et al. Global, regional, and national prevalence of overweight and obesity in children and adults during 1980–2013: a systematic analysis for the Global Burden of Disease Study 2013. *Lancet.* 2014;384(9945):766–781.

REFERENCES

1. Koplan JP, Liverman CT, Kraak VI, Committee on Prevention of Obesity in Children and Youth. Preventing childhood obesity: Health in the balance: Executive summary. *Journal of the American Dietetic Association.* 2005;105(1):131–138.
2. Is overweight the new normal weight? [blog]. *Huffingtonpost.com.* 2011. http://www.huffingtonpost.com/2011/09/11/normalizing-obesity_n_956111.html. Accessed September 6, 2013,

3. United States of overweight? *Health Buzz, Newroom.* 2011. http://www.lpollockpr .com/2011/07/12/united-states-of-overweight/. Accessed September 6, 2013.

4. IFIC Foundation Releases 2011 Food and Health Survey: Price approaches taste as top influencer for Americans when purchasing foods and beverages. *Food Insight.* 2011. http://www.foodinsight.org/Press-Release/Detail.aspx?topic=Price_Approaches_ Taste_as_Top_Influencer_for_Americans_When_Purchasing_Foods_Beverages. Accessed September 6, 2013.

5. WHO. Obesity and overweight: Fact sheet. 2013. http://www.who.int/mediacentre/ factsheets/fs311/en/index.html. Accessed September 6, 2013.

6. CDC. Overweight and obesity. 2013. http://www.cdc.gov/obesity/. Accessed September 6, 2013.

7. Kumanyika SK, Obarzanek E, Stettler N, et al. Population-based prevention of obesity: The need for comprehensive promotion of healthful eating, physical activity, and energy balance: A scientific statement from American Heart Association Council on Epidemiology and Prevention, Interdisciplinary Committee for Prevention (Formerly the Expert Panel on Population and Prevention Science). *Circulation.* 2008;118(4):428–464.

8. Ng M, Fleming T, Robinson M, et al. Global, regional, and national prevalence of overweight and obesity in children and adults during 1980–2013: A systematic analysis for the Global Burden of Disease Study 2013. *Lancet.* 2014;384(9945):766–781.

9. McGinnis JM, Foege WH. Actual causes of death in the United States. *JAMA.* 1993;270(18):2207–2212.

10. Mokdad AH, Marks JS, Stroup DF, Gerberding JL. Actual causes of death in the United States, 2000. *JAMA.* 2004;291(10):1238–1245.

11. CDC. About the National Health and Nutrition Examination Survey. 2013. http://www .cdc.gov/nchs/nhanes/about_nhanes.htm. Accessed September 5, 2013.

12. CDC. Behavioral Risk Factor Surveillance System. 2013. http://www.cdc.gov/brfss/ about/brfss_today.htm. Accessed September 5, 2013.

13. CDC. Youth Risk Behavior Surveillance System (YRBSS). 2013. http://www.cdc.gov/ HealthyYouth/yrbs/index.htm. Accessed September 6, 2013.

14. CDC. National Health Interview Survey. 2013. http://www.cdc.gov/nchs/nhis.htm. Accessed September 5, 2013.

15. CDC. Overweight and obesity: Basics about childhood obesity. 2013. http://www.cdc .gov/obesity/childhood/basics.html. Accessed September 6, 2013.

16. Fryar CD, Carroll MD, Ogden CL. Prevalence of obesity among children and adolescents: United States, trends 1963–1965 through 2009–2010. *NCHS Health E-Stat.* 2012. http://www.cdc.gov/nchs/data/hestat/obesity_child_09_10/obesity_child_09_10.htm. Accessed September 6, 2013.

17. Fryar CD, Carroll MD, Ogden CL. Prevalence of overweight, obesity, and extreme obesity among adults: United States, trends 1960–1962 through 2009–2010. *NCHS Health E-Stat.* 2012. http://www.cdc.gov/nchs/data/hestat/obesity_adult_09_10/obesity_ adult_09_10.htm. Accessed September 6, 2013.

18. CDC. Overweight and obesity: Causes and consequences. 2013. http://www.cdc.gov/ obesity/adult/causes/index.html. Accessed September 6, 2013.

19. Manson JE, Willett WC, Stampfer MJ, et al. Body weight and mortality among women. *N Engl J Med.* 1995;333(11):677–685.

20. Truesdale KP, Stevens J, Lewis CE, Schreiner PJ, Loria CM, Cai J. Changes in risk factors for cardiovascular disease by baseline weight status in young adults who

maintain or gain weight over 15 years: The CARDIA study. *Int J Obes (Lond).* 2006;30(9):1397–1407.

21. Wannamethee SG, Shaper AG, Walker M. Overweight and obesity and weight change in middle aged men: Impact on cardiovascular disease and diabetes. *J Epidemiol Commun H.* 2005;59(2):134–139.

22. Daniels SR, Arnett DK, Eckel RH, et al. Overweight in children and adolescents: Pathophysiology, consequences, prevention, and treatment. *Circulation.* 2005;111(15):1999–2012.

23. Daniels SR. The consequences of childhood overweight and obesity. *The Future of children/Center for the Future of Children, the David and Lucile Packard Foundation.* 2006;16(1):47–67.

24. Thompson DR, Obarzanek E, Franko DL, et al. Childhood overweight and cardiovascular disease risk factors: The National Heart, Lung, and Blood Institute Growth and Health Study. *J Pediatr.* 2007;150(1):18–25.

25. Field AE, Cook NR, Gillman MW. Weight status in childhood as a predictor of becoming overweight or hypertensive in early adulthood. *Obes Res.* 2005;13(1): 163–169.

26. Davison KK, Birch LL. Weight status, parent reaction, and self-concept in five-year-old girls. *Pediatrics.* 2001;107(1):46–53.

27. Hayden-Wade HA, Stein RI, Ghaderi A, Saelens BE, Zabinski MF, Wilfley DE. Prevalence, characteristics, and correlates of teasing experiences among overweight children vs. non-overweight peers. *Obes Res.* 2005;13(8):1381–1392.

28. Narayan KM, Boyle JP, Thompson TJ, Sorensen SW, Williamson DF. Lifetime risk for diabetes mellitus in the United States. *JAMA.* 2003;290(14):1884–1890.

29. Belluck P. Children's life expectancy being cut short by obesity. *The New York Times.* March 17, 2005.

30. CDC. Overweight and obesity: A growing problem: What causes childhood obesity? 2013. http://www.cdc.gov/obesity/childhood/problem.html. Accessed September 6, 2013.

31. CDC. Overweight and obesity: Causes and consequences: What causes overweight and obesity? 2013. http://www.cdc.gov/obesity/adult/causes/index.html. Accessed September 6, 2013.

32. U.S. Department of Health and Human Services. The Surgeon General's call to action to prevent and decrease overweight and obesity. 2001. http://www.ncbi.nlm.nih.gov/books/NBK44206/pdf/TOC.pdf. Accessed January 26, 2015.

33. CDC. Overweight and obesity: Adult obesity facts. 2013. http://www.cdc.gov/obesity/data/adult.html. Accessed September 6, 2013.

34. CDC. Overweight and obesity: Data, maps, and trends. 2014. http://www.cdc.gov/obesity/data/databases.html. Accessed September 11, 2014.

35. French SA, Story M, Jeffery RW. Environmental influences on eating and physical activity. *Annu Rev Publ Health.* 2001;22:309–335.

36. Handy SL, Boarnet MG, Ewing R, Killingsworth RE. How the built environment affects physical activity: Views from urban planning. *Am J Prev Med.* 2002;23(2):64–73.

37. Young LR, Nestle M. The contribution of expanding portion sizes to the US obesity epidemic. *Am J Public Health.* 2002;92(2):246–249.

38. French SA, Harnack L, Jeffery RW. Fast food restaurant use among women in the Pound of Prevention study: Dietary, behavioral and demographic correlates. *Int J Obesity.* 2000;24(10):1353–1359.

39. Pereira MA, Kartashov AI, Ebbeling CB, et al. Fast-food habits, weight gain, and insulin resistance (the CARDIA study): 15-year prospective analysis. *Lancet.* 2005;365(9453):36–42.

40. Block JP, Scribner RA, DeSalvo KB. Fast food, race/ethnicity, and income: A geographic analysis. *Am J Prev Med.* 2004;27(3):211–217.

41. Schulze MB, Manson JE, Ludwig DS, et al. Sugar-sweetened beverages, weight gain, and incidence of type 2 diabetes in young and middle-aged women. *JAMA.* 2004;292(8):927–934.

42. Kumanyika SK. Environmental influences on childhood obesity: Ethnic and cultural influences in context. *Physiol Behav.* 2008;94(1):61–70.

43. CDC. Overweight and obesity: Strategies and solutions. 2013. http://www.cdc.gov/obesity/childhood/solutions.html. Accessed September 5, 2013.

44. USDA. USDA Center for Nutrition Policy and Promotion. 2013. http://www.cnpp.usda.gov/. Accessed September 5, 2013.

45. USDA. USDA Choose MyPlate.gov. 2013. http://www.choosemyplate.gov/. Accessed September 5, 2013.

46. USDA. USDA Center for Nutrition Policy and Promotion: Dietary guidelines for Americans. 2010. http://www.cnpp.usda.gov/DietaryGuidelines.htm. Accessed September 5, 2013.

47. Let's Move: America's move to raise a healthier generation of kids. 2013. http://www.letsmove.gov/learn-facts/epidemic-childhood-obesity. Accessed September 5, 2013.

48. The Guide to Community Preventive Services: What works to promote health. 2013. http://www.thecommunityguide.org/index.html. Accessed September 6, 2013.

49. The Guide to Community Preventive Services: Obesity prevention and control. 2013. http://www.thecommunityguide.org/obesity/index.html. Accessed September 6, 2013.

50. The Guide to Community Preventive Services: Increasing physical activity. 2008. http://www.thecommunityguide.org/pa/index.html. Accessed September 6, 2013.

51. USPSTF. US Preventive Services Task Force Home. 2013. http://www.uspreventiveservicestaskforce.org/. Accessed September 6, 2013.

52. USPSTF. Screening for obesity in children and adolescents. 2010. http://www.uspreventiveservicestaskforce.org/uspstf/uspschobes.htm. Accessed September 6, 2013.

53. USPSTF. Screening for and management of obesity in adults. *USPSTF Recommendation Statement.* 2012. http://www.uspreventiveservicestaskforce.org/uspstf/uspsobes.htm. Accessed September 6, 2013.

54. Dietz WH, Gortmaker SL. Preventing obesity in children and adolescents. *Annu Rev Publ Health.* 2001;22:337–353.

55. Morland K, Diez Roux AV, Wing S. Supermarkets, other food stores, and obesity: The atherosclerosis risk in communities study. *Am J Prev Med.* 2006;30(4):333–339.

56. Morland K, Wing S, Diez Roux A, Poole C. Neighborhood characteristics associated with the location of food stores and food service places. *Am J Prev Med.* 2002;22(1):23–29.

57. Morland KB, Evenson KR. Obesity prevalence and the local food environment. *Health Place.* 2009;15(2):491–495.

58. Frank LD, Andresen MA, Schmid TL. Obesity relationships with community design, physical activity, and time spent in cars. *Am J Prev Med.* 2004;27(2):87–96.

59. Ebbeling CB, Feldman HA, Osganian SK, Chomitz VR, Ellenbogen SJ, Ludwig DS. Effects of decreasing sugar-sweetened beverage consumption on body weight in adolescents: A randomized, controlled pilot study. *Pediatrics.* 2006;117(3):673–680.

60. James J, Thomas P, Cavan D, Kerr D. Preventing childhood obesity by reducing consumption of carbonated drinks: Cluster randomised controlled trial. *BMJ.* 2004;328(7450):1237.

61. Thorndike AN, Riis J, Sonnenberg LM, Levy DE. Traffic-light labels and choice architecture: Promoting healthy food choices. *Am J Prev Med.* 2014;46(2): 143–149.

62. Flodmark CE, Marcus C, Britton M. Interventions to prevent obesity in children and adolescents: A systematic literature review. *Int J Obes (Lond).* 2006;30(4): 579–589.

63. Flynn MA, McNeil DA, Maloff B, et al. Reducing obesity and related chronic disease risk in children and youth: A synthesis of evidence with 'best practice' recommendations. *Obes Rev.* 2006;7(Suppl 1):7–66.

64. Summerbell CD, Waters E, Edmunds LD, Kelly S, Brown T, Campbell KJ. Interventions for preventing obesity in children. *Cochrane Db Syst Rev.* 2005(3):1–78.

65. Yancey AK, Fielding JE, Flores GR, Sallis JF, McCarthy WJ, Breslow L. Creating a robust public health infrastructure for physical activity promotion. *Am J Prev Med.* 2007;32(1):68–78.

66. Levi J, Segal LM, Thomas K, St. Laurent R, Lang A, Rayburn J. F as in fat: How obesity threatens America's future. 2013. http://www.rwjf.org/content/dam/farm/reports/reports/2013/rwjf407528. Accessed September 6, 2013.

67. Gates S. American obesity in 2030: Most U.S. residents will be obese within next 2 decades. *Huffingtonpost.com.* 2012. http://www.huffingtonpost.com/2012/09/18/us-obesity-2030-americans-obese_n_1893578.html. Accessed September 5, 2013.

68. Begley S. Fat and getting fatter: U.S. obesity rates to soar by 2030. *Reuters.* 2012. http://www.reuters.com/article/2012/09/18/us-obesity-us-idUSBRE88H0RA20120918. Accessed September 5, 2013.

69. Kolbert E. XXXL. *The New Yorker.* 2009. http://www.newyorker.com/arts/critics/books/2009/07/20/090720crbo_books_kolbert. Accessed September 6, 2013.

70. Xi B, Mi J, Zhao M, et al. Trends in abdominal obesity among US children and adolescents. *Pediatrics.* 2014;134(2):e334–339.

71. CDC. Progress on childhood obesity. *CDC Vital Signs.* 2013. http://www.cdc.gov/vitalsigns/childhoodobesity/. Accessed September 6, 2013.

72. Christakis NA, Fowler JH. The spread of obesity in a large social network over 32 years. *N Engl J Med.* 2007;357(4):370–379.

73. U.S. Department of Health and Human Services. National Prevention Strategy. 2011. http://www.surgeongeneral.gov/initiatives/prevention/strategy/. Accessed September 6, 2013.

74. U.S. Department of Health and Human Services. HHS.gov/Open Prevention and Public Health Fund. 2013. http://www.hhs.gov/open/recordsandreports/prevention/. Accessed September 6, 2013.

75. Hu T, Bazzano LA. The low-carbohydrate diet and cardiovascular risk factors: Evidence from epidemiologic studies. *Nutr Metab Cardiovas.* 2014;24(4):337–343.

76. Bazzano LA, Hu T, Reynolds K, et al. Effects of low-carbohydrate and low-fat diets: A randomized trial. *Ann Intern Med.* 2014;161(5):309–318.

77. Flegal KM, Kit BK, Orpana H, Graubard BI. Association of all-cause mortality with overweight and obesity using standard body mass index categories: A systematic review and meta-analysis. *JAMA.* 2013;309(1):71–82.

78. Heymsfield SB, Cefalu WT. Does body mass index adequately convey a patient's mortality risk? *JAMA*. 2013;309(1):87–88.
79. Willett WC, Hu FB, Thun M. Overweight, obesity, and all-cause mortality. *JAMA*. 24 2013;309(16):1681.
80. Campos P. Our absurd fear of fat. *The New York Times*. 2013. http://www.nytimes.com/2013/01/03/opinion/our-imaginary-weight-problem.html. Accessed September 6, 2013.
81. Hughes V. The big fat truth. *Nature*. 2013;497(7450). http://www.nature.com/news/the-big-fat-truth-1.13039. Accessed September 5, 2013.

CHAPTER 4

Preventing Obesity—Raising the Price of Sugar-Sweetened Beverages?

LEARNING OBJECTIVES

- Describe data and trends in consumption of sugar-sweetened beverages in both children and adults in the United States.
- Discuss the relationship between consumption of sugar-sweetened beverages and obesity.
- Review the evidence that raising the price of sugar-sweetened beverages will limit consumption.
- Identify opposing arguments to policy changes that would increase the price of sugar-sweetened beverages.
- Summarize the public health impact of proposed price increases.

THE CONTROVERSY

An April 2013, *U.S. News and World Report-Health* story reported that Americans were less than enthusiastic about taxing soda and candy based on the results of a Harris Interactive/HealthDay poll that found that the majority of U.S. adults oppose taxes on soda and candy.[1] According to the story, between 56 and 58% of those polled were opposed to these taxes; levels of support for the taxes was much lower, between 21 and 23%. According to the article, the chairman of Harris Interactive declared, "This is a strong vote against the 'nanny state.'"[1]

The poll itself was an online survey of 2,132 adults conducted in March and April of 2013 by Harris Interactive, drawn from individuals who have agreed to participate in their surveys.[2] Harris specifically asked consumers to react to the statement, "Some state governments have proposed charging a separate sales tax on candy and/or sodas containing sugar or corn syrup sold in that state . . . would you favor or oppose the idea of your state adopting/approving this proposal?" According to their results, 21% of all adults surveyed strongly or somewhat supported a tax on candy, and 23% supported a tax on sodas containing sugar or corn syrup.[1,2] In contrast, 58% somewhat or strongly opposed a tax on candy, and 55% opposed a tax on sodas.[1,2] They also asked respondents to react to statements about taxing sodas and candy: 67% agreed and 17% disagreed with the statement, "It should not be the role of government to influence what we eat and drink to make healthier choices."[2] Furthermore, 51% of respondents disagreed and 26% agreed with the statement, "Sales taxes on candy and sodas would help to reduce obesity."[2]

The poll was conducted and results were published during a time when states such as Vermont,[3] Texas,[4] and California[5] (after two California communities defeated such proposals in 2012) were considering proposals to raise the price of sugar-sweetened beverages to help combat childhood obesity.[2] The poll's timing also coincided with efforts by the city of New York to ban large, sugar-sweetened beverages and the subsequent state appeals court ruling that the limits in the ban were "arbitrary and capricious."[6] Meanwhile, the American Heart Association's blog optimistically stated, "Soda debate bubbling," describing recent efforts in California, New York, and Illinois to gain public support for a tax and Mexico's price hike on sugar-sweetened drinks.[7]

BACKGROUND AND SCOPE OF THE PUBLIC HEALTH AND HEALTH POLICY ISSUE

The Centers for Disease Control and Prevention (CDC) emphasize that sugar-sweetened beverages (SSBs) add both calories and sugar to the diets of children and adults, representing the largest source of added sugar.[8] The Dietary Guidelines for Americans (2010) from the U.S. Department of Agriculture (USDA) and U.S. Department of Health and Human Services (HHS) recommend reducing the intake of SSBs.[9] *Healthy People 2020*, national public health goals and objectives for the United States for the year 2020, has objectives related to SSBs in its topic area of Nutrition and Weight Status. Objectives include increasing the number of states with nutrition standards for food and beverages for children in child care and increasing the percentage of schools in the United States that do not sell or offer calorically sweetened beverages to students.[10] CDC has also published "The Guide to Strategies for Reducing the Consumption of Sugar-Sweetened Beverages," which details a variety of public health strategies.[8] CDC recommends such approaches as improving availability of drinking water, decreasing the cost of healthy beverages (relative to SSBs), including discussion of SSBs in healthcare settings, and reducing availability of SSBs in a variety of settings.[8]

Trends in Consumption

A comprehensive review of dietary sugar intake and cardiovascular health reported the consumption of sugars and sweeteners increased by 19% between 1970 and 2005, from about 400 to 476 calories per day, as noted by the USDA's Economic Research Service.[11] In addition, the USDA's 1994–1996 Continuing Survey of Food Intakes reported that added sweeteners represent 16% of total energy intake, in a large national sample, and soft drinks represented the single largest source of added sweeteners.[12] Using three national surveys, French and colleagues found that consumption of soft drinks among youth aged 6 to 17 years increased from 5 ounces to 12 ounces per day when comparing the time period 1977–1978 to 1994–1998.[13] In addition, during the study time period, the source of consumed soft drinks from restaurants and vending machines increased, although soft drinks consumed at home was still the largest source.[13] Evidence that consumption of SSBs increases rather than displaces total energy consumed is suggested by a study of 33 individuals by Flood and colleagues, who found that increasing beverage size resulted in significantly more total energy consumed during meals.[14] Other reports support these conclusions.[15]

Data from the National Health and Nutrition Examination Survey (NHANES 2005–2008) published by the National Center for Health Statistics (NCHS)[16] regarding consumption of SSBs in the United States showed that males and females consumed an average of 178 kcal and 103 kcal respectively each day (see **Figure 4–1**). According to this analysis, about 50% of the U.S. population consumes drinks with added-sugar on any day; this figure is highest for boys age 2–19 (70%) and girls age 2–19 (60%)[16] (see **Figure 4–2**).

In addition, there are racial and ethnic differences: in children and adolescents age 2–19, the percentage of total daily kilocalories consumed from SSBs was higher in non-Hispanic black children and adolescents than in both Mexican-Americans and non-Hispanic white individuals.

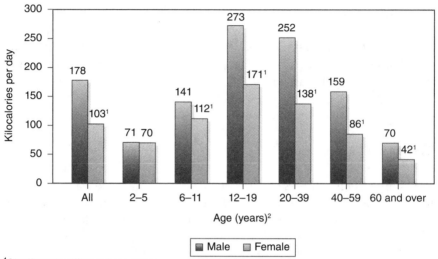

[1]Significantly different from males.
[2]Significant quadratic trend for both males and females.

Figure 4–1 Mean kilocalories from sugar drinks for ages 2 and over.

Reproduced from Ogden CL, Kit, BK, Carroll, MD, Park, S. Consumption of Sugar Drinks in the United States, 2005–2008. NCHS Data Brief, no. 71. Hyattsville, MD.: National Center for Health Statistics 2011. http://www.cdc.gov/nchs/data/databriefs/db71.pdf. Accessed September 2, 2013.

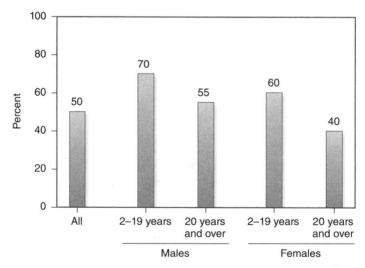

Figure 4–2 Percentage of U.S. population aged 2 and over who drink sugar drinks on a given day.

Reproduced from Ogden CL, Kit, BK, Carroll, MD, Park, S. Consumption of Sugar Drinks in the United States, 2005–2008. NCHS Data Brief, no. 71. Hyattsville, MD.: National Center for Health Statistics 2011. http://www.cdc.gov/nchs/data/databriefs/db71.pdf. Accessed September 2, 2013.

For those aged 20 and older, consumption was lowest in non-Hispanic white individuals.[16] The percentage of total daily kilocalories from SSBs varied by poverty level as well: there was greater consumption in people with lower incomes and differences were most pronounced in adults over the age of 20.[16] More than half the calories from SSBs were consumed at home, and of these, more than 90% were bought in stores.[16] These statistics are directly relevant to the policy discussion about raising prices of SSBs.

Kumar and colleagues used data from CDC's Behavioral Risk Factor Surveillance System (BRFSS) to calculate how often SSBs were consumed by U.S. adults in 18 states.[17] They included both soda and fruit drinks that contained sugar. More than one-quarter (26.3%) of people responding to the survey said they drank either soda, fruit drinks, or both one or more times per day.[17] Soda consumption was highest in Mississippi (32.4%) and Tennessee (30.2%) and consumption of fruit drinks was highest in Nevada (18.7%), Mississippi (17.0%), and Tennessee (16.5%).[17] For all respondents, reported daily consumption of soda (17.1%) was higher than for fruit drinks (11.6%). There were differences in consumption by age, with individuals age 18 to 34 reporting the highest percentages of daily consumption of soda or fruit drinks; men consumed more daily soda than women, and black non-Hispanic and Hispanic respondents reported higher fruit drink and soda consumption than white respondents.[17] Although results were self-reported and not all 50 states were included, the authors wondered whether reported geographic differences in SSB marketing[18] might be a contributing factor[17] (see **Figure 4–3**).

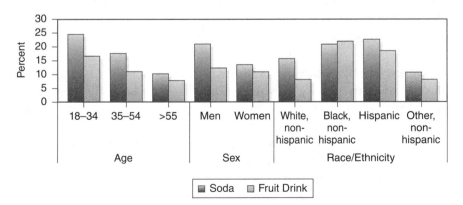

Figure 4–3 Regular soda and fruit drink consumption in 18 states, 2012.

Data from Kumar GS, Pan L, Park S, et al. Sugar-sweetened beverage consumption among adults - 18 States, 2012. MMWR Morb Mortal Wkly Rep. Aug 15 2014;63(32):686–690. http://www.cdc.gov/mmwr/preview/mmwrhtml/mm6332a2.htm

Does SSB Consumption Contribute to Obesity and Chronic Diseases?

To investigate the relationship between soft drink consumption and health outcomes, Vartanian and colleagues performed a meta-analysis of 88 studies.[19] In their analysis, soft drink consumption was associated with increases in energy intake, body weight, and chronic health conditions such as type 2 diabetes, and these relationships were stronger in prospective and experimental studies.[19] A review of 30 high-quality studies that evaluated the relationship between SSBs and obesity found higher intakes of SSBs were related to weight gain and obesity in children and adults.[20]

In an analysis of the Health Professionals Follow-Up Study (HPFS) of 42,883 men, de Koning and colleagues found that SSBs (but not artificially sweetened beverages) were associated with a significantly increased risk for coronary heart disease.[21] Ludwig and colleagues followed 548 elementary-school children from Massachusetts schools to determine whether increases in SSB consumption were related to subsequent weight gain and risk of obesity. After 19 months, in this widely quoted study, the authors noted an increase in BMI and a 60% increased risk (odds ratio) of obesity for each additional daily serving of a SSB.[22] In 2013, DeBoer and colleagues, in a large observational study, found that higher BMIs were also associated with SSB consumption in very young children (age 2–5), with an increased risk of obesity seen in children as young as 5 years.[23] Another comprehensive review relates increasing SSB consumption with increased obesity, type 2 diabetes mellitus, and cardiovascular disease, in both the United States and globally.[15]

Interventions to Reduce Soda Consumption—What Do They Tell Us?

A randomized controlled trial, conducted in schools in England, included 644 elementary schoolchildren, and was designed to determine whether childhood obesity could be prevented by reducing soda consumption through an educational campaign.[24] The year-long educational program was designed to discourage soda consumption and promote a healthy diet. In addition to increased water consumption in both groups, the study showed a reduction in carbonated drink consumption and prevalence of overweight and obese children after one year.[24]

A randomized controlled pilot study in Massachusetts studied the relationship between decreasing SSB consumption and the subsequent impact on adolescents' weights.[25] Researchers randomized 103 adolescents to receive weekly home deliveries of non-caloric beverages and compared them to a control group who followed their usual soft drink consumption habits. After the 25-week study period, there was a 82% reduction in SSB consumption in the group receiving home delivery of non-caloric beverages, and body mass index (BMI) decreased only in the group with the highest BMI at the beginning of the study.[25] Associations between reduced consumption of SSBs and subsequent decrease in BMI were also seen in overweight girls in Brazil in another randomized trial.[26]

In another category of studies, investigators looked at the impact of federal or state policies and regulations concerning "competitive foods and beverages," which are foods and drinks sold in schools in addition to (in competition with) school meal programs and are more likely to be high in fat, calories, and added sugar.[27–29] A review of 19 states that implemented restrictive policies between 2004 and 2007 showed significant reported declines in access to soft drinks and less-nutritious snacks.[28] Another study of more than 16,000 children aged 11 to 14, examined the relationship between the strength of state competitive food and beverage laws and obesity. These investigators found that children in states with weaker laws were more likely to be overweight or obese.[29] A systematic review of school competitive food and beverage policies, noted that they were often associated with changes in availability and consumption. However investigators noted limitations in the study designs and felt that more and higher quality research is needed.[27]

EVIDENCE BASE FOR PREVENTION AND PRACTICE

What Is the Evidence that Raising Price Will Limit Consumption?

The strongest evidence that raising price will reduce consumption and actually translate to public health benefits comes from success in tobacco prevention and control.[30,31] Evidence of the effectiveness of increased tobacco excise taxes in reducing consumption, reducing initiation of smoking and prevalence of smoking in young people, and encouraging cessation is extensively documented.[32] In addition, there is consensus that such strategies, in the area of tobacco policy, improve public health.[32] Arguments supporting public health and economic benefits of raising the price of SSBs through taxation cite potential mechanisms and studies relating increased consumption to adverse health outcomes[15,33,34] and medical costs related to overweight and obesity.[33] Estimates of medical costs related to obesity have risen from $78.5 billion in 1998 to $147 billion in 2008.[35] About 50%

of these costs are publically funded through the Medicare and Medicaid programs,[35] bolstering arguments for public policy interventions.[34]

In 2009, Brownell and colleagues, proposed a 1 cent per ounce excise tax for beverages containing added caloric sweeteners.[33] Why use an excise tax rather than simply raising the sales tax? Arguments in favor of excise taxes relate to the effectiveness of this type of taxation in influencing buying and consumption. In addition, concerns that raising other taxes, such as sales taxes, could have the unintended consequence of encouraging consumers to buy larger (and potentially less expensive per volume) containers of SSBs; such price increases would not be noticed until consumers were already in store check-out lines, resulting in little influence on their decisions regarding whether and how much to buy.[33] There would not likely be a tax when refillable fountain beverages are purchased, and as such, the overall approach of increasing sales taxes, an approach already used by more than 30 states, would have little or no impact on reducing consumption of SSBs.[33] In contrast, excise taxes would more likely result in higher retail prices that consumers would actually see *before* their purchase decisions, contributing to less SSB purchasing and ultimately less consumption.[33] Raising the price of SSBs by 1 cent per ounce would result in a price increase in a 20-ounce soda from 15–20%.[33]

But what is the relationship between price increases and consumption of SSBs? To answer this, Andreyeva and colleagues reviewed 160 studies of food pricing and elasticity of demand, defined as the "expected proportional change in product demand for a given percentage change in price"[31] to determine estimates of elasticity for 16 food and beverage groups. Categories of "food away from home" and "soft drinks" had some of the highest price elasticity in their extensive review, suggesting that a 10% tax on SSBs could result in an 8% to 10% reduction in consumer buying.[31] Evidence from national studies showing that about one-half of SSB consumption happens at home, with more than 90% of the beverages bought in stores,[16] supports the public health impact of proposed price increases.

Additional Supporting Arguments

Another argument for increasing excise taxes is to generate additional revenue to strengthen public health efforts to prevent obesity.[33,34] For example, raising the tax on SSBs nationally by 1 cent per ounce would result in $14.9 billion of revenue annually, which could be used to fund public health and healthcare programs; similar approaches could be utilized at the state level.[33] Public support is increasing, but not universally,[2] and it is likely to be much higher when funds are directly used for programs to prevent obesity. A poll conducted in New York State in 2008 noted that 52% of respondents supported a soda tax, and support increased to 72% if the revenue generated was used for obesity prevention programs for children and adults.[33,34] Similarly, a Vermont poll conducted in 2011 showed that support for a tax on SSBs rose from 42% to 77% when revenue would be used for health and dental care for children.[36] A growing list of national health care and public health organizations have policy statements, resolutions, or reports recommending SSB taxes, such as the American Academy of Pediatrics, American Public Health Association, and others.[37]

Wang and colleagues estimated the public health effect of a 1 cent per ounce price increase on SSBs in the United States. They estimated that consumption of SSBs in U.S. adults between the ages of 25 to 64 would decrease by 15%, and risk of diabetes would drop.[38] Additionally, 95,000 heart attacks, 8,000 strokes, and 26,000 premature deaths might be prevented and $17 billion in healthcare costs might be saved, in a 10-year period.[38]

What Are Opposing Arguments?

The American Beverage Association (ABA) is "the trade association that represents America's non-alcoholic beverage industry. Today the ABA represents hundreds of beverage producers, distributors, franchise companies, and support industries."[39] In 2009, the ABA formed Americans Against Food Taxes (AAFT) at a time when a SSB tax was being considered as part of the potential financing strategy for the Patient Protection and Affordable Care Act (ACA).[6] The industry collectively (21 organizations) spent more than $24 million on congressional lobbying against a potential national excise tax on SSBs; $5 million was spent on a national marketing campaign to support AAFT.[40] A television ad, created by AAFT, called "Grocery," shows a mother grocery shopping, emphasizing that families are unable to afford such taxes.[41] Ultimately, the proposed tax was not part of later financing strategies for the ACA.[40] Later videos from AAFT, such as "Give Me a Break," take issue with government intrusion and politicians' efforts to control what Americans eat, drink, and buy.[42]

Another example is the formation in 2010 of the No D.C. Beverage Tax coalition, a "local coalition of citizens, businesses, and associations,"[43] in opposition to a proposed tax on sugar-sweetened juices, energy drinks, and sodas in Washington, DC.[44] This coalition argued that the government should not have such a role, taxes are already too high, and that such taxes are not effective in promoting health, will hurt jobs, and are "discriminatory and regressive."[43]

In addition, the beverage industry actively critiques scientific studies related to public health benefits of taxing SSBs. The ABA publishes news releases and statements and published a formal response[45] to the 2013 *Pediatrics* study "Sugar-sweetened beverages and weight gain in 2- to 5-year-old children,"[23] The ABA criticized methodology, highlighted study limitations, and specifically noted, "This group of children was studied at a time when they would normally gain weight and grow."[45]

Who are the Americans supporting AAFT? They are described as "a coalition of concerned citizens—responsible individuals, financially strapped families, small and large businesses in communities across the country—who are opposed to the government tax hikes on food and beverages."[46] Although designed to appear as a grassroots group of concerned citizens, some authors call for the need to identify the sources of funding and financial ties in organizations such as AAFT that are playing roles in policy debates. These same authors further identified participating groups and membership of AAFT.[46] They found that over 90% of participating community organizations were either "sponsored by or associated with the food and beverage industry," and highlighted connections to community groups that serve vulnerable populations, such as low income and minority populations.[46] Financial connections between the beverage industry and numerous minority organizations have been observed nationally, and were recently highlighted in New York City, as controversy erupted over the Bloomberg administration's proposed soda ban.[6] One *New York Times* writer in "The Battle Over Taxing Soda," suggested these fierce arguments over taxing SSBs will likely continue in the short term, but predicts that "Someday, we will probably look back on our gallon-a-week soda habit the way we now look back on allowing children to ride without seat belts . . . We will wonder what we were thinking."[44]

DISCUSSION QUESTIONS: TEMPLATE FOR DISCUSSION

1. Significance of this public health issue:
    a. Why is this health issue important?
    b. How many people does it impact?
    c. How serious is it?
    d. Is it preventable?

2. What is the evidence base for prevention?
3. What specific strategies should be used to achieve progress on this health issue?
    a. What evidence-based approach would you use?
    b. Where would you start if you are an individual citizen; public health professional; healthcare professional; community, state, or federal policymaker?
4. Specific questions for this topic:
    a. What is the evidence that SSBs contribute to obesity?
    b. What is the evidence that raising the price will limit consumption?
    c. What are the opposing arguments?
5. What is the controversy?
    a. Define the controversy.
    b. Is controversy a good or bad thing? (Does it help or hinder progress?)
6. *Why* is this health issue controversial?
    a. What specific factors are involved?
    b. Do economics, government, scientific uncertainty, or politics play a role?
    c. What is the role of the media?
7. How would you respond to the controversy?

PERSPECTIVES TO CONSIDER

Policy strategies are often controversial. This is not surprising, as they often leverage laws, ordinances, changes in price, or other means to impact entire populations, whether communities, states, or an entire country. Obesity is a pressing public health issue, impacting children and adults, contributing to chronic conditions and current and future healthcare costs. The evidence for the contribution of SSBs is compelling, when looking at consumption rates, weight, health outcomes, and studies that reduce soft drink consumption. Likewise, the argument that raising the price of SSBs though excise taxes (that actually raise the price for consumers and impact buying decisions) on reducing consumption is strong. Although a different public health issue, lessons learned from tobacco prevention and control—using a combination of strategies including education, media campaigns, community programs, connections to health care, and policy initiatives, such as raising the price of tobacco products, has been effective.[30,32] Based on evidence, similar strategies to prevent obesity will likely help.

So why is there so much controversy? If there is so much evidence, why have such proposals not been uniformly successful? Some hints are contained in the Harris poll,[1,2] revealing that of those sampled, there is not good agreement (or understanding) that raising the prices of items such as SSBs can reduce consumption. Would more people agree with and support such proposals if they had confidence in the evidence for substantial public health benefits? The arguments against—that people cannot afford new "taxes," and that government intrusion into the food choices of individual citizens is unwanted, have been successful, creating a distraction from the public health issue itself.

Whereas physicians, nurses, public health professionals, teachers, and advocates use "evidence" that this policy option will succeed, opponents ask whether this is indeed the proper role for public health agencies and our government. In addition, when such debates occur, each policy initiative is debated and argued against as if it stood alone, when in reality, it is just one strategy used in combination with other evidence-based approaches. Public support for SSB price increases is highest when the revenue generated will be used for the health issue itself.[33,34] To be successful, advocacy strategies must also address public concerns, in order to stem the controversy and strengthen support.

FOR ADDITIONAL STUDY

Chaloupka J, Powell LM, Chriqui JF. Sugar-sweetened beverage taxes and public health. *Robert Wood Johnson Foundation Research and Publications.* 2009.

Friedman RR, Brownell KD. Sugar-sweetened beverages taxes: An updated policy brief. *Rudd Report.* 2012.

Chokshi DA, Stine NW. Reconsidering the politics of public health. *JAMA.* 2013; 310(10):1025–1026.

Malik VS, Popkin BM, Bray GA, Despres JP, Hu FB. Sugar-sweetened beverages, obesity, type 2 diabetes mellitus, and cardiovascular disease risk. *Circulation.* 2010;121(11):1356–1364.

REFERENCES

1. Norton A. Most Americans oppose soda, candy taxes. *US News & World Report: Health.* 2013. http://health.usnews.com/health-news/news/articles/2013/04/25/most-americans-oppose-soda-candy-taxes. Accessed April 25, 2013.
2. Norton A. Most Americans oppose soda, candy taxes. 2013. http://www.harrisinteractive.com/NewsRoom/PressReleases/tabid/446/ctl/ReadCustom%20Default/mid/1506/ArticleId/1185/Default.aspx. Accessed August 28, 2013.

3. Rudarakanchana N. Coalition pushes for sugar-sweetened beverage tax. *VTDigger.org.* 2013. http://vtdigger.org/2013/02/07/sugar-sweetened-beverage-tax-introduced/. Published February 7, 2013.Accessed September 1, 2013.

4. Michael and Susan Dell Center for Healthy Living. Should Texas consider a tax on sugar-sweetened beverages? [blog]. 2013. http://msdcenter.blogspot.com/2013/03/should-texas-consider-tax-on-sugar.html. Published March 21, 2013. Accessed September 1, 2013.

5. Sankin A. New California soda-tax bill under consideration. *Huffington Post.com.* 2013. http://www.huffingtonpost.com/2013/04/26/california-soda-tax_n_3165417.html. Published April 26, 2013. Accessed September 2, 2013.

6. Confessore N. Minority groups and bottlers team up in battles over soda. *The New York Times.* 2013. http://www.nytimes.com/2013/03/13/nyregion/behind-soda-industrys-win-a-phalanx-of-sponsored-minority-groups.html?pagewanted=all&_r=0. Published March 12, 2013. Accessed September 2, 2013.

7. Soda debate bubbling across the country. [blog]. American Heart Association. 2014. http://blog.heart.org/soda-debate-bubbling-across-the-country/. Accessed September 1, 2014.

8. CDC. The CDC guide to strategies for reducing the consumption of sugar-sweetened beverages. 2010. http://www.cdph.ca.gov/SiteCollectionDocuments/StratstoReduce_Sugar_Sweetened_Bevs.pdf. Accessed September 1, 2014.

9. Dietary Guidelines for Americans 2010. http://www.health.gov/dietaryguidelines/dga2010/DietaryGuidelines2010.pdf. Accessed September 1, 2014.

10. *Healthy People 2020.* 2011. http://www.healthypeople.gov/2020. Accessed January 30, 2014.

11. Johnson RK, Appel LJ, Brands M, et al. Dietary sugars intake and cardiovascular health: A scientific statement from the American Heart Association. *Circulation.* 2009;120(11):1011–1020.

12. Guthrie JF, Morton JF. Food sources of added sweeteners in the diets of Americans. *J Amn Diet Assoc.* 2000;100(1):43–51.

13. French SA, Lin BH, Guthrie JF. National trends in soft drink consumption among children and adolescents age 6 to 17 years: Prevalence, amounts, and sources, 1977/1978 to 1994/1998. *J Am Diet Assoc.* 2003;103(10):1326–1331.

14. Flood JE, Roe LS, Rolls BJ. The effect of increased beverage portion size on energy intake at a meal. *J Am Diet Assoc.* 2006;106(12):1984–1990.

15. Malik VS, Popkin BM, Bray GA, Despres JP, Hu FB. Sugar-sweetened beverages, obesity, type 2 diabetes mellitus, and cardiovascular disease risk. *Circulation.* 2010;121(11):1356–1364.

16. Ogden C, Kit BK, Carroll MD, Park S. Consumption of sugar drinks in the United States, 2005–2008. *NCHS Data Brief.* 2011:1-8. http://www.cdc.gov/nchs/data/databriefs/db71.pdf. Accessed September 2, 2013.

17. Kumar GS, Pan L, Park S, et al. Sugar-sweetened beverage consumption among adults - 18 States, 2012. *MMWR Morb Mortal Wkly Rep.* 2014;63(32):686–690.

18. Martin-Biggers J, Yorkin M, Aljallad C, et al. What foods are US supermarkets promoting? A content analysis of supermarket sales circulars. *Appetite.* 2013;62:160–165.

19. Vartanian LR, Schwartz MB, Brownell KD. Effects of soft drink consumption on nutrition and health: A systematic review and meta-analysis. *Am J Public Health.* 2007;97(4):667–675.

20. Malik VS, Schulze MB, Hu FB. Intake of sugar-sweetened beverages and weight gain: A systematic review. *Am J Clin Nutr.* 2006;84(2):274–288.
21. de Koning L, Malik VS, Kellogg MD, Rimm EB, Willett WC, Hu FB. Sweetened beverage consumption, incident coronary heart disease, and biomarkers of risk in men. *Circulation.* 2012;125(14):1735–1741, S1731.
22. Ludwig DS, Peterson KE, Gortmaker SL. Relation between consumption of sugar-sweetened drinks and childhood obesity: A prospective, observational analysis. *Lancet.* 2001;357(9255):505–508.
23. Deboer MD, Scharf RJ, Demmer RT. Sugar-sweetened beverages and weight gain in 2- to 5-year-old children. *Pediatrics.* 2013;132(3):413–420.
24. James J, Thomas P, Cavan D, Kerr D. Preventing childhood obesity by reducing consumption of carbonated drinks: Cluster randomised controlled trial. *BMJ.* 2004; 328(7450):1237.
25. Ebbeling CB, Feldman HA, Osganian SK, Chomitz VR, Ellenbogen SJ, Ludwig DS. Effects of decreasing sugar-sweetened beverage consumption on body weight in adolescents: A randomized, controlled pilot study. *Pediatrics.* 2006;117(3):673–680.
26. Sichieri R, Paula Trotte A, de Souza RA, Veiga GV. School randomised trial on prevention of excessive weight gain by discouraging students from drinking sodas. *Public Health Nutr.* 2009;12(2):197–202.
27. Chriqui JF, Pickel M, Story M. Influence of school competitive food and beverage policies on obesity, consumption, and availability: A systematic review. *JAMA Pediatrics.* Mar 2014;168(3):279–286.
28. Fernandes MM. A national evaluation of the impact of state policies on competitive foods in schools. *J School Health.* 2013;83(4):249–255.
29. Hennessy E, Oh A, Agurs-Collins T, et al. State-level school competitive food and beverage laws are associated with children's weight status. *J School Health.* 2014;84(9):609–616.
30. Chaloupka FJ, Powell LM, Chriqui JF. Sugar-sweetened beverage taxation as public health policy: Lessons from tobacco. *Choices.* 2011;26(3):1–6.
31. Andreyeva T, Long MW, Brownell KD. The impact of food prices on consumption: A systematic review of research on the price elasticity of demand for food. *Am J Public Health.* 2010;100(2):216–222.
32. Chaloupka FJ, Straif K, Leon ME. Effectiveness of tax and price policies in tobacco control. *Tobacco Control.* 2011;20(3):235–238.
33. Brownell KD, Farley T, Willett WC, et al. The public health and economic benefits of taxing sugar-sweetened severages. *N Engl J Med.* 2009;361(16):1599–1605.
34. Brownell KD, Frieden TR. Ounces of prevention: The public policy case for taxes on sugared beverages. *N Engl J Med.* 2009;360(18):1805–1808.
35. Finkelstein EA, Trogdon JG, Cohen JW, Dietz W. Annual medical spending attributable to obesity: Payer-and service-specific estimates. *Health Aff (Millwood).* 2009;28(5): w822-831.
36. Friedman RR, Brownell KD. Sugar-sweetened beverages taxes: An updated policy brief. *Rudd Report.* 2012. http://www.yaleruddcenter.org/resources/upload/docs/what/reports/Rudd_Policy_Brief_Sugar_Sweetened_Beverage_Taxes.pdf. Accessed September 2, 2013.

37. Yale Rudd Center. Sugar-sweetened beverage taxes and sugar intake: Policy statements, endorsements, and recommendations. 2012. http://www.yaleruddcenter.org/resources/upload/docs/what/policy/SSBtaxes/SSBTaxStatements.pdf. Accessed September 2, 2013.

38. Wang YC, Coxson P, Shen YM, Goldman L, Bibbins-Domingo K. A penny-per-ounce tax on sugar-sweetened beverages would cut health and cost burdens of diabetes. *Health Aff (Millwood)*. 2012;31(1):199–207.

39. American Beverage Association. 2013. http://www.ameribev.org/about-aba/history/. Accessed September 3, 2013.

40. Spolar C, Eaton J. Food lobby mobilizes, as soda tax bubbles up. *Huffington Post. com*. 2010. http://www.huffingtonpost.com/2009/11/04/soda-tax-mobilizes-food-l_n_345840.html. Published March 18, 2010. Updated May 25, 2011. Accessed September 2, 2103.

41. Americans Against Food Taxes. Grocery. [video]. 2009. http://www.youtube.com/watch?v=NYrOxsWrss8&list=UUc3OU0UO8B3TXw3TU_G-YqQ. Accessed September 3, 2013.

42. Americans Against Food Taxes. Give me a break. [video]. 2011. http://www.youtube.com/watch?v=NQrIH1opr1I&list=UUc3OU0UO8B3TXw3TU_G-YqQ. Accessed September 3, 2013.

43. No DC Beverage Tax coalition. No DC beverage tax. 2010. http://www.nodcbevtax.com/. Accessed September 1, 2014.

44. Leonhardt D. The battle over taxing soda. *The New York Times*. 2010. http://www.nytimes.com/2010/05/19/business/economy/19leonhardt.html. Accessed September 1, 2014.

45. American Beverage Association. News releases and statements: American Beverage Association statement on children and sugar-sweetened beverages study. [online]. 2013. http://www.ameribev.org/news-media/news-releases-statements/more/311/. Accessed September 2, 2013.

46. Yanamadala S, Bragg MA, Roberto CA, Brownell KD. Food industry front groups and conflicts of interest: The case of Americans Against Food Taxes. *Public Health Nutr.* 2012;15(8):1331–1332.

CHAPTER 5

Tobacco: E-Cigarettes—
Help or Hazard?

LEARNING OBJECTIVES

- Discuss the data about e-cigarette use and trends in the United States.
- Describe strategies used to promote e-cigarettes to children and adults.
- Given current data and research, assess the public health impact of e-cigarettes in children and adults in the United States.
- Identify policies related to tobacco products and e-cigarettes that would be effective in protecting and promoting public health.

THE CONTROVERSY

According to the Centers for Disease Control and Prevention (CDC), e-cigarette use in middle and high school students in the United States has doubled in just a year. Among high school students, from 2011 to 2012, those who had ever used e-cigarettes went from 4.7% to 10.0%.[1] Sales of electronic cigarettes have rocketed in recent years, and are predicted to reach $1.7 billion by the end of 2013.[2] On September 24, 2013, U.S. Attorneys General from 40 states petitioned the U.S. Food and Drug Administration (FDA) to regulate e-cigarettes under the authority granted in the 2009 Family Smoking Prevention and Tobacco Control Act by October 31, 2013.[2] Meanwhile, the CEO of R.J. Reynolds Vapor, which manufactures electronic cigarettes said, "If the FDA wants to improve or remove the risk to public health, this is the FDA's dream product."[3]

BACKGROUND AND SCOPE OF THE PUBLIC HEALTH AND HEALTH POLICY ISSUE

Trends in Tobacco Use and Public Health Strategies

According to CDC, despite our progress, "tobacco use remains the single largest preventable cause of disease, disability, and death in the United States."[4] Despite declines since the 1960s, as of 2010, nearly 20% of adults in the United States continue to smoke cigarettes, which translates to about 45.3 million adults, with men smoking slightly more than women (22% vs. 17%). Smoking is more common in American Indian/Alaska Native populations (31.4%), in adults with lower incomes, and those without a college degree. Smoking rates vary by state from a low of 9.1% to a high of 26.8% across the United States.[4] CDC further estimates that about 50% of adults who continue smoking will die from diseases such as lung cancer, chronic obstructive pulmonary disease, ischemic heart disease, stroke, and other cancers related to their smoking,[4] and that cigarette smoking is responsible for an estimated 443,000 deaths in the United States each year.[5] On a global level, the World Health Organization (WHO) estimates there are about 6 million annual deaths from tobacco and projects as many as a billion deaths by the end of this century if evidence-based tobacco control policies are not implemented.[6]

Since most adults who smoke began smoking when they were young (88% by age 18 and 99% by age 26),[7,8] strategies to keep adolescents and young adults from starting a smoking habit are essential for long-term prevention. Continued efforts to help smokers to quit are also a priority for current smokers, with both of these strategies necessary for substantial long-term reductions in population tobacco use[7] (see **Figure 5–1**).

From 2000 to 2011, smoking declined dramatically in middle and high school students, but despite these trends, an estimated 4,000 adolescents try cigarettes each day and 1,000 become daily smokers.[9] The U.S. Surgeon General reminds us of the health risks, "Of every three young smokers, only one will quit, and one of those remaining smokers will die from tobacco-related causes."[8] Nicotine, the highly addictive drug contained in tobacco products, is responsible for dependence on tobacco products and is the reason why smokers have such difficulty quitting. Furthermore, experts note that nicotine may be as addictive as cocaine or heroin.[10]

In 2014, CDC updated their guide, "Best Practice for Comprehensive Tobacco Control Programs." The guide recommends comprehensive and sustained efforts that include state and community programs and policies;

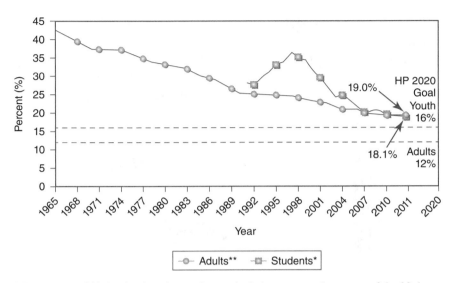

* Percentage of high school students who smoked cigarettes on 1 or more of the 30 days preceding the survey. Data first collected in 1991. (Youth Risk Behavior Survey, 1991–2011).

** Percentage of adults who are current cigarette smokers (National Health Interview Survey, 1965–2011).

Figure 5–1 Trends in current cigarette smoking by high school students and adults.

Reproduced from Centers for Disease Control and Prevention, Smoking and Tobacco Use (2013). Trends in Current Cigarette Smoking Among High School Students and Adults, United States, 1965–2011. http://www.cdc.gov/tobacco/data_statistics/tables/trends/cig_smoking. Accessed September 28, 2013.

health communication and media efforts; cessation interventions; and surveillance and ongoing evaluation to effectively reduce smoking and its related health consequences.[7]

What Are E-Cigarettes?

Electronic cigarettes (or e-cigarettes) are rechargeable battery-powered devices that heat liquid nicotine and a chemical (often propylene glycol) to create a vapor that is inhaled by the user.[11] Rather than *smoking*, use of e-cigarettes is called *vaping*, and the heated cloud of nicotine-containing vapor is exhaled as a puff of vapor smoke. These devices were first patented in 2004 by Ruyan Group, Ltd. in Beijing, China, and are available in the

United States in many retail outlets and on the Internet.[11] The WHO calls e-cigarettes a type of electronic nicotine delivery system (ENDS), which may also contain flavoring, including candy and fruit flavors.[2,12] They sometimes look like cigarettes, and when used, e-cigarette use generally looks like smoking. However, there are many different types and styles

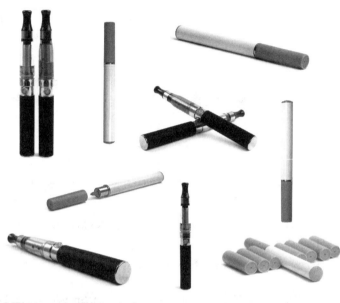

© GeorgeMPhotography/Shutterstock

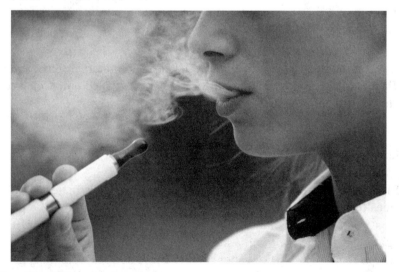

© Diego Cervo/Shutterstock

of e-cigarettes, and some even look like pens or USB memory sticks, depending on the manufacturer.[12] Levels of nicotine may range from 6 to 24 mg of nicotine per cartridge, but some may contain 100 mg or more,[12] and some authors note that "no standard definition of ENDS exists."[13,14]

Trends in E-Cigarette Use

Use of e-cigarettes has increased dramatically in both adults and children. CDC reports that 6% of all U.S. adults have tried e-cigarettes in 2011, and 21% of cigarette smokers used e-cigarettes in 2011, more than double the rate from the previous year.[15] Data from the National Youth Tobacco Survey showed that e-cigarette use in high school students increased significantly in one year, from 4.7% in 2011 to 10% in 2012[1] (see **Figure 5–2**). In addition, CDC notes that the increase in use of e-cigarettes was not just in adolescents who already smoke regular cigarettes; about 160,000 middle and high school students who do not smoke cigarettes

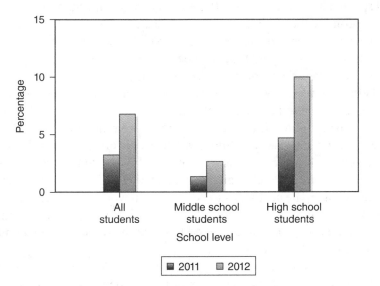

Figure 5–2 Ever electronic cigarette use among middle and high school students, by year—National Youth Tobacco Survey, United States, 2011–2012.

Reproduced from Centers for Disease Control and Prevention (2013). Electronic Cigarette Use Among Middle and High School Students—United States, 2011–2012. Morbidity and Mortality Weekly Report (MMWR) 2013: 62(35); 729–730. http://www.cdc.gov/mmwr/preview/mmwrhtml/mm6235a6.htm. Accessed September 28, 2013.

used e-cigarettes in 2012, raising concerns about the potential for nicotine addiction in adolescents.[1]

Since 2010, about half of all states in the United States have attempted to ban sales to minors because of gaps in federal regulations.[16] In contrast to the United States, electronic cigarettes have been heavily regulated or banned in other countries such as Brazil, Australia, Canada, Norway, Singapore, and Panama.[11,13,17]

Advertising and Promotion

Along with the increase in popularity of e-cigarettes, there has been a sharp increase in companies, brands, and interest by financial investors since 2006.[18,19] Critics compare the style of mass advertising and promotion of e-cigarettes (currently unregulated by federal tobacco laws), to decades-earlier advertising campaigns by tobacco companies that promoted cigarette smoking.[20] For example, after spending $12.4 million during the first quarter of 2013, blu eCigs brand (from Lorillard tobacco company) will spend $30 million during 2013 to reach target audiences, using celebrities to promote their products.[20] Their website states that their e-cigarettes "duplicate the true size and feel of traditional cigarettes for a wonderfully rich user experience" and they include "hygiene," "durability," and "social features" in starter pack promotions on the Internet.[21] Another brand uses a marketing theme of "rewrite the rules" to promote the social acceptability of e-cigarettes in today's environment.[20]

Advertising on the Internet is especially prominent: authors of a 2010 study note that Google searching for "electronic cigarette" results in many top search results for companies and brands.[11] These authors note marketing of e-cigarettes as "green," availability of a variety of flavors, and marketing strategies that invite customers to become "real world promoters" or "online affiliates" (as long as they do not make health, therapeutic, or smoking cessation claims),[22] are all designed to reach the rapidly growing number of people using the Internet.[11]

In their September 24, 2013 letter to FDA Commissioner Margaret Hamburg, 40 U.S. Attorneys General cite evidence that a 30-second Super Bowl ad from one e-cigarette brand reached more than 10 million viewers and sales later increased by 30–40%.[2] With a combination of smaller and larger tobacco companies now participating with huge marketing budgets, sales of e-cigarettes are projected to reach $1.7 billion by the end of 2013.[2,20]

EVIDENCE BASE FOR PREVENTION AND PRACTICE

Public Health Concerns

As e-cigarette use increases rapidly, concerns about potential impacts on public health fall into general categories related to quality control and potential impurities, social perceptions of smoking, and lack of research. Nicotine levels and impurities, including potential toxins, are not well quantified. Another concern is that e-cigarettes may create a path to tobacco use among users who do not currently smoke cigarettes. In addition, research is sparse regarding whether e-cigarettes have a potential role in smoking cessation.[11,13,14,23]

In 2009, the FDA warned the public about contaminants of electronic cigarettes, after conducting a laboratory analysis of 18 e-cigarette cartridges.[24,25] In the analysis, FDA researchers found detectable levels of carcinogens such as nitrosamines and other substances such as diethylene glycol, a component of antifreeze, which is toxic to humans, as well as additional potentially harmful compounds from tobacco. Surprisingly, they noted that nicotine levels varied widely, with "smoke" from one e-cigarette cartridge containing nicotine levels that were more than twice the amount found in an FDA-regulated nicotine-containing product used for smoking cessation.[25]

Additionally, long-term effects of regularly inhaling one of the chemicals commonly used to help create the vapor from e-cigarettes, propylene glycol, is not known.[13] Nicotine is addictive, as addictive as cocaine or heroin, and is one reason why quitting smoking is so difficult, especially for long-term cigarette smokers.[10] Nicotine-containing products designed for use in smoking cessation are regulated by the FDA, and other products containing nicotine that were potentially intended for use in smoking cessation that do not meet these standards have been removed from the market.[13]

In a 2013 report from CDC documenting the doubling of use of e-cigarettes by high school students in a single year, investigators also raised health concerns about the effects of nicotine on the still-developing adolescent brain, as well as the potential for nicotine addiction in adolescents using e-cigarettes.[1] Whether the use of e-cigarettes at a young age and subsequent nicotine addiction may later increase use of other tobacco products, such as cigarettes, is another concern.[1] Part of this worry stems from CDC data that reported, in 2012, nearly 1.8 million middle and high school students have ever tried e-cigarettes in a single year, and that 20% of the youngest survey respondents—middle school aged children—who had tried e-cigarettes, had never smoked a regular cigarette before.[26]

Flavors and cartoon characters that may make e-cigarettes more attractive to children and adolescents create yet another layer of intense discussion among public health officials about the marketing of e-cigarettes to children; such marketing strategies have been banned for cigarettes.[2] Ease of access (especially through the Internet), marketing strategies that may appeal to children and adolescents, potentially harmful contaminants, variable levels of nicotine, and concerns that widespread use of e-cigarettes may again "normalize" smoking behavior after dramatic progress, all contribute to public health concerns as e-cigarettes gain more widespread use in both children and adults.[17,27,28]

Nicotine poisoning was reported in a 10-month-old child who drank a small amount of liquid nicotine used to refill e-cigarettes.[29] CDC analyzed and reported the types and numbers of calls (September 2010 to February 2014) to U.S. poison centers from e-cigarette-related poisonings.[30] During the time of the study, poison centers in the U.S. received a total of 2,405 e-cigarette exposure calls. Calls increased dramatically from one call per month in September 2010 to 215 calls per month in February 2014.[30] About half of the calls were about children under 5 years of age who had an e-cigarette exposure (such as inhalation, eye or skin exposure, or ingestion of the liquid nicotine), and 42% were in people older than 20. The most common complaints that precipitated calls to the poison centers were nausea, vomiting, and eye irritation. One suicide from liquid nicotine injected intravenously was also reported during this time.[30] In response, the American Academy of Pediatrics, an organization of 62,000 pediatricians, immediately released a statement calling for government action to protect the health of children.[31]

Quitting Smoking: Do E-Cigarettes Help?

Effective evidence-based smoking cessation strategies include: brief interventions in a healthcare setting, counseling (whether by phone, in person, or in groups), behavior-change strategies, or medications (nicotine replacement or other prescription medications). Medications proven to be effective (FDA regulated) used in combination with some form of evidence-based counseling works best.[10] Marketers of e-cigarettes have avoided overt claims of effectiveness for smoking cessation, and thus the

FDA regulatory requirements for such products, with e-cigarettes carefully marketed to consumers as an "alternative to cigarettes."[13]

However, consumers, especially current smokers, are using them for help in quitting smoking. In 179 e-cigarette users in Poland, nearly 90% used them as cessation aids and perceived them to be less harmful than cigarettes, but despite their widespread use for this purpose, 85% of people participating in the study did not believe they were safe.[32] A survey of nearly 6,000 current and former smokers in the United States, Canada, United Kingdom (UK), and Australia, from 2010–2011, found that awareness of ENDS among smokers was high overall (US, 73%; UK, 54%; Canada, 40%; Australia, 20%) and higher in smokers who lived in countries with fewer legal restrictions. Of those smokers who knew about them, 16% had actually tried an e-cigarette.[33] In addition, 85.1% used ENDS to help them quit and three-quarters used them to help them cut down; nearly 80% used ENDS because they believed they were safer than cigarettes.[33]

Evidence of Effectiveness of E-Cigarettes for Smoking Cessation

To date, there is sparse research on the effectiveness of electronic cigarettes when used for smoking cessation. Some studies are limited by the use of smokers' *perception* of benefit using surveys as the research method,[32] but lack biochemical verification that smoking cessation has actually occurred. A 2011 online cross-sectional survey of first-time users of one brand of e-cigarettes, found self-reported quit rates of 31% after 6 months, and higher rates in those using e-cigarettes more than 20 times per day; however, the survey response rate was 4.5% and self-reported quit rates were not biochemically verified.[34] In a 2013 randomized controlled trial conducted in New Zealand to study use of e-cigarettes for smoking cessation (compared with nicotine patches and placebo e-cigarettes), investigators found a percentage of e-cigarette users had quit smoking (7.3%) verified by levels of exhaled carbon monoxide. However, overall levels of quitting were low in the study, and the authors were unable to statistically compare e-cigarettes to placebo e-cigarettes or nicotine patches.[35] An accompanying editorial noted that both the European Union and United Kingdom intended to regulate e-cigarettes as "medicinal devices," and more research was urgently needed to determine whether or not e-cigarettes were effective in smoking cessation.[36]

Others express concerns that because of variability in nicotine content, smokers using e-cigarettes for cessation purposes may prolong their addiction; these authors recommend that clinicians advise patients to use FDA-approved nicotine replacement therapies.[14] Whether or not e-cigarettes may help smokers to quit remains an ongoing research question, despite public perception, continued controversy, rising popularity, and celebrity endorsement.[37] A large cross-sectional study published in 2014 of U.S. middle and high school students from the National Youth Tobacco Survey in 2011 and 2012 found associations between e-cigarette use and cigarette smoking, and concluded that e-cigarette use may actually promote cigarette use.[38] A 2014 scientific review published by the American Heart Association (AHA) described a meta-analysis of e-cigarette use and quitting smoking, concluding "e-cigarette use in the real world is associated with significantly lower odds of quitting smoking cigarettes."[23]

Popular media also suggests pregnant women may be using e-cigarettes in lieu of cigarettes.[39] An estimated 25% of women of child-bearing age smoke cigarettes, with many continuing to smoke while pregnant.[40] Use of cigarettes during pregnancy is associated with a variety of pregnancy complications: babies born at low birth weight (LBW) or small for gestational weight (SGA), and increased later risk for sudden infant death syndrome (SIDS).[41] Research from both animal and human studies suggests nicotine, a component of nicotine replacement therapy (NRT) used for smoking cessation, may cause harm to the normal development of the fetal nervous system.[40] Despite the widespread health consequences of smoking during pregnancy, some experts recommend complete avoidance of nicotine during pregnancy because of potential adverse health effects attributed specifically to nicotine.[40,42]

Health Policy and Regulatory Strategies—The U.S. Food and Drug Administration

On April 25, 2011 the FDA announced to the public its intent to regulate e-cigarettes under the authority granted to them in the Family Smoking Prevention and Tobacco Control Act of 2009.[43] This law gave them the ability to regulate "tobacco products," defined as any product "made or derived from tobacco" that is not a "drug," "device," or a combination of these under the Federal Food, Drug, and Cosmetic Act.[43]

The 2009 Family Smoking Prevention and Tobacco Control Act provides regulatory authority for the FDA Center for Tobacco Products; smoking cessation products using nicotine are regulated by the FDA Center for Drug

Evaluation and Research (CDER).[13] This announcement came in the wake of a U.S. Court of Appeals for the District of Columbia decision (Sottera, Inc. v. Food & Drug Administration, 627 F.3d 891). In this decision, the court concluded that e-cigarettes cannot be regulated as therapeutic drugs or devices (unless marketed for this purpose) and should instead be regulated under the 2009 Tobacco Control Act, as they are products "made or derived from tobacco."[43] The lawsuit and subsequent appeals court decision came in response to the FDA's efforts to halt e-cigarette entry by some manufacturers into the United States.[44] The FDA, in an April 2011 public statement, said it would issue a regulation under its ability to regulate "tobacco products" under the 2009 law.[43]

The Nation's Attorneys General Call for Regulation

As of 2013, the FDA had not issued regulations, and on September 24, 2013, U.S. Attorneys General from 40 states petitioned the FDA to regulate e-cigarettes under the authority granted in the 2009 Family Smoking Prevention and Tobacco Control Act by October 31, 2013.[2] In the absence of federal oversight, about half the states in the United States had already banned sales to minors, but FDA regulation as allowed in the 2009 Tobacco Control Act had not yet materialized. One FDA official was quoted as characterizing the regulation of e-cigarettes as "the wild, wild West."[18]

On April 24, 2014, the FDA issued a press release announcing its long-awaited proposed new regulations over tobacco products, including e-cigarettes, cigars, pipe tobacco, nicotine gels, and other tobacco products not currently regulated by FDA.[45] Specifics included requirements to register products, marketing review, a requirement that claims of reduced risk be backed by scientific evidence, prohibitions on providing free samples, minimum age rules, vending machine prohibitions, and health warnings.[45]

How Do E-Cigarettes Fit with Tobacco Prevention and Control Policy?

Based on the near-exponential growth in use of e-cigarettes, some experts are calling for banning sales and marketing to children and eliminating the use of flavors that might appeal to children.[46] Others are calling on the FDA to issue regulations citing the dangers of electronic cigarette use, particularly to children.[14] Tobacco prevention and control has a long history, and the most recent CDC guide, "Best Practices for Comprehensive Tobacco Control Programs"[7] emphasizes the importance of programs and policies that support "tobacco-free" norms as well as tracking and evaluating progress towards health goals.[7]

How do these recommendations relate to electronic cigarettes? Although tobacco products are taxed at the federal and state levels, and increasing the price of tobacco products can promote cessation and prevent smoking in children and adolescents,[47] as of 2013, only Minnesota had a tax on e-cigarettes.[48] Ads and marketing strategies for e-cigarettes are currently permissible in ways that promotion of other tobacco products is not. Other effective tobacco prevention and control policies to reduce the harmful effects of tobacco products have included restricting access by children and adolescents under 18; smoke-free policies, regulations, ordinances, and laws; and insurance coverage of evidence-based cessation methods.[47] Such policies are not currently universally applied to e-cigarettes, and a growing group of scientists, physicians, and prominent national health organizations are supporting the FDA's regulatory efforts and calling for careful monitoring and additional research.[31,49]

In 2014, the AHA published an extensive scientific review of electronic cigarettes,[23] followed by a comprehensive policy statement.[49] The AHA expressed concerns similar to other public health organizations that widespread use of e-cigarettes might "normalize" smoking, become a gateway to tobacco use by children or former smokers, and reverse many years of progress in tobacco prevention and control.[49] They supported FDA oversight and efforts to prevent access by minors, restrictions on marketing and advertising to youth, including e-cigarettes both in smoke-free air laws and in the definition of tobacco-products and smoking in state laws, and taxing e-cigarettes.[49] In addition, they recommend that clinicians include e-cigarettes when asking patients about their smoking status. They call for extensive monitoring of the public health effects and suggest an extensive research agenda for the future.[49]

Controversy Within the Public Health Community

Despite the ongoing worry that e-cigarette use will "renormalize" smoking,[28] the growing use of e-cigarettes is complex and controversial, even among researchers, clinicians, and public health experts, with some considering a role for e-cigarettes as a way to reducing harm from cigarette smoking.[28,50] Bell and Keane note the challenge of providing a consistent public message about the harms of tobacco use, considering the role of nicotine "as both a poison and remedy."[50] Users of electronic cigarettes give a near-identical visual perception of smoking, despite the fact they are *vaping* and not actually *smoking* cigarettes. However, as these authors point out, harm reduction strategies are already used in other public health settings, such as drug addiction, and needle-exchange programs to prevent HIV.[50]

However, there is much disagreement, almost polarization, on this point. While CDC data shows a doubling of e-cigarette use by middle and high school students in one year's time,[1] *The Wall Street Journal* reports that a former U.S. Surgeon General has joined the board of a large e-cigarette company.[48] There is, however, near consensus that the government urgently must regulate e-cigarettes, they should be made inaccessible to minors, and the harms (and any potential benefits) clearly understood, through rigorous oversight and research.[2,28,49] In the meantime, the WHO takes a hard line on the current state of the evidence, stating that "smokers will obtain the maximum health benefit if they completely quit both tobacco and nicotine use."[51] The WHO in 2014 wrote that regulation is needed to both protect the public and enable research studies to determine potential benefits and harms from ENDS. They further outline the need for specific regulation in such areas as advertising and promotion, sales to minors, banning fruit and candy flavorings that appeal to children, and prohibiting unsubstantiated health claims.[51,52]

DISCUSSION QUESTIONS: TEMPLATE FOR DISCUSSION

1. Significance of this public health issue:
   a. Why is this health issue important?
   b. How many people does it impact?
   c. How serious is it?
   d. Is it preventable?
2. What is the evidence base for prevention?
3. What specific strategies should be used to achieve progress on this health issue?
   a. What evidence-based approach would you use?
   b. Where would you start if you are an individual citizen; public health professional; healthcare professional; community, state, or federal policymaker?

4. Specific questions for this topic:
   a. Are e-cigarettes harmful to individuals? To the public's health? Why or why not?
   b. With sparse available research data, what should government agencies do to protect the public?
   c. What are the arguments for and against e-cigarettes as a harm-reduction strategy?
5. What is the controversy?
   a. Define the controversy.
   b. Is controversy a good or bad thing? (Does it help or hinder progress?)
6. *Why* is this health issue controversial?
   a. What specific factors are involved?
   b. Do economics, government, scientific uncertainty, or politics play a role?
   c. What is the role of the media?
7. How would you respond to the controversy?

PERSPECTIVES TO CONSIDER

Since the 1964 Surgeon General's report was first published, tobacco prevention and control has been a public health priority. Although progress has been made in both children and adults in the United States, tobacco use is still widely recognized as the leading preventable cause of disease and death.[4] The meteoric rise in the promotion, sales, and use of electronic cigarettes poses an immediate challenge for public health officials at all levels. New e-cigarette "bars" create a promotional image of vaping as a healthier alternative to cigarette smoking, with e-cigarettes sold alongside healthy beverages and food, all enjoyed in a social tavern atmosphere.[53] The rapid rise in use and potential health risks are not well known to the public.

How did this happen? As of 2014, restrictions on the advertising and marketing of tobacco products do not apply to e-cigarettes in the United States, despite the fact that the FDA is actively proposing broad changes. Further confounding this controversial issue is the widely held perception that e-cigarettes are less harmful than smoking traditional cigarettes and can actually help quit smoking. There are still huge gaps in our knowledge, with potentially serious consequences. Because use of e-cigarettes is rising so fast, health concerns are increasingly recognized (especially for children) and research gaps are plentiful; thus, the risks of *not* having a framework to protect children and to evaluate needed research has grown in urgency. Many smokers, including pregnant women,[39] are already using ENDS as a way to reduce or quit smoking. In the meantime, public health officials, health professionals, and the media can educate the public on this critical and controversial issue, while far too many questions remain.

FOR ADDITIONAL STUDY

Grana R, Benowitz N, Glantz SA. E-cigarettes: A scientific review. *Circulation.* 2014; 129:1972–1986.
Bhatnagar A, Whitsel LP, Ribisl KM, et al. Electronic cigarettes: A policy statement from the American Heart Association. *Circulation.* 2014.

REFERENCES

1. CDC. Electronic cigarette use among middle and high school students - United States, 2011–2012. *MMWR.* 2013;62(35):729–730.
2. National Association of Attorneys General. Letter to U.S. Food and Drug Administration. 2013. http://www.naag.org/assets/files/pdf/E%20Cigarette%20Final%20Letter%20(5)(1).pdf. Accessed September 30, 2013.
3. Burritt C. E-cigarette pioneers holding breath as big firms invade. *Bloomberg.* 2013. http://www.bloomberg.com/news/2013-06-20/e-cigarette-pioneers-holding-breath-as-big-firms-invade-retail.html. Accessed September 30, 2013.
4. CDC. Adult Smoking in the US. *Vital Signs.* 2011. http://www.cdc.gov/vitalsigns/AdultSmoking/index.html. Accessed September 28, 2013.
5. CDC. Smoking and tobacco use: Annual deaths attributable to cigarette smoking–United States, 2000–2004. 2008. http://www.cdc.gov/tobacco/data_statistics/tables/health/attrdeaths/index.htm. Accessed September 30, 2013.
6. WHO. WHO report on the global tobacco epidemic, 2013: Enforcing bans on tobacco advertising, promotion, and sponsorship. 2013. http://www.who.int/tobacco/global_report/2013/en/. Accessed September 28, 2013.
7. CDC. Best practrices for comprehensive tobacco control programs, 2014. http://www.cdc.gov/tobacco/stateandcommunity/best_practices/index.htm. Accessed February 24, 2015.
8. U.S. Department of Health and Human Services. 2012 Surgeon General's report: Preventing tobacco use among youth and young adults. 2012. http://www.cdc.gov/tobacco/data_statistics/sgr/2012/. Accessed September 28, 2013.
9. CDC. Smoking and tobacco use: Youth and tobacco use. 2013. http://www.cdc.gov/tobacco/data_statistics/fact_sheets/youth_data/tobacco_use/index.htm. Accessed September 30, 2013.

10. CDC. Smoking and tobacco use: Smoking cessation. 2013. http://www.cdc.gov/tobacco/data_statistics/fact_sheets/cessation/quitting/. Accessed September 30, 2013.

11. Yamin CK, Bitton A, Bates DW. E-cigarettes: A rapidly growing Internet phenomenon. *Ann Intern Med.* 2010;153(9):607–609.

12. WHO. Questions and answers on electronic cigarettes or electronic nicotine delivery systems (ENDS). 2013. http://www.who.int/tobacco/communications/statements/eletronic_cigarettes/en/. Accessed September 28, 2013.

13. Cobb NK, Byron MJ, Abrams DB, Shields PG. Novel nicotine delivery systems and public health: The rise of the "e-cigarette". *Am J Public Health.* 2010;100(12):2340–2342.

14. Cobb NK, Abrams DB. E-cigarette or drug-delivery device? Regulating novel nicotine products. *N Engl J Med.* 2011;365(3):193–195.

15. CDC. About one in five U.S. adult cigarette smokers have tried an electronic cigarette. [press release]. 2013. http://www.cdc.gov/media/releases/2013/p0228_electronic_cigarettes.html. Accessed September 28, 2013.

16. Esterl M. E-cigarette use rising among youth, study says. *The Wall Street Journal Online.* 2013. http://online.wsj.com/article/SB10001424127887323893004579057080653155754.html. Accessed September 20, 2013.

17. Kelland K, Hirschlet B. E-cigarettes gain steam, but health experts wary it could serve as "gateway" to tobacco smoking. *Huffpost.* 2013. http://www.huffingtonpost.com/2013/06/13/e-cigarettes-electronic-tobacco-smoking-help-smokers-quit_n_3433791.html. Accessed September 28, 2013.

18. Esterl M. E-cigarettes fire up investors, regulators. *Wall Street Journal Online.* 2013. http://online.wsj.com/article/SB10001424127887324904004578535362153026902.html. Accessed September 30, 2013.

19. Montopoli B. Tobacco companies bet on electronic cigarettes. 2013. http://www.cbsnews.com/8301-201_162-57588583/tobacco-companies-bet-on-electronic-cigarettes/. Accessed September 30, 2013.

20. Elliot S. E-cigarette makers' ads echo tobacco's heyday. *The New York Times.* 2013. http://www.nytimes.com/2013/08/30/business/media/e-cigarette-makers-ads-echo-tobaccos-heyday.html. Accessed September 28, 2013.

21. Blu. [advertisement]. 2013. http://www.blucigs.com/. Accessed September 28, 2013.

22. Greensmoke. Planet Green Smoke: Your source for all things affiliate. 2013. https://earn.greensmoke.com/home/. Accessed September 30, 2013.

23. Grana R, Benowitz N, Glantz SA. E-cigarettes: A scientific review. *Circulation.* 2014;129(19):1972–1986.

24. FDA. FDA and public health experts warn about electronic cigarettes. 2009. http://www.fda.gov/newsevents/newsroom/pressannouncements/ucm173222.htm. Accessed September 28, 2013.

25. FDA. Summary of results: Laboratory analysis of electronic cigarettes conducted by FDA. 2009. http://www.fda.gov/newsevents/publichealthfocus/ucm173146.htm. Accessed September 28, 2013.

26. Tavernise S. Rise is seen in students who use e-cigarettes. *The New York Times.* 2013. http://www.nytimes.com/2013/09/06/health/e-cigarette-use-doubles-among-students-survey-shows.html?_r=0. Accessed September 30, 2013.

27. Nine terribly disturbing things about electronic cigarettes. *The Huffington Post.* 2013. http://www.huffingtonpost.com/2013/09/03/electronic-cigarettes_n_3818941.html. Accessed September 30, 2013.

28. Fairchild AL, Bayer R, Colgrove J. The renormalization of smoking? E-cigarettes and the tobacco "endgame". *N Engl J Med.* 2014;370(4):293–295.
29. Bassett RA, Osterhoudt K, Brabazon T. Nicotine poisoning in an infant. *N Engl J Med.* 2014;370(23):2249–2250.
30. Chatham-Stephens K, Law R, Taylor E, et al. Notes from the field: Calls to poison centers for exposures to electronic cigarettes—United States, September 2010–February 2014. *MMWR Morb Mortal Wkly Rep.* 2014;63(13):292–293.
31. Perrin JM. AAP Statement on new e-cigarette poisoning data, need for government action. [press release]. American Academy of Arts and Sciences. 2014. http://www.aap.org/en-us/about-the-aap/aap-press-room/Pages/EcigarettePoisoning.aspx#sthash.PRzDynAe.dpuf. http://www.aap.org/en-us/about-the-aap/aap-press-room/Pages/EcigarettePoisoning.aspx. Accessed September 14, 2014.
32. Goniewicz ML, Lingas EO, Hajek P. Patterns of electronic cigarette use and user beliefs about their safety and benefits: an Internet survey. *Drug Alcohol Rev.* 2013;32(2): 133–140.
33. Adkison SE, O'Connor RJ, Bansal-Travers M, et al. Electronic nicotine delivery systems: international tobacco control four-country survey. *Am J Prev Med.* 2013;44(3): 207–215.
34. Siegel MB, Tanwar KL, Wood KS. Electronic cigarettes as a smoking-cessation tool: Rsults from an online survey. *Am J Prev Med.* 2011;40(4):472–475.
35. Bullen C, Howe C, Laugesen M, et al. Electronic cigarettes for smoking cessation: A randomised controlled trial. *Lancet.* 2013;382(9905):1629–1637.
36. Hajek P. Electronic cigarettes for smoking cessation. *Lancet.* 2013;382(9905):1614–1616.
37. Cole D. Are e-cigarettes a boon or a menace? *Natl Geogr Daily News.* 2013. http://news.nationalgeographic.com/news/2013/09/130916-electronic-cigarettes-smoking-nicotine-science/. Accessed November 1, 2013.
38. Dutra LM, Glantz SA. Electronic cigarettes and conventional cigarette use among U.S. adolescents: a cross-sectional study. *JAMA Pediatrics.* 2014;168(7):610–617.
39. Nightcap. E cigarettes: Some are 'vaping' instead of smoking while pregnant. [video]. Aol.com. On Parenting. 2013. http://on.aol.com/video/e-cigarettes--some-are-vaping-instead-of-smoking-while-pregnant-517916510. Accessed November 1, 2013.
40. Pauly JR, Slotkin TA. Maternal tobacco smoking, nicotine replacement and neurobehavioural development. *Acta Paediatr.* 2008;97(10):1331–1337.
41. Murin S, Rafii R, Bilello K. Smoking and smoking cessation in pregnancy. *Clin Chest Med.* 2011;32(1):75-91, viii.
42. Wickstrom R. Effects of nicotine during pregnancy: Human and experimental evidence. *Curr Neuropharmacol.* 2007;5(3):213–222.
43. FDA. Regulation of e-cigarettes and other tobacco products. 2011. http://www.fda.gov/newsevents/publichealthfocus/ucm252360.htm. Accessed September 28, 2013.
44. Shelton D, Mullin S. E-cigarettes get a "smoking" break: D.C. circuit clarifies scope of FDA's authority over e-cigarettes, Vol 2013. FDA. 2011. http://www.fdalawblog.com/2011/01/articles/legislation/e-cigarettes-get-a-smoking-break-d-c-circuit-clarifies-scope-of-fdas-authority-over-e-cigarettes/ Accessed September 28, 2013.
45. FDA. FDA proposes to extend its tobacco authority to additional tobacco products, including e-cigarettes. [news release]. 2014. http://www.fda.gov/newsevents/newsroom/pressannouncements/ucm394667.htm. Accessed September 4, 2014.
46. Editorial Board. E-Smoking among teenagers. *The New York Times.* 2013. http://www.nytimes.com/2013/09/16/opinion/e-smoking-among-teenagers.html. Accessed September 28, 2013.

47. CDC. Chronic disease prevention and health promotion: Tobacco use. 2011. http://www.cdc.gov/chronicdisease/resources/publications/aag/osh.htm. Accessed September 30, 2013.
48. Esterl M. States urge FDA to regulate e-cigarettes. *Wall Street Journal Online.* September 24, 2013. http://online.wsj.com/article/SB100014240527023037596045 79095461997304256.html. Accessed September 30, 2013.
49. Bhatnagar A, Whitsel LP, Ribisl KM, et al. Electronic cigarettes: A policy statement from the American Heart Association. *Circulation.* 2014. http://circ.ahajournals.org/content/130/16/1418.long Accessed September 16, 2014.
50. Bell K, Keane H. Nicotine control: E-cigarettes, smoking and addiction. *Intl J Drug Policy.* 2012;23(3):242–247.
51. WHO. Electronic nicotine delivery systems: World Health Organization. July 21, 2014. http://apps.who.int/gb/fctc/PDF/cop6/FCTC_COP6_10-en.pdf?ua=1 Accessed September 16, 2014.
52. Jolly D, Tavernise S. World Health Organization urges stronger regulation of electronic cigarettes. *The New York Times.* 2014. http://www.nytimes.com/2014/08/27/business/international/world-health-organization-urges-stronger-regulation-of-electronic-cigarettes.html?_r=0. Accessed September 16, 2014.
53. Terbush J. The vapologist will see you now: Inside New York's first e-cigarette bar. *The Week.* 2013. http://theweek.com/article/index/251049/the-vapologist-will-see-you-now-inside-new-yorks-first-e-cigarette-bar. Accessed November 1, 2013.

CHAPTER 6

Tobacco: Reducing Exposure to Secondhand Smoke

LEARNING OBJECTIVES

- Describe the scientific evidence linking exposure to secondhand smoke to adverse health effects in children and adults.
- Discuss trends in exposure to secondhand smoke in the United States and globally.
- Examine and discuss research supporting the effectiveness of smoke-free policies in reducing health risks.
- Prepare arguments for and against smoke-free policies in outdoor settings.
- Formulate strategies to eliminate exposure to and health consequences from secondhand smoke in the United States and worldwide.

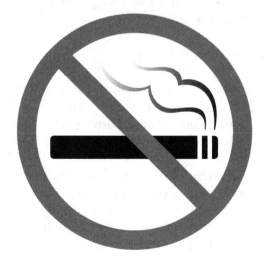

THE CONTROVERSY

In just 5 years, the number of outdoor smoking bans has doubled.[1] In July 2013, Woodruff Park in Atlanta, GA became another outdoor location that banned smoking, despite some local skepticism about the need or health benefits.[1] Experts from the U.S. Centers for Disease Control and Prevention in Atlanta argue against any safe level of exposure to secondhand smoke.[2] This is the same conclusion reached by the 2006 Surgeon General's report, "The Health Consequences of Involuntary Exposure to Tobacco Smoke" which states: "The scientific evidence indicates that there is no risk-free level of exposure to secondhand smoke."[3] More outdoor locations are becoming smoke free, including beaches and college campuses. However, as the New York State Supreme Court halts an outdoor smoking ban in New York state parks,[4] some academic experts are questioning these policies. A Columbia University professor declared: "The evidence of a risk to people in open-air settings is flimsy."[1] While health advocates cite research showing positive health benefits from such policies,[2] the smokers' advocacy group, New York Citizens Lobbying Against Smoker Harassment (CLASH) sued and successfully argued against the ban in New York state parks, claiming the resulting judicial decision is "a wake-up call for those looking to restrict smoker's rights."[4]

BACKGROUND AND SCOPE OF THE PUBLIC HEALTH AND HEALTH POLICY ISSUE

Secondhand Smoke: Health Effects

Secondhand smoke (SHS), sometimes also called environmental tobacco smoke (ETS), as the name implies, contains smoke exhaled by a smoker and also smoke from a lit and burning cigarette or other tobacco product, all of which is potentially inhaled by other people.[5] In addition to secondhand smoking, exposure to environmental tobacco smoke may also be called "passive or involuntary smoking,"[5] because individuals who are nonsmokers may be exposed to harmful components of SHS, especially in indoor settings, even when they do not smoke cigarettes. National and international public health agencies and experts have concluded there are potentially serious health risks from exposure to SHS.[3,5-7] The U.S. Environmental Protection Agency (EPA) estimates that SHS contains more than 4,000 substances, some of which are carcinogenic.[5]

After many years of accumulating scientific evidence, the EPA determined in 1993, in a 530-page report, that SHS (called ETS or passive smoking) was classified a "Class A" or "known human carcinogen," responsible for causing lung cancer in about 3,000 U.S. nonsmokers each year.[8] The landmark report stated that ETS was responsible for respiratory disease in children, causing asthma in healthy children (and making symptoms worse in children who already have asthma), and causing severe respiratory tract infections in both infants and young children.[8]

More recently, CDC estimated that about 88 million nonsmokers (which represents about 40% of nonsmoking adults) in the United States are exposed to SHS, which can cause heart disease and lung cancer in adults who do not smoke.[6] Although the level of population exposure to SHS represents a dramatic reduction since 1988–1991 (before the EPA's 1993 classification), when it was estimated that 88% of nonsmokers were exposed to SHS, rates of exposure for adults and children remain high, with about half of all children currently exposed to SHS.[6] In infants and children, additional research about health effects shows that SHS is a causative factor in sudden infant death syndrome (SIDS) and middle ear infections, in addition to previously known associations with asthma and severe respiratory infections.[6]

Even the science linking exposure to secondhand smoke with adverse health consequences has been controversial. Barnes and Bero critically evaluated 106 review articles to try and determine why different articles have reached different conclusions about the health effects of SHS.[9] Of all the factors relating to research quality the studies, only an author's affiliation with the tobacco industry was significantly associated with the article's conclusion that secondhand smoke was *not* harmful to human health.[9] In a more detailed review of tobacco industry documents, Tong and Glantz wrote that industry-sponsored research questioning the "biologic plausibility" of research findings and promoting "stress" as a reason for adverse health effects from secondhand smoke, were just some of the strategies that contributed to scientific controversy during this time.[10]

Public Health Perspective: Preventing Exposure to Secondhand Smoke

From a public health perspective, preventing nonsmokers from exposure to SHS requires laws and policies that ban smoking in indoor settings,

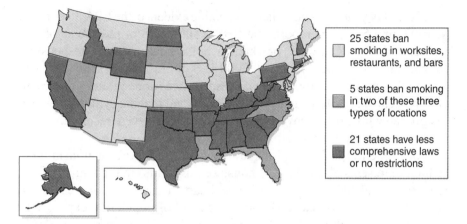

25 states ban smoking in worksites, restaurants, and bars

5 states ban smoking in two of these three types of locations

21 states have less comprehensive laws or no restrictions

Figure 6–1 Tobacco use policies: Secondhand smoke, United States.
Reproduced from Centers for Disease Control and Prevention: Vital Signs.
http://www.cdc.gov/vitalsigns/tobaccouse/secondhandsmoke/infographic.html

and CDC estimates that 21 states in the United States have either no restrictions or weaker smoke-free indoor air quality laws[6] (see **Figure 6–1**).

Exposure to secondhand smoke often occurs in homes and worksites, but also happens in cars and in public indoor places that have not enacted smoke-free policies.[11] Globally, the World Health Organization (WHO) uses the MPOWER strategy for tobacco: *Monitor* tobacco use and prevention policies, *Protect* people from tobacco smoke, *Offer* help to quit, *Warn* about the dangers of tobacco use, *Enforce* bans on tobacco advertising, and *Raise* taxes on tobacco.[6,7] Although secondhand smoke is responsible for an estimated 600,000 annual deaths worldwide,[12,13] the WHO estimates in 2012, just 16% of the world's population has a smoke-free environment, despite the state of scientific knowledge about SHS and effectiveness of smoke-free laws and policies[7] (see **Figure 6–2**).

EVIDENCE BASE FOR PREVENTION AND PRACTICE

Public Health Policies to Reduce Exposure to Secondhand Smoke

The 2006 Surgeon General's Report, "The Health Consequences of Involuntary Exposure to Tobacco Smoke," reaffirmed the health consequences of exposure to secondhand smoke, confirmed that millions

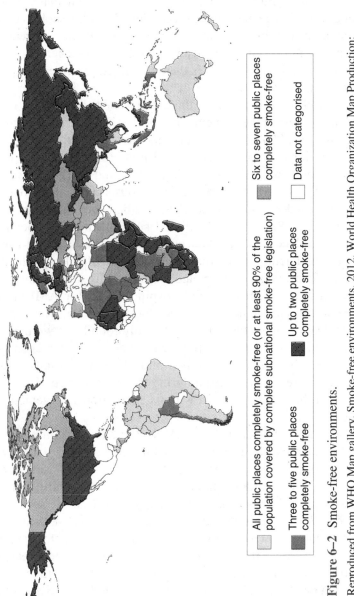

Figure 6–2 Smoke-free environments.

Reproduced from WHO Map gallery. Smoke-free environments, 2012. World Health Organization Map Production: Public Health Information and Geographic Information Systems (GIS) World Health Organization © 2013 http://gamapserver.who.int/mapLibrary/Files/Maps/SmokeFreeEnvironments_2012.png

of children and adults in the United States have ongoing secondhand smoke exposure and stated scientific findings confirming there is "no risk-free level of exposure."[3] Furthermore, the report reinforced that previously used strategies to reduce exposure to secondhand smoke, such as creating separate smoking areas in restaurants, air filtering, and increasing ventilation are not effective in preventing exposure. The Surgeon General concluded that *not* smoking in indoor spaces is the only effective strategy to prevent exposure to SHS in nonsmokers.[3]

Other research has centered on the effectiveness of policies to limit SHS exposure. Some of the first evidence for health benefits of a smoking ban came from a 2004 study that documented a significant decline in hospital admissions for acute myocardial infarction, following passage and enforcement of a local law banning public and workplace smoking in Helena, MT.[14] Using "before-and-after" observational methods and a population-based registry, researchers studied the impact of a 2006 smoke-free law in Spain that prohibited smoking in all indoor public places and workplaces (except some commercial establishments) and the subsequent rate of acute myocardial infarctions (AMIs), hospitalizations, and deaths.[15] The investigators noted a statistically significant decline in the overall AMI occurrence and hospitalization for AMI after the smoke-free law was implemented.[15] When looking further at demographic variables and smoking status, they additionally found that women, older individuals, and passive smokers (defined as never and former smokers) had the greatest benefits, and women and older individuals also had significant decreases in AMI death during the study period. The authors concluded that the 2006 law, even with its exemptions, prevented AMIs in this population.[15]

In another study in Olmsted County, MN, Hurt and colleagues measured the impact of a smoke-free restaurant ordinance and workplace laws on subsequent myocardial infarctions and sudden cardiac deaths using a before-and-after study.[16] Myocardial infarctions dropped by one-third, 18 months after the workplace law began, a statistically significant decrease, while the observed 17% decrease in sudden cardiac deaths was not statistically significant.[16] Other known cardiovascular risk factors (except for smoking) showed no decline over this same time period, suggesting that reductions in myocardial infarctions were associated with implementation of these laws.[16] New York State's 2003 smoking ban resulted in an 8% decline in hospitalizations for AMI by 2004.[17]

Studies have also compared total vs. partial smoking bans. Researchers in Argentina compared hospital admissions for AMI in two cities,

Santa Fe, which implemented a 100% smoke-free law, and Buenos Aires, whose smoke-free law had exceptions and allowed smoking areas.[18] The investigators found significant decreases in AMI hospital admissions in Santa Fe, which began after the law was implemented and continued over time. This same decline was not found in Buenos Aires, suggesting the benefits of a more restrictive policy.[18] In 2013, the American Heart Association (AHA) noted that smoke-free laws in Colorado resulted in fewer ambulance calls to public places, including casinos, after casinos were added to their no-smoking law.[19]

Meta-Analyses of Smoking Bans

Several large analyses of multiple research studies, called meta-analyses, have evaluated health impacts of smoke-free policies on populations. One meta-analysis included twelve published studies from areas in the United States, Canada, Italy, and Ireland, finding a significant decrease in hospital admission rates for acute myocardial infarction one year after the laws had been implemented.[20] Another meta-analysis including 17 studies from North America, Italy, Great Britain, and New Zealand demonstrated a 10% reduction in risk for acute myocardial infarction following the implementation of comprehensive smoke-free laws.[21] A report of 11 studies spanning the period 2004 through 2009 in the United States, Canada, Italy, and Scotland, found an overall decline of 17% in AMIs in areas with workplace and public smoking bans, with benefits increasing over time.[22]

A meta-analysis from the United States, Italy, Canada, Switzerland, Great Britain, and New Zealand, between 2004 and 2011, used 18 different studies to determine the relationship between implementation of smoke-free laws and subsequent risk of acute myocardial infarction (AMI).[23] When combining all studies, the investigators found a significant (13%) decrease in the risk of AMI after implementation of these laws.[23] In addition, they noted that results varied by geographic location and one of the most important contributors to AMI reduction was whether there was a decrease in smoking rates; larger drops in smoking rates were associated with steeper declines in the risk for AMI (called a dose-response relationship) adding strength to the argument that these findings were cause and effect.[23] In addition to health benefits from reducing exposure to secondhand smoke, this study provided evidence that at least some of the positive health impact of the laws was directly due to subsequent declines in smoking.[23] A meta-analysis of 45 studies analyzing the relationship between smoke-free laws and subsequent hospitalizations for heart disease, strokes, and lung diseases showed a significant drop in hospital admissions for all of these conditions, and more comprehensive laws resulted in stronger benefits.[24]

Research studies have also looked at hospitalization for a range of diseases associated with exposure to secondhand smoke following implementation of statewide smoking laws. In a study of the impact of Arizona's 2007 comprehensive statewide law, hospitalizations for conditions associated with exposure to SHS, including AMI, angina, stoke, and asthma, declined significantly following the statewide ban, while no decline was seen in hospitalizations for medical conditions *not* associated with SHS.[25] A study in Scotland, which followed implementation of a smoke-free law, showed a significant decline (18.2%) in hospital admissions for asthma in children younger than 15.[26] Comprehensive smoke-free laws are considered by experts to be an essential public health approach to reducing the impact of cardiovascular disease on a global basis.[12]

Economic Impact

During attempts to pass smoke-free indoor laws and policies, opponents of smoke-free policies have cited potentially negative effects on businesses; some of these have been "anecdotal" reports that did not use actual sales data.[27] One early report in West Lake Hills, TX, used sales data to evaluate restaurant sales before and after implementation of a local smoke-free ordinance. Findings suggested sales were not adversely impacted by the ordinance.[27] In another example published in 2010, Klein and colleagues studied the impact of smoke-free indoor policies on employment in bars and restaurants in two Minnesota cities.[28] Over a 5-year period, investigators found restaurant employment increased by 3–4%, but findings varied between bars in both cities, with a 5–6% increase in one city and a 1% decrease in the other.[28]

Evidence of positive economic impact at a state level in the United States comes from a study of sales in all Washington bars and taverns following the implementation of a statewide smoke-free law passed by ballot initiative in November 2005 and implemented a month later.[29] Investigators developed a mathematical model to project sales revenues, taking into account background seasonal trends. Although in the first 3 months after the law was implemented there was no change in sales, further study projected large increases in sales (estimated at $105.5 million) 2 years after the law was implemented.[29]

The American Lung Association regularly updates the status of U.S. efforts to enact statewide smoke-free laws. As of 2014, they reported that 28 states and the District of Columbia have comprehensive laws (that include most public places, workplaces, restaurants and bars).[30] In addition, they annually grade states from A to F on the strength of their efforts to reduce exposure to SHS. In 2014, states such as California, Washington, Oregon, Vermont, New York, and Nebraska received an "A," whereas states such as Alaska, Texas, North Carolina, South Carolina, and Kentucky all received an "F."[30]

Smoking Bans: Indoors vs. Outdoors

Bans on smoking have extended to outdoor public spaces. Americans for Nonsmokers' Rights, a national lobbying organization formed in 1976, regularly updates its website with tobacco policies implemented in a variety of settings, such as casinos, healthcare facilities, outdoor dining, and colleges and universities.[31] As of October 1, 2014, 1,478 college or university campuses are 100% smoke-free, 976 are 100% tobacco-free campuses, and nearly 300 include e-cigarettes in their restrictions. This represents a substantial increase from the 446 U.S. campuses with such restrictions in 2010.[31] Parks, beaches, and Starbucks are just some of the locations where smoking restrictions outdoors are expanding.[32] The New York City Council voted to ban smoking in parks, public beaches, and outdoor pedestrian malls on May 23, 2011, including places such as Central Park and Times Square.[33] Some of the evidence presented in support of this proposal by the New York City Health Commissioner included the finding that even though only 16% of NYC residents smoked, 57% tested positive for cotinine (which correlates with exposure to cigarette smoke).[33] In June 2013, a company banned smoking nationwide in 40,000 rental units to "create healthier living conditions," beginning their efforts in New York locations in 2009.[34] However not all policy makers are on board: in September 2014, New Jersey Governor Chris Christie vetoed a widely supported bill banning smoking in public parks and New Jersey beaches, citing the need to preserve "local control" in policymaking.[35]

How close is too close to smokers? In 2007, researchers from Stanford conducted an experiment in 10 locations near the Stanford campus.[36] They measured specific airborne particles, called particulate matter-2.5 (PM2.5), in cigarette smoke from actual smokers in outdoor settings, using portable electronic devices. Investigators found that risks for exposure to these particles was higher the closer you were to smokers, and it was possible for nonsmokers to be exposed to significant amounts of cigarette smoke depending how far away they were and whether they were upwind or downwind. Exposure levels were lower when they moved 6 feet away from the burning cigarette.[36] In contrast to patrons, other experts note that servers (wait staff) in some types of outdoor restaurant and bar seating may accumulate substantial exposure to SHS because of the long hours worked in this environment.[33]

Will Smoking Bans Result in More Smoking at Home?

Some arguments against outdoor smoking bans have included the concern that such bans will increase smoking in cars and homes, potentially exposing children and adults to harmful levels of secondhand smoke.[37] A national study provided data showing that the opposite occurred: smoke-free laws actually increased the chances that smoke-free policies were put into effect in homes. Data from the Tobacco Use Supplement to the Current Population Survey (TUS-CPS) was used in combination with information about smoke-free indoor air laws, to determine whether living in areas with these laws impacted whether or not there was a smoke-free policy at home.[37] Investigators found that people living in areas with strong smoke-free indoor air laws (covering public places and worksites) were much more likely to have a voluntary smoke-free policy in the home, and this was true whether smokers or nonsmokers lived in the household.[37] In addition, voluntary smoke-free home policies were even more likely in areas where smoke-free laws were stronger.[37] According to the authors, their findings were consistent with the concepts of nonsmoking "norm-spreading" as a result of comprehensive smoking bans in indoor places.[37] Although the percentages of homes with nonsmoking policies has increased three-fold since the early 1990s, in U.S. homes where both children and smokers live, only 50% of homes had policies that banned smoking.[38] Smoke-free homes were also less likely in African American and non-Hispanic white households, as well as in households where adults had less education and income. Home smoking bans, however, were *more* likely in states with lower adult smoking rates.[38]

How Far Can Outdoor Bans Go?

In February 2013, New York's Office of Parks, Recreation and Historic Preservation banned outdoor smoking in state parks, including beaches and picnic areas, to protect the public from exposure to secondhand smoke.[39] They were subsequently sued in April of the same year by New York City Citizens Lobbying Against Smoker Harassment (CLASH),[40] and on October 8, 2013, the New York State Supreme Court stopped the ban, determining in its ruling that the parks office had overstepped its authority.[39]

DISCUSSION QUESTIONS: TEMPLATE FOR DISCUSSION

1. Significance of this public health issue:
   a. Why is this health issue important?
   b. How many people does it impact?
   c. How serious is it?
   d. Is it preventable?
2. What is the evidence base for prevention?
3. What specific strategies should be used to achieve progress on this health issue?
   a. What evidence-based approach would you use?
   b. Where would you start if you are an individual citizen; public health professional; healthcare professional; community, state, or federal policymaker?
4. Specific questions for this topic:
   a. What is the evidence that secondhand smoke causes adverse health effects?
   b. What is the evidence that policies creating smoke-free environments protects public health and improves health outcomes?
   c. How strong is the evidence for restricting smoking in outdoor locations? Are there health benefits in addition to reducing exposure to secondhand smoke?
5. What is the controversy?
   a. Define the controversy.
   b. Is controversy a good or bad thing? (Does it help or hinder progress?)

6. *Why* is this health issue controversial?
   a. What specific factors are involved?
   b. Do economics, government, scientific uncertainty, or politics play a role?
   c. What is the role of the media?
7. How would you respond to the controversy?

PERSPECTIVES TO CONSIDER

It's difficult to now image an earlier time when smoking was everywhere—indoors, in hospitals, stores and shopping malls, in schools and public buildings. Gradual declines in smoking rates in adults and the important determination by the EPA in 1993 that environmental tobacco smoke (secondhand smoke) was a human carcinogen (in the same categories as asbestos and benzene) have helped reduce exposure to SHS in the United States.[8] The 1993 EPA report propelled public attention, debate, and subsequent passage and implementation and of many laws and policies at local and state levels, all designed to protect the public from adverse health effects from SHS.[30]

Subsequently, many studies of health benefits (and some on economic impact) were published. Several large combined studies (meta-analyses) showed reductions in acute myocardial infarctions (and in some studies cerebrovascular events [strokes] and respiratory disease) after smoke-free policies were implemented in different geographic settings.[20–24] What was remarkable was how fast positive effects could be documented in entire populations following the passage of comprehensive smoke-free laws, often in a matter of months. Observed smoking declines and improved health outcomes are important findings. They suggest that creating an environment in which *not smoking* is the stated norm may be important in changing behavior, something also implied in the relationship between living in areas covered by smoke-free laws or policies and having a smoke-free policy in the home.[37]

This is highly relevant today in the context of smoking rates in young adults, many of college age, and national efforts to ban smoking or tobacco products altogether (including e-cigarettes) on college campuses. It seems logical that *not* being able to smoke in a location might indeed be like jumping over hurdle after hurdle, becoming just nuisance enough to encourage someone to consider making a quit attempt, or not to start smoking at all. What is the magnitude of the impact that public smoking bans have on decisions to quit smoking? Or never to start? Additional research could help to further quantify this.

But here is the controversy: where do we draw the line? How far can and should government and other entities go in policymaking to "encourage" people to quit smoking? Do benefits to the health of the entire population, scientific research, and social norms support such strategies? Eliminating SHS exposure in indoor settings and resultant evidence of health benefits is compelling, but the WHO tells us that only a small percentage of the world's population is covered by such policies. The rationale and impact of restrictions on *outdoor* smoking rely on the assertion that exposure to ETS is a risk at any level, and also on the potential positive impact on reducing smoking rates of entire populations. Given the public health impact of tobacco use (including SHS) in the United States and worldwide and current controversy when restrictions in outdoor settings are proposed, additional policy research could help. Defining the policy impact on decision making by smokers to quit or nonsmokers to continue not smoking would help advance the scientific foundation.

FOR ADDITIONAL STUDY

Tong EK, Glantz SA. Tobacco industry efforts undermining evidence linking secondhand smoke with cardiovascular disease. *Circulation.* 2007;116(16):1845–1854.

Lin H, Wang H, Wu W, Lang L, Wang Q, Tian L. The effects of smoke-free legislation on acute myocardial infarction: A systematic review and meta-analysis. *BMC Public Health.* 2013;13:529.

Tan CE, Glantz SA. Association between smoke-free legislation and hospitalizations for cardiac, cerebrovascular, and respiratory diseases: A meta-analysis. *Circulation.* 2012;126(18):2177–2183.

REFERENCES

1. Associated Press. Outdoor smoking bans double in U.S. past 5 years. *CBS News.* 2013. http://www.cbsnews.com/8301-204_162-57597699/. Accessed October 20, 2013.
2. Associated Press. Anti-smoking battle moves outdoors, bans increase. 2013. http://www.foxnews.com/health/2013/08/08/anti-smoking-battle-moves-outdoors-bans-increase/. Accessed October 20, 2013.
3. USDHHS. The health consequences of involuntary exposure to tobacco smoke: A report of the Surgeon General. 2006. http://www.ncbi.nlm.nih.gov/books/NBK44324/. Accessed October 15, 2013.
4. Hupfl A. Smokers' rights group challenged consitutionality of the regulation. *USA Today.* 2013. http://www.usatoday.com/story/news/nation/2013/10/11/new-york-state-park-smoking-ban/2967991/. Accessed October 20, 2013.

5. EPA. Health effects of exposure to seondhand smoke. 2013. http://www.epa.gov/smokefree/healtheffects.html. Accessed October 15, 2013.

6. CDC. Tobacco use: Smoking and secondhand smoke. *CDC Vital Signs*. 2010. http://www.cdc.gov/vitalsigns/TobaccoUse/SecondhandSmoke/index.html. Accessed October 15, 2013.

7. WHO. WHO report on the global tobacco epidemic, 2013: Enforcing bans on tobacco advertising, promotion, and sponsorship. 2013. http://www.who.int/tobacco/global_report/2013/en/. Accessed September 28, 2013.

8. EPA. EPA designates passive smoking a "Class A" or known human carcinogen. 1993. http://www2.epa.gov/aboutepa/epa-designates-passive-smoking-class-or-known-human-carcinogen. Accessed October 15, 2013.

9. Barnes DE, Bero LA. Why review articles on the health effects of passive smoking reach different conclusions. *JAMA*. 1998;279(19):1566–1570.

10. Tong EK, Glantz SA. Tobacco industry efforts undermining evidence linking secondhand smoke with cardiovascular disease. *Circulation*. 2007;116(16):1845–1854.

11. CDC. Smoking and tobacco use: Secondhand smoke (SHS) facts. 2013. http://www.cdc.gov/tobacco/data_statistics/fact_sheets/secondhand_smoke/general_facts/. Accessed October 20, 2013.

12. Tan CE, Glantz SA. Smokefree air: An important strategy to reducing heart attacks around the world. *Glob Heart*. 2012;7(2):189–191.

13. Oberg M, Jaakkola MS, Woodward A, Peruga A, Pruss-Ustun A. Worldwide burden of disease from exposure to second-hand smoke: A retrospective analysis of data from 192 countries. *Lancet*. 2011;377(9760):139–146.

14. Sargent RP, Shepard RM, Glantz SA. Reduced incidence of admissions for myocardial infarction associated with public smoking ban: Before and after study. *BMJ*. 2004;328(7446):977–980.

15. Aguero F, Degano IR, Subirana I, et al. Impact of a partial smoke-free legislation on myocardial infarction incidence, mortality and case-fatality in a population-based registry: the REGICOR study. *PLoS One*. 2013;8(1):e53722.

16. Hurt RD, Weston SA, Ebbert JO, et al. Myocardial infarction and sudden cardiac death in Olmsted County, Minnesota, before and after smoke-free workplace laws. *Arch Intern Med*. 2012;172(21):1635–1641.

17. Juster HR, Loomis BR, Hinman TM, et al. Declines in hospital admissions for acute myocardial infarction in New York state after implementation of a comprehensive smoking ban. *Am J Public Health*. 2007;97(11):2035–2039.

18. Ferrante D, Linetzky B, Virgolini M, Schoj V, Apelberg B. Reduction in hospital admissions for acute coronary syndrome after the successful implementation of 100% smoke-free legislation in Argentina: A comparison with partial smoking restrictions. *Tob Control*. 2012;21(4):402–406.

19. American Heart Association. No-smoking law in Colorado casinos led to fewer ambulance calls. 2013. http://newsroom.heart.org/news/no-smoking-law-in-colorado-casinos-led-to-fewer-ambulance-calls. Accessed October 20, 2013.

20. Lightwood JM, Glantz SA. Declines in acute myocardial infarction after smoke-free laws and individual risk attributable to secondhand smoke. *Circulation*. 2009;120(14):1373–1379.

21. Mackay DF, Irfan MO, Haw S, Pell JP. Meta-analysis of the effect of comprehensive smoke-free legislation on acute coronary events. *Heart*. 2010;96(19): 1525–1530.

22. Meyers DG, Neuberger JS, He J. Cardiovascular effect of bans on smoking in public places: A systematic review and meta-analysis. *J Am Coll Cardiol*. 2009;54(14):1249–1255.

23. Lin H, Wang H, Wu W, Lang L, Wang Q, Tian L. The effects of smoke-free legislation on acute myocardial infarction: A systematic review and meta-analysis. *BMC Public Health*. 2013;13:529.

24. Tan CE, Glantz SA. Association between smoke-free legislation and hospitalizations for cardiac, cerebrovascular, and respiratory diseases: A meta-analysis. *Circulation*. 2012;126(18):2177–2183.

25. Herman PM, Walsh ME. Hospital admissions for acute myocardial infarction, angina, stroke, and asthma after implementation of Arizona's comprehensive statewide smoking ban. *Am J Public Health*. 2011;101(3):491–496.

26. Mackay D, Haw S, Ayres JG, Fischbacher C, Pell JP. Smoke-free legislation and hospitalizations for childhood asthma. *N Engl J Med*. 2010;363(12):1139–1145.

27. Assessment of the impact of a 100% smoke-free ordinance on restaurant sales— West Lake Hills, Texas, 1992–1994. *MMWR Morb Mortal Wkly Rep*. 1995;44(19): 370–372.

28. Klein EG, Forster JL, Erickson DJ, Lytle LA, Schillo B. Economic effects of clean indoor air policies on bar and restaurant employment in Minneapolis and St Paul, Minnesota. *J Public Health Manag Pract*. 2010;16(4):285–293.

29. Boles M, Dilley J, Maher JE, Boysun MJ, Reid T. Smoke-free law associated with higher-than-expected taxable retail sales for bars and taverns in Washington state. *Prev Chronic Dis*. 2010;7(4):A79.

30. American Lung Association. State grades: Smokefree air laws. 2014. http://www .stateoftobaccocontrol.org/state-grades/state-rankings/smokefree-air-laws.html. Accessed September 24, 2014.

31. ANR. Americans for Nonsmokers' Rights. [website]. 2014. http://www.no-smoke.org/ aboutus.php?id=436. Accessed September 28, 2014.

32. Smoking bans. *The Huffington Post*. 2013. http://www.huffingtonpost.com/tag/ smoking-bans. Accessed October 20, 2013.

33. Colgrove J, Bayer R, Bachynski KE. Nowhere left to hide? The banishment of smoking from public spaces. *N Engl J Med*. 2011;364(25):2375–2377.

34. Hughes CJ. A smoking ban in all related companies rentals. *The New York Times*. 2013. http://www.nytimes.com/2013/06/16/realestate/a-smoking-ban-in-all-related-companies-rentals.html?_r=0. Accessed October 20, 2013.

35. Sheppard K. Chris Christie to Jersey Shore crowd: Smoke 'em if ya got 'em. *The Huffington Post*. 2014. http://www.huffingtonpost.com/2014/09/11/christie-smoking-ban-veto_n_5806806.html. Accessed September 28, 2014.

36. Shwartz M. Study confirms the risk of exposure to secondhand tobacco smoke at sidewalk cafes and other outdoor settings. *Stanford News Service*. 2007. http://news .stanford.edu/pr/2007/pr-smoke-050907.html. Accessed October 14, 2013.

37. Cheng KW, Glantz SA, Lightwood JM. Association between smokefree laws and voluntary smokefree-home rules. *Am J Prev Med*. 2011;41(6):566–572.

38. Mills AL, White MM, Pierce JP, Messer K. Home smoking bans among U.S. households with children and smokers: Opportunities for intervention. *Am J Prev Med.* 2011;41(6):559–565.
39. Dolmetsch C. N.Y. state parks outdoor smoking ban is blocked by court. *Bloomberg. com News.* 2013. http://www.bloomberg.com/news/2013-10-11/new-york-state-parks-outdoor-smoking-ban-blocked.html. Accessed October 20, 2013.
40. New York City CLASH. New York City Citizens Lobbying Against Smoker Harassment (CLASH). [website]. 2013. http://www.nycclash.com/. Accessed October 20, 2013.

CHAPTER 7

Alcohol: Binge Drinking on College Campuses

LEARNING OBJECTIVES

- Discuss the data and trends in binge drinking on college campuses in the United States.
- Describe the health effects of binge drinking on individuals and the "secondhand" effects on others.
- Critically assess the evidence for the effectiveness of lowering the minimum legal drinking age (MLDA) in reducing binge drinking.
- Predict the public health consequences of changing the MLDA on a state-by-state basis.
- Identify evidence-based policies that are effective in preventing binge drinking in young adults.
- Propose evidence-based strategies to reduce binge drinking in young adults and related adverse health effects in this population.

THE CONTROVERSY

"We should prepare young adults to make responsible decisions about alcohol in the same way we prepare them to operate a motor vehicle . . ." said John M. McCardell Jr., president emeritus of Middlebury college and current vice chancellor of the University of the South in Sewanee, TN.[1] In an opinion piece for *The New York Times*, McCardell suggested that similar to the approach used to get a driver's license, after successful completion of an alcohol education course, we should issue permits—followed by licenses—to drink alcohol, as long as state laws were obeyed.[1] There could be specific requirements determined by individual states whose role would become "laboratories of experimentation" related to changes in current age-restrictions.[1]

McCardell was the founder of the Amethyst Initiative (Choose Responsibility), a group of more than 130 signatory university presidents calling for public debate on the current minimum legal drinking age of 21 in the United States.[2] However Boston University president, Robert A. Brown (*not* a signatory), counters, "I worry about the consequences of lowering the age on the large number of teenagers not in college, as well as the environment for students in high school who would experience increased exposure to alcohol."[3] Another university professor argues that "Policy decisions should be based on science and research, not politics and self-serving interests,"[4] and further remarked that, "Given the high stakes—student health and academic performance—as well as the overwhelming research supporting the MLDA [minimum legal drinking age], it is surprising that any university president would sign the Amethyst Initiative."[4] Other academic experts editorialize, "There is no scientific evidence to suggest that a lower minimum legal drinking age would create conditions for responsible drinking or would lead young adults aged 18–20 years to make healthy decisions about drinking."[5]

One *U.S. News & World Report* writer cited the experience of Britain, where the drinking age is 18 and 40% of British teens begin drinking at age 13 or even younger, as a warning for this proposal.[6] The *New York Times* editorial board, in response to the Amethyst Initiative, wrote: "Whatever the causes, the solutions almost certainly lie mostly within the colleges—perhaps with better counseling or stronger bans on under-age drinking—not by lowering the legal drinking age.[7]

BACKGROUND AND SCOPE OF THE PUBLIC HEALTH AND HEALTH POLICY ISSUE

Health Effects and Trends in Binge Drinking in Young Adults

Alcohol is the third leading "actual cause of death" in the United States, with an estimated 85,000 deaths attributed to health consequences of excess alcohol use in 2000.[8] This estimate increased to 88,000 deaths per year in 2006–2010.[9] The Centers for Disease Control and Prevention (CDC) estimates that for each person dying from too much alcohol use, their lives were shortened by about 30 years.[9]

CDC defines binge drinking as drinking five or more alcoholic drinks in a short time period (about 2 hours) for men, and four or more drinks for women.[10] Binge drinking is responsible for at least 79,000 annual U.S.

deaths, and using data from the U.S. Behavioral Risk Factor Surveillance System (BRFSS), binge drinking is generally more common in men, adults aged 18–34 (26% report binge drinking), and those with household incomes of at least $75,000 (19% report binge drinking).[10] About 38 million adults in the United States binge drink—although the amount varies, to as much as 8 drinks each time.[11]

Furthermore, CDC estimates 90% of the alcohol used by young people is from binge drinking, compared to a figure just over 50% for all adult alcohol use in the United States.[11] Although people aged 18–34 as a group have the most binge drinkers, people age 65 and older binge drink more often.[11] Binge drinking rates also vary by household income: although people with household incomes of at least $75,000 comprise the highest percentage of binge drinkers (20.2%), people in households earning incomes less than $25,000 also have a higher number of monthly binges (5.0 vs. 3.7) and drink more drinks each time they binge drink (an average of 8.5 drinks vs. 7.2 drinks) than those in the highest income category.[11] Across the United States, reported rates of binge drinking vary widely, from a low of 10.9% (reported in Utah) to a high of 25.6% reported in Wisconsin[11] (see **Figure 7–1**).

Binge drinking is associated with increased risk for a variety of unplanned, serious, or even fatal conditions including: motor vehicle crashes, violence, and risk of pregnancy, sexually transmitted diseases, and HIV, due to

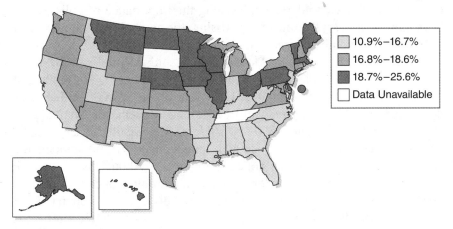

☐	10.9%–16.7%
▨	16.8%–18.6%
■	18.7%–25.6%
☐	Data Unavailable

Figure 7–1 United States: Percent of adults who binge drink.

Reproduced from Centers for Disease Control and Prevention. Vital Signs: Binge Drinking, January 2012. http://www.cdc.gov/vitalsigns/BingeDrinking/index.html

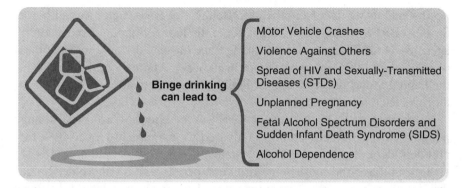

Figure 7–2 Public health consequences of binge drinking.
Reproduced from Centers for Disease Control and Prevention. Vital Signs: Binge Drinking, January 2012. http://www.cdc.gov/vitalsigns/BingeDrinking/index.html

impaired judgment related to rapid, excessive alcohol consumption. Binge drinking also increases later risk for alcohol dependence, and for women who are pregnant, binge drinking increases risk for fetal alcohol disorders and also sudden infant death syndrome (SIDS)[9,10] (see **Figure 7–2**).

In 2007, because of the magnitude of this public health problem in the United States, the U.S. Surgeon General issued a "call to action" to prevent underage drinking and its consequences.[12] Another comprehensive report from the Institute of Medicine (IOM), "Reducing Underage Drinking: A Collective Responsibility," highlights collective roles and responsibilities of a variety of stakeholders, emphasizing the importance of policies and laws limiting access; the role of advertising; the alcohol and entertainment industries; and youth-focused and community interventions.[13]

The National Institute on Alcohol Abuse and Alcoholism (NIAAA) reports on the magnitude of health and social impacts of excessive alcohol consumption on college campuses Each year about 599,000 college students (aged 18–24) are injured and 1,825 college students die from injuries related to alcohol.[14] Nearly 700,000 students are assaulted each year by another student who has used alcohol; an estimated 97,000 students are rape victims each year across college campuses.[14] About 25% of college students report academic problems related to their alcohol consumption.[14] Furthermore, although alcohol consumption levels are high enough to meet definitions for alcohol abuse or dependence, few students recognize this as a problem. Nearly one-fifth (19%) of college students are considered by clinical definitions to be abusing or dependent on alcohol, but only a small percentage (5%) of students get treatment.[14]

Harvard School of Public Health College Alcohol Study

Some of the most extensive research about alcohol consumption on college campuses, including data about health effects, "secondhand" impacts on other students, risk factors for binge drinking, and potential preventive strategies comes from Harvard researchers who conducted the Harvard School of Public Health College Alcohol Study (CAS) from 1992 to 2006.[15] These investigators sampled more than 50,000 students at 120 colleges to gather data from a national perspective, in contrast to previous studies on one or a few college campuses.[15] Researchers used definitions of binge drinking similar to that of CDC[10] and World Health Organization (WHO),[16] defining binge drinking as "five or more drinks in a row" for men and four for women, in the prior two weeks, levels that were related to most of the harmful consequences from drinking in this population.[15] They further defined "frequent binge drinking" as binge drinking three times or more in the past two weeks, and documented these and other measures of alcohol consumption to assess consequences, risks, and preventive factors.[15]

The Harvard researchers found, in surveys conducted from 1993 to 2001, that 44% of U.S. 4-year college students were binge drinking, a figure similar to other national surveys of alcohol consumption in the United States.[15] Although this overall statistic changed little during this time period, the authors noted that both the numbers of college students who report totally abstaining from alcohol and the numbers reporting frequent binge drinking increased, with almost half of all students surveyed (48%) reported "drinking to get drunk" as a reason for drinking.[15] About 50% of college students who binge drink have previously consumed alcohol at this level, prior to entering college, and the rest start binge drinking after they arrive.[15]

Consistent with other studies, the CAS found binge drinking associated with adverse health, academic, and social problems, including 13% of students reporting driving after consuming at least five drinks and nearly one-quarter reporting riding with such a driver.[15] The CAS also commonly noted drinking levels that met clinical criteria for alcohol abuse or dependence. In their national sample, nearly one-third of college students and 60% of students who were frequently binge drinking, met the clinical definition of "alcohol abuse."[15] Furthermore, contrary to common perceptions of risks related to college drinking, researchers found that 1 in 17 of all college students and 20% of "frequent binge drinkers" met clinical criteria for "alcohol dependence."[15] Similar to other reports, in the CAS, fewer than 3% of college students who reported frequent binge drinking had gotten help, and the vast majority of students drinking at this level were not at all concerned about their alcohol use.[15]

In addition to health, social, and academic effects on the drinkers themselves, the Harvard CAS noted effects on others in the same environment. Such "secondhand effects" as damage to personal property, injury, noise, or violence (including insults, arguments, and physical and sexual violence) were all extensively documented.[15]

Factors Associated with College Student Drinking

Results from the CAS also imply that environmental factors may relate to differences in binge drinking rates. For example, in these studies, binge drinking rates varied in colleges in different geographic regions of the United States.[15] Among the more than 100 colleges participating, rates of reported binge drinking varied dramatically, from 1% to 76%, but were consistent within individual college environments over the duration of the study.[15] Factors associated with binge drinking in college freshmen included fraternity and sorority membership, availability and reduced cost of alcoholic beverages, the state in which the college was located, and the college's binge drinking rate.[15] Conversely, less binge drinking was seen in colleges with more ethnic and racial diversity, female students, older students, and campuses where more students were involved in volunteering.[15] Substance-free living environments and the strength and number of local and state alcohol-related policies were also associated with less binge drinking.[15,17]

One intriguing analysis used data from the BRFSS and the CAS to study college binge drinking rates and whether or not they were related to binge drinking rates in the state where the college was located.[17] In addition, the same investigators studied the influence of the type and number of alcohol control policies in place on the amount of binge drinking.[17] They found a strong statistical relationship between overall adult binge drinking rates and college binge drinking rates in a particular state. For example, students attending college in states with a lower adult binge drinking rate were less likely to binge drink than those attending college in states where adult binge drinking rates were higher, highlighting the role of the surrounding environment in college drinking behavior.[17]

Investigators also studied the relationship between binge drinking and alcohol control policies such as keg registration, drinking and driving laws, restrictions on reduced-price promotions and advertising, by using additional data from Mothers Against Drunk Driving (MADD). Attending college in a state with a greater number (4 or more) and stronger alcohol control policies was associated with lower binge drinking rates.[17] These studies reinforced the important impact of the surrounding environment, cultural factors, and local or statewide laws and policies on how much binge drinking actually happens on college campuses.[17]

EVIDENCE BASE FOR PREVENTION AND PRACTICE

Evidence-based policies that are effective in reducing binge drinking include raising the price of alcohol, enforcing legal drinking age laws, and restricting numbers and density of locations that sell alcohol.[17] A frequently used approach on college campuses (about half of the colleges in the CAS) to prevent binge drinking and reduce alcohol use is called "social-norms marketing," designed to reinforce less harmful levels of drinking using media and other communication channels. However, the CAS found no evidence of decreased alcohol use in colleges using this approach.[15] These results were controversial and ultimately, additional study to look further at program details in different locations was called for.[15]

Evidence-Based Strategies to Reduce Alcohol Consumption

The Community Preventive Services Task Force, an independent group of scientific experts, reviews and publishes recommendations for community prevention. Their recommendations are based on scientific evidence about "what works" on a population level to improve public health in a variety of areas.[18] The Task Force conducts "systematic reviews," reporting the effectiveness of various programs, policies, and interventions designed to improve public health; they characterize interventions as "strong" and "sufficient" reflecting the panels' confidence in the strength of the scientific evidence.[18] In their review of interventions to prevent excessive alcohol use, they recommend interventions directed to the general public, such as "dram shop liability," where the alcohol establishment has legal liability for harm caused by intoxicated patrons.[19] Other recommended evidence-based interventions include increasing the price of alcoholic beverages through taxes, limiting days and hours of alcohol sales, and regulating the numbers of locations selling or serving alcohol through zoning or licensing.[19]

The Task Force noted there was not enough scientific evidence to determine the effectiveness of such common practices as training alcoholic beverage servers. They recommend increased enforcement, such as using "decoys" to prevent sales of alcohol to minors.[19]

In addition, the Task Force reviewed interventions to reduce drinking and driving, recommending 0.08% blood alcohol concentration (BAC) laws, with lower BAC laws for younger drivers,[20] and maintaining the current MLDA, based on the evidence of decreased alcohol-related crashes and injuries.[20,21] They noted in 14 studies, raising the MLDA from age 18 to 21 decreased "crash-related outcomes" in 16–17-year-olds by an average of 16% and, conversely, lowering the MLDA increased harm from motor vehicle crashes by 10%.[21] The Task Force determined there was not enough scientific evidence to recommend such interventions as "designated drivers" and "social norming" campaigns.[20]

Many, if not all, colleges and universities use alcohol education. In a survey of 747 college presidents, nearly all colleges used alcohol education, especially among first-year students.[15] A randomized controlled study involving 30 universities evaluated the impact of AlcoholEdu, a 2- to 3-hour online course to prevent and reduce harm from excessive alcohol use, in new college freshmen.[22] Compared to schools in the study not using AlcoholEdu, investigators found significant decreases in alcohol-related problems during the fall semester after students had just completed AlcoholEdu. Furthermore, for schools where at least 70% of students completed AlcoholEdu, the benefits were greater.[22]

Unfortunately, in this study the curriculum did not improve academic difficulties related to alcohol use, risky sexual behavior related to alcohol use, or drinking and driving (or being a passenger in a car with someone who had been drinking), and the benefits seen in the fall, following course completion, did not last into the spring semester.[22] Researchers acknowledged the need for colleges and universities to utilize a comprehensive and evidence-based approach that includes the college and surrounding community.[22]

In a separate publication, Paschall and colleagues reported statistically significant decreases in use of alcohol in the past 30 days, as well as binge drinking during the fall semester immediately following completion of AlcoholEdu; however, these reductions were not seen later, in the spring semester.[23] The authors concluded AlcoholEdu had a positive impact on alcohol use by new freshmen college students, but also concluded this educational approach needs additional support from broader prevention approaches.[23]

How well have colleges in the United States responded to national recommendations for prevention of alcohol misuse? The NIAAA published evidence-based recommendations in 2002 from a task force on college drinking.[24] Nelson and colleagues surveyed 351 college administrators 6 years later to determine progress. They found that 98% of colleges used educational programs, about two-thirds had intervention programs for students with alcohol-related problems, and about half used programs that were evidence based.[24] However, 21% of college administrators surveyed were not aware of the NIAAA recommendations, and most were not aware of or involved with prevention activities in their local communities, such as mandatory beverage service training policies, density of locations selling or serving alcohol, enforcement of laws prohibiting sales to underage students, or increasing the price of alcohol, all evidence-based approaches.[24]

Minimum Legal Drinking Age in the United States

In the United States, data from national surveys demonstrate that risks of alcohol dependence overall, becoming alcohol dependent by age 25, and long-term alcohol dependence are all increased with younger ages of alcohol use; risks increase for every year before age 21 a person begins to use alcohol.[25] In 1984, the U.S. Congress passed a law that withheld federal highway construction funds if states did not enact age 21 as the MLDA; by 1988 this had passed in all 50 states.[25]

In addition to reviews conducted by the Community Preventive Services Task Force,[21] the MLDA is one of the most studied policies in public health. Wagenaar and Toomey reviewed MLDA laws from 1960 to 2000, conducting an extensive and critical review of the literature, and specifically reported on the best-designed studies.[26] Their review concluded that a higher MLDA was associated with both reduced alcohol consumption and reduced motor vehicle crashes.[26] Thirty-three studies examining the relationship between MLDA and alcohol consumption were reviewed and one-third found reduced consumption associated with increased MLDA.[26]

In the review of 79 studies examining the relationship of MLDA and motor vehicle crashes, 58% noted higher MLDA was associated with reduced crashes. The only caveat of their extensive review was the lack of high-quality studies specifically evaluating college student populations; only 9% of the 64 studies targeting this population were of sufficient quality to be used for their review and no statistically significant associations were noted.[26]

Comparing Drinking in Europe and the United States

Although researchers note challenges of international comparisons of alcohol consumption, such as differences in drinking cultures, differences in drink sizes and amount of alcohol, and survey and research methods, much current information is available about international alcohol consumption in different geographic areas, age populations, and levels of consumption.[27] As any alcohol use in young people is associated with an increased risk of adverse health effects or alcohol dependence in adulthood, some surveys (such as ones looking at international consumption), specifically measure drinking rates before age 13.[25]

People commonly believe that in European countries, where minimum purchasing ages for alcohol are frequently lower than in the United States, there is less problem drinking, because alcohol is allowed and introduced at younger ages.[28] Minimum purchasing ages, often compared with our MLDA of 21 in the United Stated, range from a low of age 14 (for beer and wine in Switzerland) and age 15 in Belgium to 21 in Russia and Ukraine.[28]

Data from the European School Survey Project on Alcohol and Other Drugs (ESPAD) from 2007 (that surveyed 15- and 16-year-olds from 35 European countries) are often compared to the Monitoring the Future (MTF) survey, which is a yearly survey of 8th, 10th, and 12th graders in the United States. Published data argue against the notion that drinking rates and excess consumption are lower in European countries.[28] For example, more youth in European countries report drinking during the past month (which is often used as a measure of current alcohol use) than do young people in the United States.[28] In addition, rates of "intoxication" in European youth, including those younger than age 13, are higher than those in the United States for a majority of European countries.[28] For the United States, in 2007, one-third of 10th graders reported consuming alcohol in the past 30 days, a rate lower than in 15 European countries included in the 2007 ESPAD (including Germany, France, Denmark, Netherlands, Norway, Spain, Switzerland, UK, and others), with the exception of Iceland, where 31% reported drinking in the past month.[28] In addition, these two surveys asked 15–16-year-olds about being "intoxicated" in the past 30 days, and found 18% of U.S. students surveyed reporting being intoxicated, and 10 of 15 European countries surveyed reported rates equal to or higher, with Austria (31%), the UK (33%), and Denmark (49%) reporting the highest figures.[28]

The 2011 ESPAD survey included more than 100,000 students and reported data about alcohol consumption in 15- and to 16-year-old students from 36 European countries.[29,30] Overall, with the exception of Iceland, 57% of those aged 15–16 years from these countries drank alcohol in the past month, with rates similar among boys and girls, although boys reported drinking about one-third greater average amounts than girls. Although there were no clear geographic trends, substantial differences were seen between the countries surveyed. Higher past 30-day consumption rates were noted in students from Denmark and the Czech Republic (both 75%), and lowest in Albania (32%) and Iceland (17%). Furthermore, when students were asked about their "most recent drinking day," Danish students drank more than students from Albania, Moldova, Montenegro, and Romania.[29,30]

One particular measure from the 2011 ESPAD is similar to measures used in alcohol surveys in the United States. When assessing "heavy episodic drinking" in the ESPAD survey, students were asked about drinking five or more drinks on one occasion during the past month, the definition of "binge drinking" used in the United States. Overall, in European countries, the percentage of students reporting heavy episodic drinking increased in *girls* from 29% in 1995 to 41% in 2007, and was 38% in 2011, along with 43% of *boys* reporting this level of drinking in 2011.[29,30] Rates of reported heavy episodic drinking varied in different countries, from 13% of students in Iceland to 56% in Denmark. In Sweden, rates of heavy episodic drinking were higher in girls than boys, in contrast to 22 other counties, where rates in boys were higher. In addition, in all countries together, almost 60% had consumed alcohol by age 13 and 12% reported having been intoxicated by that age[29,30] (see **Figure 7–3**).

Policy Experiments: Lowering the Minimum Age—Evidence from New Zealand

In 1999 in New Zealand, following passage of the Sale of Liquor Amendment Act, the minimum legal purchasing age for alcohol was reduced from age 20 to age 18.[31] Researchers subsequently compared rates of alcohol-related crashes and hospitalizations in both 18–19 and 15–17-year-olds, compared to 20–24-year-olds, before and after the law went into effect. They found that both alcohol-related crash and hospitalization rates in young men aged 15–19 years and young women increased following the law change.[31] For example, following the law

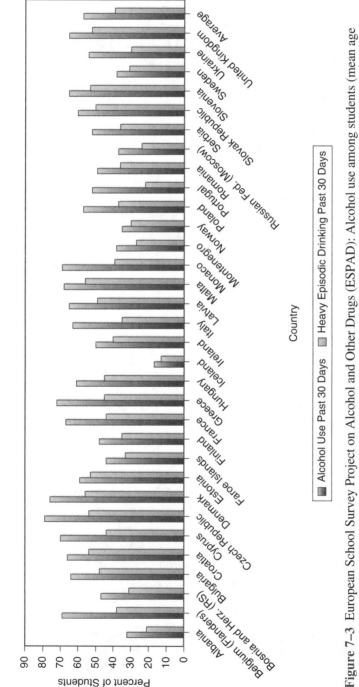

Figure 7-3 European School Survey Project on Alcohol and Other Drugs (ESPAD): Alcohol use among students (mean age 15.8 years), by country, 2011.

Data from the Summary 2011 ESPAD Report: Substance use Among Students in 36 European Countries.

change, in young men, the alcohol-related crash rate was 12% higher for 18–19-year-olds and 14% higher for 15–17-year-olds. In young women, the increases were even higher: in women aged 18–19 years, there was a 51% increase and in women aged 15–17 years, the rate was 24% higher.[31] Other investigators looked at patients coming to a city emergency department in New Zealand for the year following the law change.[32] They noted a 50% (statistically significant) increase in intoxicated 18–19-year-olds coming to the emergency room, an increasing (but not statistically significant) trend in the intoxicated 15–17-year-olds, and no change in 19-year-olds coming to the emergency department for intoxication in the same time period. Results were attributed to changes in the minimum purchasing age law (reduced from age 20 to age 18) one year prior.[32]

DISCUSSION QUESTIONS: TEMPLATE FOR DISCUSSION

1. Significance of this public health issue:
   a. Why is this health issue important?
   b. How many people does it impact?
   c. How serious is it?
   d. Is it preventable?
2. What is the evidence base for prevention?
3. What specific strategies should be used to achieve progress on this health issue?
   a. What evidence-based approach would you use?
   b. Where would you start if you are an individual citizen; public health professional; healthcare professional; community, state, or federal policymaker?
4. Specific questions for this topic:
   a. What is the evidence for the effectiveness of the current MLDA? For the proposed reduced MLDA?
   b. What specific, evidence-based policies, if systematically applied, could result in reductions in binge drinking and related health consequences?
   c. What barriers prevent such evidence-based policies from being implemented on a community, statewide, or national level?
5. What is the controversy?
   a. Define the controversy.
   b. Is controversy a good or bad thing? (Does it help or hinder progress?)

6. *Why* is this health issue controversial?
   a. What specific factors are involved?
   b. Do economics, government, scientific uncertainty, or politics play a role?
   c. What is the role of the media?
7. How would you respond to the controversy?

PERSPECTIVES TO CONSIDER

Why are some college presidents so enamored with the Amethyst Initiative? Why are some skeptical? Would such "state experiments" be dangerous? Many wish that a single policy change could be effective, but evidence shows that comprehensive, sustained, evidence-based approaches, including policy changes, have resulted in substantial reductions in harm from alcohol.[11,15,17,19]

How many colleges in the United States have actually implemented the policies shown to be effective? Few.[24] Relationships with local communities and businesses, required to implement successful policies such as reducing density of liquor outlets, are sometimes challenging. One of the lessons from the CAS that is infrequently cited and rarely heard in the public debate, is the percentage of college-age students already drinking to levels of clinical concern, i.e., alcohol dependence.[15]

College campuses are not islands, and the CAS showed that the drinking environment where colleges are located is an important factor.[15,17] This is not surprising, but makes preventing health consequences of excess alcohol consumption even more challenging in some geographic areas. Published studies also show that evidence-based strategies are under-utilized, especially those that connect college campuses with the local community.[15,17] For alcohol prevention policy, strategies such as raising alcohol prices, and reducing the density of locations selling or serving alcohol are very effective, but hard to implement in practice. Based on what is effective in reducing binge drinking on college campuses, the fact that so few of these evidence-based strategies are widely implemented, represents missed opportunities for prevention. Even stronger relationships and partnerships are needed between college and university officials, public health agencies, healthcare organizations, social service agencies, and policy makers to put the evidence into practice to improve this area of public health.

FOR ADDITIONAL STUDY

This intriguing study evaluates how changes in alcohol consumption in an individual's social network influences alcohol consumption:[33]

Rosenquist JN, Murabito J, Fowler JH, Christakis NA. The spread of alcohol consumption behavior in a large social network. *Ann Intern Med.* 2010;152(7):426–433, W141.

REFERENCES

1. McCardell JM. Let them drink at 18, with a learner's permit. *The New York Times.* 2012. http://www.nytimes.com/roomfordebate/2012/05/28/do-we-need-to-redefine-adulthood/let-them-drink-at-18-with-a-learners-permit. Accessed October 28, 2013.
2. Amethyst Initiative: Rethink the Drinking Age. [website]. 2013. http://www.theamethystinitiative.org/. Accessed October 28, 2013.
3. Daniloff C. Drinking: 18 vs. 21. *BU Today.* 2010. http://www.bu.edu/today/2010/drinking-18-vs-21/. Accessed October 28, 2013.
4. Glassman T. Is the glass half empty, half full or dry? *J Global Drug Policy Pract* 2008;2(4):16–18.
5. Wechsler H, Nelson TF. Will increasing alcohol availability by lowering the minimum legal drinking age decrease drinking and related consequences among youths? *Am J Public Health.* 2010;100(6):986–992.
6. Ewers J. Bid by college presidents to lower the drinking age remains a long shot: Binge drinking may be worsening on campus, but the British experience is a cautionary tale. *U.S. News.* 2008. http://www.usnews.com/news/national/articles/2008/08/25/bid-by-college-presidents-to-lower-the-drinking-age-remains-a-long-shot. Accessed October 28, 2013.
7. Editorial Board. Binge drinking on campus. *The New York Times.* 2009. http://www.nytimes.com/2009/07/01/opinion/01wed3.html?_r=0. Accessed November 1, 2013.
8. Mokdad AH, Marks JS, Stroup DF, Gerberding JL. Actual causes of death in the United States, 2000. *JAMA.* 2004;291(10):1238–1245.
9. CDC. Fact sheets: Alcohol use and health. 2012. http://www.cdc.gov/alcohol/fact-sheets/alcohol-use.htm. Accessed October 28, 2013.
10. CDC. Binge drinking. *CDC Vital Signs.* 2010. http://www.cdc.gov/vitalsigns/pdf/2010-10-vitalsigns.pdf. Accessed October 28, 2013.
11. CDC. Binge drinking: Nationwide problem, local solutions. *CDC Vital Signs.* 2012. http://www.cdc.gov/vitalsigns/bingedrinking/. Accessed October 28, 2013.
12. USDHHS. Surgeon General's call to action to prevent and reduce underage drinking. 2007. http://www.ncbi.nlm.nih.gov/books/NBK44360/. Accessed October 28, 2013.
13. Bonnie RJ, O'Connell ME, Eds. Reducing underage drinking: A collective responsibility. National Academies Press. 2004. http://www.iom.edu/Reports/2003/Reducing-Underage-Drinking-A-Collective-Responsibility.aspx. Accessed November 1, 2013.
14. NIAAA. College drinking: Fact sheet. 2013. http://pubs.niaaa.nih.gov/publications/CollegeFactSheet/CollegeFactSheet.pdf. Accessed October 28, 2013.
15. Wechsler H, Nelson TF. What we have learned from the Harvard School Of Public Health College Alcohol Study: Focusing attention on college student alcohol consumption and the environmental conditions that promote it. *J Stud Alcohol Drugs.* 2008;69(4):481–490.

16. WHO. Global status report on alcohol and health. 2011. http://www.who.int/substance_abuse/publications/global_alcohol_report/msbgsruprofiles.pdf. Accessed November 1, 2013.

17. Nelson TF, Naimi TS, Brewer RD, Wechsler H. The state sets the rate: The relationship among state-specific college binge drinking, state binge drinking rates, and selected state alcohol control policies. *Am J Public Health.* 2005;95(3):441–446.

18. The Guide to Community Preventive Services. [website]. http://www.thecommunityguide.org/index.html. Accessed November 1, 2013.

19. The Community Guide: Preventing excessive alcohol consumption. http://www.thecommunityguide.org/alcohol/index.html. Accessed November 1, 2013.

20. The Community Guide: Motor vehicle-related injury prevention: Reducing alcohol-impaired driving. http://www.thecommunityguide.org/mvoi/AID/index.html. Accessed November 1, 2013.

21. The Community Guide: Reducing alcohol-impaired driving: Maintaining current minimum legal drinking age (MLDA) laws. http://www.thecommunityguide.org/mvoi/AID/mlda-laws.html. Accessed November 1, 2013.

22. Paschall MJ, Antin T, Ringwalt CL, Saltz RF. Effects of AlcoholEdu for college on alcohol-related problems among freshmen: A randomized multicampus trial. *J Stud Alcohol Drugs.* 2011;72(4):642–650.

23. Paschall MJ, Antin T, Ringwalt CL, Saltz RF. Evaluation of an Internet-based alcohol misuse prevention course for college freshmen: Findings of a randomized multi-campus trial. *Am J Prev Med.* 2011;41(3):300–308.

24. Nelson TF, Toomey TL, Lenk KM, Erickson DJ, Winters KC. Implementation of NIAAA College Drinking Task Force recommendations: How are colleges doing 6 years later? *Alcohol Clin Exp Res.* 2010;34(10):1687–1693.

25. Hingson RW. The legal drinking age and underage drinking in the United States. *Arch Pediatr Adolesc Med.* 2009;163(7):598–600.

26. Wagenaar AC, Toomey TL. Effects of minimum drinking age laws: Review and analyses of the literature from 1960 to 2000. *J Stud Alcohol Suppl.* 2002(14):206–225.

27. Bloomfield K, Stockwell T, Gmel G, Rehn N. International comparisons of alcohol consumption. *Alcohol Res Health.* 2003;27(1):95–109.

28. Friese B, Grube JW. Youth drinking rates and problems: A comparison of European countries and the United States. 2007. http://resources.prev.org/documents/ESPAD.pdf. Accessed October 28, 2013.

29. The 2011 European School Survey Project on Alcohol and Other Drugs (ESPAD) Report. 2012. http://www.espad.org/Uploads/ESPAD_reports/2011/The_2011_ESPAD_Report_SUMMARY.pdf. Accessed October 28, 2013.

30. European Monitoring Centre for Drugs and Drug Addiction. Summary 2011 ESPAD report: Substance use among students in 36 European countries. 2012. http://www.espad.org/Uploads/ESPAD_reports/2011/Extended_EMCDDA_2011_ESPAD_Summary_EN.pdf. Accessed October 28, 2013.

31. Kypri K, Voas RB, Langley JD, et al. Minimum purchasing age for alcohol and traffic crash injuries among 15- to 19-year-olds in New Zealand. *Am J Public Health.* 2006; 96(1):126–131.

32. Everitt R, Jones P. Changing the minimum legal drinking age—its effect on a central city emergency department. *NZMJ.* 2002;115(1146):9–11.

33. Rosenquist JN, Murabito J, Fowler JH, Christakis NA. The spread of alcohol consumption behavior in a large social network. *Ann Intern Med.* 2010;152(7):426–433, W141.

CHAPTER 8

Health Reform: Controlling Costs

LEARNING OBJECTIVES

- Identify contributors to healthcare spending in the United States.
- Describe system barriers to controlling costs, while improving access and quality of health care.
- Discuss the public health impact of rising healthcare costs in the United States.
- Identify geographic differences in healthcare spending and contributing factors.
- Identify evidence-based strategies to improve the efficiency and effectiveness of the healthcare delivery system in the United States.
- Propose effective strategies to control healthcare costs that involve health professionals and consumers.

THE CONTROVERSY

On March 23, 2010, President Obama signed the Patient Protection and Affordable Care Act (ACA), an expansive law designed to expand access to health insurance coverage, control costs, improve quality, and promote access to primary and preventative care.[1] The law itself passed amid controversy, partisan politics, and compromise, for example, allowing coverage only of U.S. citizens and legal residents, and beginning Consumer Operated and Oriented Plans (CO-OP) in lieu of additional government programs.[2] The bill added a 10% tax on indoor tanning services as part of the comprehensive financing strategy, inserted at the last minute in exchange for removing a 5% tax on elective cosmetic surgery, called the "Botax."[3] Since its passage, the ACA has remained controversial, with 53% of 1,506 *USA Today* and Pew poll respondents disapproving of the law.[4] In April 2014, the Kaiser Family Foundation (KFF) noted that even though 8 million people signed up for health insurance through the new "exchanges," their Tracking Poll still found 46% of respondents had an "unfavorable view" of the law, and 57% of respondents felt the ACA was not working as originally intended.[5] Just 3 months later, KFF's poll reported more than half of the respondents (53%) still had a negative opinion of the ACA.[5]

Healthcare costs are an area of intense concern. The 2000 World Health Report ranked the United States health care system overall as 37th in the world.[6] In 2006, the U.S. ranked number 1 in per capita healthcare spending, but far lower on measures of population health status: 39th in infant mortality, 42nd and 43rd for adult male and female mortality, and 36th in life expectancy.[6] These authors and many others continue to raise the same question: "Why do we spend so much to get so little?"[6] After achieving several years of lower growth in healthcare expenditures (attributed in part to the poor economy and increased co-pays and deductibles, which serve as barriers to health care), the picture in 2013, following rising healthcare enrollment from the ACA, was quite different. One healthcare company reported increased prescription medication use, visits to doctors' offices, and hospital use, and data from government sources reported the highest growth rate since 2004.[7]

A 2013 *New York Times* series, "The $2.7 Trillion Medical Bill," lamented the role of colonoscopies, a recommended colon cancer screening test for healthy individuals, in our total annual U.S. healthcare expenditures.[8] The average U.S. price for colonoscopy is more than $1,000 in the United States, with figures as high as $6,385 reported in Long Island, NY and $7,563 in Keene, NH, compared to $655 for the same test in Switzerland.[8] When comparing the United States to Canada, Spain, or the Netherlands, similar price disparities are found for coronary angiograms, hip replacements, and MRI scans respectively.[8]

And how might patients know healthcare prices in advance? With great difficulty, as most hospitals (in one study in Philadelphia, PA) were able to answer questions about the price of parking but not about common medical procedures.[9,10] In addition, income of medical specialists (such as dermatologists), who may order additional tests or perform procedures, far exceeds that of medical generalists providing primary care.[11] One cancer epidemiologist wonders, "Is there a true epidemic or is there an epidemic of biopsies and treatments that are not needed?"[11] Another health economics professor, when analyzing medical tests, treatments, and reimbursements in the United States, simply quipped, "Each patient is like an ATM machine."[11]

BACKGROUND AND SCOPE OF THE PUBLIC HEALTH AND HEALTH POLICY ISSUE

What Contributes to Rising Healthcare Costs?

There is no disagreement about the enormity of U.S. healthcare spending. Many authors agree that the United States, compared to other countries, spends a large absolute amount, estimated in recent years, at $2.6 trillion, which translates to about 18% of the gross domestic product (GDP).[12,13] This figure increased further to $2.8 trillion in 2012, with average healthcare spending reaching $8,915 for each person in the United States, according to data from the U.S. Centers for Medicare and Medicaid Services (CMS).[14] CMS currently projects total U.S. health expenditures to exceed $5.1 trillion in 2023[15] (see **Figure 8–1**).

Kaiser Health News and the PBS NewsHour reported on seven factors contributing to trends in current healthcare spending, termed the "seven drivers of U.S. healthcare costs."[12] First, healthcare providers and hospitals are paid for individual services (called "fee-for-service" payment), creating incentives that may result in more, not less, health care.[12] Aging of the population and increasing obesity rates contribute to more chronic conditions, such as diabetes, which ultimately require more health care. Chronic

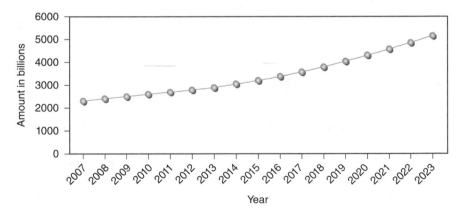

Figure 8–1 Total projected National Health Expenditures, United States.

Data from Centers for Medicare and Medicaid Services. National Health Expenditure Data. NHE Projections 2013–2023; Table 1, National Health Expenditures and Selected Economic Indicators, Levels and Annual Percent Change: Calendar Years 2007–2013. Available at http://www.cms.gov/Research-Statistics-Data-and-Systems/Statistics-Trends-and-Reports/NationalHealthExpendData/NationalHealthAccountsProjected.html

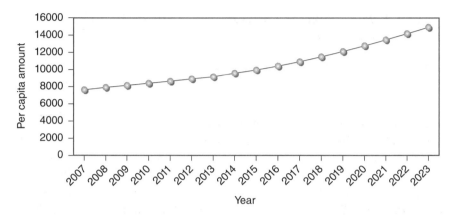

Figure 8–2 Projected per capita National Health Expenditures, United States.

Data from Centers for Medicare and Medicaid Services. National Health Expenditure Data. NHE Projections 2013–2023; Table 1, National Health Expenditures and Selected Economic Indicators, Levels and Annual Percent Change: Calendar Years 2007–2013. Available at http://www.cms.gov/Research-Statistics-Data-and-Systems/Statistics-Trends-and-Reports/NationalHealthExpendData/NationalHealthAccountsProjected.html

conditions are known contributors to healthcare spending: one report from 2010 estimates that 84% of all healthcare spending in the United States is related to health care for people with chronic conditions, and for Medicare spending, this figure is even higher, an estimated 99%.[12] CMS projects continued health expenditure increases, reaching nearly $15,000 per capita in 2023[15] (see **Figure 8–2**).

Another factor is the availability and demand for new medical technology, treatments, and pharmaceuticals (medications), that may or may not result in better outcomes for patients.[12] Other cited factors include a lack of transparency in healthcare costs, which are not readily available or obvious to consumers, as many people have health insurance coverage through their workplace.[12] Scientific evidence (evidence-based medicine) is lacking in some areas of health care, and may result in variation in the amount of care provided in different geographic locations. In addition, expanding hospital and health provider networks may either decrease or increase prices; fear of malpractice as well as ratios of primary vs. specialty healthcare professionals may also influence healthcare spending.[12]

The Robert Wood Johnson Foundation's Synthesis Project reports that provision of hospital care and health professional services together contributed to 52% of healthcare spending in 2006, and estimate that medical technology is responsible for 50–66% of increases in healthcare spending in recent years.[16] Factors such as inefficiency in healthcare delivery, worsening health status of the population, and lack of competition, also contribute to rising health-related spending.[16] Others report similar findings, especially the huge contribution of medical technology to increased spending, high administrative costs, and the role of health disparities in racial and ethnic minorities in driving additional healthcare spending.[17] The role of chronic conditions (many associated with preventable risk factors) is paramount: 20% of U.S. healthcare spending is from 1% of patients—patients with three or more chronic conditions.[17]

According to the KFF, healthcare spending in 2010 included an average of $8,402 spent per person in the United States.[18] Since 1970, health care's contribution to the Gross Domestic Product (GDP) has increased from 7.2% to nearly 18% in 2010, although there has been a slowing in the *rate* of increase since 2002.[18] As of 2012, total U.S. healthcare spending reached $2.8 trillion.[14] KFF estimates that 5% of people account for one-half of all healthcare spending.[18] Comparisons between the United States and peer countries shows U.S. per capita healthcare spending is more than double the amount of many comparison countries[19] (see **Figure 8–3**).

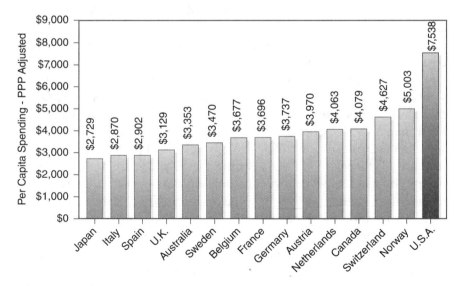

Figure 8–3 Total health expenditure per capita, U.S. and selected countries, 2008.

Reproduced from Kaiser Family Foundation: Snapshots: Health Care Spending in the United States & Selected OECD Countries. Available at http://kff.org/health-costs/issue-brief/snapshots-health-care-spending-in-the-united-states-selected-oecd-countries/

What types of services contribute to healthcare spending? About half of healthcare spending is for hospital care and clinical care provided by physicians.[18] Prescription medications comprise 10% of healthcare spending, and this has increased in the last decade.[18] Other contributing factors include the aging of the population, increases in (often preventable) chronic diseases (among people of all ages) such as health conditions related to obesity.[18]

Declines in the proportion of health care paid for by individuals (as opposed to insurance, whether public or private) helps people utilize more health care; facilitating access also increases population healthcare spending.[18,20] Since 1980, Medicare, Medicaid, and private insurance spending have all increased, while personal health care (out-of-pocket) spending has decreased by 50%.[20] However, in 2011 and 2012, out-of-pocket consumer spending increased between 3% and 4%, as ACA changes took place, resulting in some increases in cost-sharing with enrollment in some types of health plans.[14] Experts estimate that at least 20% of healthcare spending can be attributed to a combination of unnecessary or redundant care, fraud, and lack of coordinated and efficient delivery systems.[18] However, some authors argue that since 2000, the increase in prices of such services as pharmaceuticals and hospital care, rather than population demographics, are the most important factors in increased health spending.[20]

Perhaps even more controversial is the discussion about healthcare costs (and Medicare spending) during the end of life, sometimes called "the third rail" of U.S. healthcare policy.[21] The Dartmouth Atlas of Health Care reports that among the Medicare population, 90% of deaths are due to nine chronic conditions, for example such diseases as diabetes; dementia; heart, lung or kidney disease; or cancer.[22] Nearly one-third of Medicare spending (32%) can be attributed to physician and hospital-related costs for care of chronic conditions during the last 2 years of life.[22] Many patients may not, however, want the intensity of hospital-based care they receive near the end of life; the type and intensity of care they receive varies by location and depends on the usual type of care provided in their own geographic area.[22]

A comparison of care provided to Medicare patients in 2003 and 2007 concluded that, despite improvements, patients may still not be receiving the level of care they want. In 2007, patients spent fewer days in the hospital at the end of their lives (but more time in the intensive care unit [ICU]), were less likely to die in the hospital, and more likely to receive hospice care.[23] However, rather than the level of care being determined by a patient's wishes, it was related to the specific geographic region where the care was delivered. Whether or not patients died in the hospital varied fourfold, depending on where they lived and received health care.[23]

Specifically, for patients with advanced cancer who may prefer supportive, nonhospital care, the intensity of their care near the end of life depended on which medical center provided their health care, and varied tremendously. For example, in 2010, an advanced cancer patient's chance of dying in the hospital varied from 50% to 13%, depending which medical center (including cancer specialty hospitals) provided their care.[24] Whether or not patients were admitted to ICUs or received hospice care (sometimes in the last 3 days of life) also varied dramatically by geographic location. The authors highlight the importance of and gaps in communication between patients and healthcare professionals for patients with advanced cancer, and the need for earlier end-of-life conversations with a trusted physician, to ensure patients' wishes for care are followed.[24] However, these conversations are also controversial. Discussions about "death panels" during the debate over components of the ACA resulted in a huge public outcry and resulted in deleting language about end-of-life discussions.[25]

What Is the Cost Shift?

Experts disagree about the major contributing factors to healthcare cost shifting. For example, some argue that hospitals, in setting their prices, consider both the volume of a particular service and the mix of private and public (government) sources of payment for that particular service, as public payments are often lower for healthcare services.[26] On one side of the argument, insurance companies (private payers) and others in the healthcare industry argue that such practices "shift costs" of health care to private payers.[26] On the other side of this argument are health economists, who instead believe that hospitals decrease delivery of "unprofitable services" and aggressively manage their costs as coping strategies against low government reimbursement. Economists argue that current and expanding "market power" of hospitals and lack of competition are primary drivers of cost shifting.[26] Although, the question remains as to the major factor(s) in healthcare cost shifting, this debate will be increasingly relevant as provisions of the ACA and such system-wide changes, such as the creation of Accountable Care Organizations become more widespread.

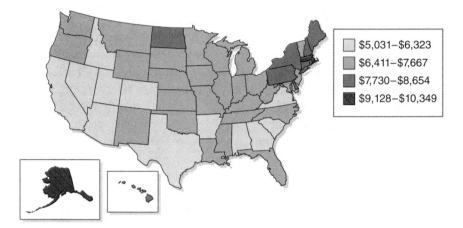

☐	$5,031–$6,323
◻	$6,411–$7,667
◼	$7,730–$8,654
◼	$9,128–$10,349

Figure 8–4 Healthcare expenditures per capita by state of residence, 2009.

Reproduced from Kaiser Family Foundation: Snapshots: Health Care Spending in the United States & Selected OECD Countries. Available at http://kff.org/other/state-indicator/health-spending-per-capita/#map

Geographic Variation: What We Have Learned from the Dartmouth Atlas and Others

Variation in healthcare expenditures in the United States by state and region is well documented[27] (see **Figure 8–4**). The Dartmouth Atlas, using Medicare data, has published geographic variations in health care across the United States for more than 20 years.[22] One of the earliest examples and one highlighted on their interactive atlas studied rates of tonsillectomies per 1,000 children, finding huge variations, even within northern New England. Tonsillectomy rates in Burlington, VT were 2.9 per 1,000 children, whereas rates in Berlin, NH were 10.4, and 4.0 in Portland, ME.[22] These data raised important questions related to delivery and costs of health care. For example, do these difference reflect real differences in children's health or are they more likely due to differences in medical opinion or lack of consensus on what works best? The Dartmouth Atlas allows geographic comparisons among such topics as surgical procedures, end-of-life care, prescription medication use, children's health care, hospitalizations, and distribution of hospitals and physicians, all to highlight geographic variation, provide data, and raise questions related to healthcare access, spending, quality, and patient outcomes.[22]

In 2014, the Center for Medicare and Medicaid Services (CMS) released extensive data to the public, in the form of a public data set, containing information about healthcare services delivered by physicians and other healthcare professionals to Medicare patients across the United States.[28] Reaction to this data, described as the largest public release of such data in 35 years, included a storm of national media reports about physicians in parts of the United States who receive the highest Medicare payments.[29] Other reports highlighted even higher salaries of healthcare administrators, whether healthcare or insurance executives, and emphasized as much as 20–30% of U.S. healthcare spending is tied to administrative costs.[30] CMS has also released Medicare data and a dashboard to help researchers examine geographic differences in Medicare spending in patients with multiple chronic conditions and emphasizes the burden of chronic conditions in different geographic areas.[31] The Commonwealth Fund describes regional variations across the United State in per capita Medicare spending, such as differences seen in two different Florida counties. In Miami-Dade County, in 2012, $14,905 was spent on each Medicare patient, compared to $7,678 in Monroe County.[32] In contrast, for the same time period, Medicare spending was $6,402 for each patient in Oregon.[32] In addition, Florida and New Jersey have the highest percentage of Medicare patients with six or more chronic conditions and Alaska and Wyoming have the fewest, factors related to overall healthcare spending.[32] Using data from all of these sources helps to identify differences in population health status, healthcare access, and practice patterns, and is important to both researchers and policymakers, especially as system-wide changes from the ACA are implemented.

Healthcare Prices: Why the Secret?

It may not be easy for consumers to determine the price of healthcare services in advance. A research study was performed to determine the availability of prices for a common orthopedic procedure, total hip replacement, in hospitals (two per state) across the United States, as well as 20 selected "top-rated" orthopedic hospitals.[33] The researchers found that 45% of the top-rated hospitals and only 10% of the others could give a price for hospital and physician services needed to perform a hip replacement, and when prices were available, they ranged from $11,100 to $125,798 for the same procedure.[33] In another study in Philadelphia, PA, researchers tried to find out the price of an electrocardiogram in 20 hospitals. Only 3 of 20 hospitals could provide the price, but 19 of 20 could recall the price for hospital parking.[9,10]

A *New York Times* author tried to trace the price and actual costs of IV saline administered to patients during a 2012 food poisoning outbreak in

New York. She found that although the cost of a bag of saline was between $.44 and $1.00, charges for "IV therapy" were nearly 1,000 times higher.[34] Lamenting the lack of pricing transparency to patients, the author opined that "the real cost of a bag of normal saline, like the true cost of medical supplies from gauze to heart implants, disappears into an opaque realm of byzantine contracts, confidential rebates, and fees . . ."[34] There is scant information or scientific research available about how prices of hospital services and goods are actually set.[35] One professor asks, "How do hospitals set prices? They set prices to maximize revenue, and they raise prices as much as they can—all the research supports that."[35] The "charge master" is an extensive list of prices of goods and services used by hospitals to determine charges to patients. Although in most U.S. locations, these prices are not publically available, California requires their reporting to government health regulators.[35]

More information is becoming available to patients and consumers, for example, the Kaiser Family Foundation publishes a "subsidy calculator" to help consumers who are buying insurance through health insurance exchanges as a result of the ACA.[36] And CMS provides a website, called Hospital Compare that allows consumers to compare hospitals on a variety of measures, such as types of services provided, patient satisfaction, complications and deaths, as well as quality measures for "timely and effective care" for a range of medical conditions and healthcare services.[37]

EVIDENCE BASE FOR PREVENTION AND PRACTICE

Two fundamental financial issues plague the U.S. healthcare system. First, when compared to peer countries, the amount spent for each person is high in the United States.[13,18] Second, compared to U.S. economic indicators, healthcare spending has increased in the United States over many years, not just in the recent past.[18] As a result of the ACA, many changes are currently occurring in healthcare settings, such as consolidation (mergers) among various components of the healthcare delivery system—hospitals, medical practices, pharmacies, and insurance companies—with potential for both risks and benefits.[20] On one hand, there is a potential for efficiency and volume-related cost savings in healthcare delivery through these consolidations; on the other hand, there may be the potential for less competition in any geographic area, including less choice for patients and uncertain impact on costs.[20] Other recent changes include substantial investments in healthcare information technology, and the changing role of patients as consumers, whether in choosing healthcare coverage (such as through the newly created health exchanges), comparing hospitals through increasingly available public data, or directly seeking healthcare information online.[20]

Some authors argue that these rapid and cumulative changes create confusion among patient, physician, and payer goals in our changing healthcare system.[20] One *New York Times* article highlights the forecast that 20% of U.S. hospitals may attempt mergers with other hospitals in the next 5 years in reaction to the ACA.[38] From 2009 to 2012, the number of mergers in U.S. hospitals has more than doubled.[38] Current policy changes promoting hospital and health system accountability for patients' health, create incentives to build better and more efficient systems to keep patients' care in less-costly outpatient settings and manage their overall health.[38] However, some believe that larger organizations, through improved negotiating strength, may actually drive prices higher. The Federal Trade Commission has reviewed and occasionally stopped some mergers from taking larger and larger shares of local or regional healthcare markets.[35,38] Some predict increased overall healthcare costs from the U.S. merger trend. The organization Catalyst for Payment Reform claims that private insurance company payments to hospitals may increase 3% as a result of mergers.[39] Another report from Nevada used the example of the fourfold increase in the price of a commonly used heart test, the echocardiogram, after a medical practice became part of a larger hospital network.[17]

Furthermore, in addition to the population-level variation in healthcare delivery and costs demonstrated by the Dartmouth Atlas,[22] stories abound of differences in healthcare costs and spending in different geographic areas of the United States.[40] There are also compelling local initiatives, such as those in Camden, NJ to identify patients with the highest costs and most extensive needs (called "hot spotters") and develop creative approaches to meet both medical and social needs.[41] Some authors note opportunities to improve "population health" as states experiment with different care models as a result of the ACA, linking health care to the health of the community.[42] However, challenges remain in systematically tailoring such approaches to diverse populations, healthcare settings, and geographic areas.

Federal and State-Based Innovations

Consumers Union and the Robert Wood Johnson Foundation have published summaries of state-based innovations, all with a goal of improving healthcare quality and reducing costs.[43] Examples from seven states: Colorado, Maryland, Minnesota, New York, Oregon, Rhode Island, and Vermont describe a variety of approaches used in these states, some already demonstrating substantial cost savings, while other innovations are still early in their implementation.[43] For example, Rhode Island uses insurance rate review as one cost containment strategy, as well as patient-centered medical homes and pay-for-performance.[43]

In 2008, Rhode Island initiated a patient-centered medical home pilot project that included five independent primary care medical practices.[44] One of the unique features of this pilot project was that Rhode Island's three largest insurance companies provided the funding. Researchers used insurance claims data to evaluate such measures as hospital admissions, emergency department visits, and quality of care measures, comparing the time period before the project began and 2 years after. After only 2 years, emergency department visits for medical conditions that could have been safely treated in primary care settings significantly decreased in the primary care practices participating in the pilot project, from 6.9 visits for every 1,000 member-months to less than 1 visit per 1,000 member-months.[44] However, substantial changes were not seen in healthcare quality measures.[44]

Accountable Care Organizations (ACOs) are geographically located, large groups of hospitals, physicians, and other health professionals who provide care to an entire patient population of Medicare patients.[45] This new model was part of the ACA, which gave the CMS the ability to create and provide funding to these new models of care. The overall goal is to provide coordinated and high-quality health care to Medicare patients, through new payment incentives and different way of delivering health care, supporting team-based health care, standardized measurement of healthcare quality, and promoting use of compatible information systems (electronic health records).[45,46] If healthcare spending targets are met and quality measures achieved, the ACO will share in the cost savings, providing financial incentives to provide more efficient and high-quality care.[45,46] As of 2014, CMS has provided funding to an estimated 287 ACOs across the United States, and encouraged the creation of about 250 ACOs in the private sector.[46]

Oregon is using Medicaid Coordinated Care Organizations, which operate similarly to ACOs, following their receipt of a federal waiver in 2012.[47] Evaluation of this initiative is pending, but one challenge faced by Oregon is a documented increase in emergency department use, following an expansion of their Medicaid program (which provides health insurance coverage for adults with limited incomes). This increase in emergency department visits included medical conditions often treated in primary care offices.[47] Colorado, another state that uses a Medicaid Accountable Care Collaborative, had a different experience, seeing an estimated $2 to $3 million net saving in its first year.[43] Vermont's goal is to implement a single-payer strategy with enabling state legislation, but a required federal waiver has not yet been submitted. ACOs and patient-centered medical homes are other features of Vermont's reform approach.[43]

Maryland uses a rigorous system of reviewing and setting rates of hospital prices, with oversight from a legislatively created Health Services Cost Review Commission.[43,48] Prior to the current system, Maryland's hospital costs exceeded the national average by 25% in 1976, but following years of implementing their regulatory seven-commissioner review system (including a Medicare waiver that provides them higher Medicare payment rates and helps pay for charity care), Maryland's overall costs were 2% lower than the national average in 2007.[48]

In addition, Western Maryland Health System, near the Appalachians, has an overall budget set by the commission and takes on responsibility for health care in the surrounding community. They have experienced a 15% decline in hospital admissions and a healthier financial profile, after emphasizing primary care and new approaches to treating chronically ill patients and health conditions common in their community.[49] However, critics note that it may not be that simple or effective to try to extend this type of system across the nation.[49] Some authors describe unique challenges faced by academic medical centers (AMCs).[50] AMCs, in addition to providing specialized clinical care ("tertiary" care), are often affiliated with undergraduate and post-graduate educational programs for physicians, nurses, and other health professionals, have a research mission and also provide health care to local community populations.[50]

But are these new models really promoting system change? One study investigated whether a commercial ACO in Massachusetts (called the Alternative Quality Contract or AQC) reduced healthcare spending, improved quality, and compared these outcomes to any changes seen in other Medicare patients in Massachusetts who were not formally part of this ACO.[51] The investigators evaluated healthcare spending for each Medicare patient as well as measures of healthcare quality, such as being readmitted to a hospital within 30 days after being discharged. They found that healthcare spending decreased in ACQ patients; however, only some quality measures were improved.[51] The investigators also noted that improvements were seen outside of the formal network, implying such ACO programs may already be promoting systematic changes in the way health care is delivered to some patient populations.[51]

Choosing Wisely

Choosing Wisely, an initiative of the American Board of Internal Medicine (ABIM), began in 2012 and now involves more than 60 medical specialty societies.[52] The goal of this initiative is to improve healthcare quality by promoting dialog between patients and physicians about medical care characterized by four principles: evidence-based, really needed, not redundant, and care that does not cause harm to the patient.[52] The Congressional Budget Office estimates nearly one-third of U.S. health care delivered is unnecessary, a finding confirmed by physicians, with nearly half of primary care physicians, in one survey, in agreement.[53] In 2011, the American College of Physicians (ACP), the second-largest physician organization in the United States, published clinical guidelines, and the rationale for *high-value, cost-conscious health care*.[54] With escalating healthcare costs, the ACP felt three steps were needed to determine if health care was "high value." These included whether health care actually provided benefits to patients, whether there was potential for harm, and what short-term and long-term costs resulted from certain types of care.[54]

The ACP developed a list of "Five Things Physicians and Patients Should Question," to focus patient care on diagnostic tests and treatments that are backed by scientific evidence (called "evidence-based" care).[55] Some of the five items include questioning the use of tests such as electrocardiograms in patients who are at "low risk" for coronary heart disease; chest x-rays in patients prior to surgery unless there is a specific indication; or x-ray, CT, or other imaging scans in patients with low back pain.[55] Other medical specialty societies have created lists specific to their specialty.[55]

A list of 45 diagnostic tests and medical treatments that may be "overused" were also compiled by nine medical specialty societies.[56] In addition to eliminating the use of unnecessary care or care that is not "evidence-based," the Choosing Wisely project aims to facilitate better discussions and decision making between physicians and patients, with both physicians and patients asking these questions.[56] In addition, to better communicate with patients and the general public, the ABIM worked closely with *Consumer Reports*, in order to make this information, based on scientific research, widely available through print and video formats.[53] Information for the public is available in areas such as allergies, cancer, heart disease, chronic pain, women's health, and which diagnostic tests are recommended for patients prior to surgery.[53]

In terms of overall policy changes, the Commonwealth Fund published a report with recommendations for a healthcare system that works better and contains costs.[57] They recommend providing incentives through payment structures to healthcare providers, ways to encourage more active engagement by patients and consumers, high-quality information about quality and costs, reducing administrative costs, and setting healthcare spending targets.[57] Such reforms, Commonwealth Fund authors write, would improve care coordination, strengthen primary care, address current malpractice policy, and make healthcare administration simpler.[57]

DISCUSSION QUESTIONS: TEMPLATE FOR DISCUSSION

1. Significance of this public health issue:
   a. Why is this health issue important?
   b. How many people does it impact?
   c. How serious is it?
   d. Is it preventable?
2. What is the evidence base for prevention?
3. What specific strategies should be used to achieve progress on this health issue?
   a. What evidence-based approach would you use?
   b. Where would you start if you are an individual citizen; public health professional; healthcare professional; community, state, or federal policymaker?
4. Specific questions for this topic:
   a. What are the most important contributing factors to rising healthcare spending?
   b. What is the role of transparency in healthcare prices, quality, and outcomes, for both patients and healthcare professionals?
   c. Do you think changes related to the ACA will result in decreased or increased healthcare spending?
5. What is the controversy?
   a. Define the controversy.
   b. Is controversy a good or bad thing? (Does it help or hinder progress?)
6. *Why* is this health issue controversial?
   a. What specific factors are involved?
   b. Do economics, government, scientific uncertainty, or politics play a role?
   c. What is the role of the media?
7. How would you respond to the controversy?

PERSPECTIVES TO CONSIDER

There is consensus that U.S. healthcare spending is too high and our population health status measures lag way behind other comparable countries.[13] Geographic variation in healthcare delivery and spending is well documented.[22] The passage of the ACA provides opportunities for innovative models of care for entire populations, including the use of ACOs in many locations.[45] Using states as laboratories for new ways to deliver health care emphasizing primary care, patient-centered medical homes, and team-based health care hold promise, but evaluations of their effectiveness in reducing costs and improving quality are still in their early stages.[43] Controversy surrounds increases in health system mergers (what some are calling "supersizing hospitals"),[38] causing some to question whether there will be more benefits or unintended consequences, such as increased costs.[20,39]

Efforts to provide evidence-based care, prevent unnecessary care, and improve decision making between patients and health professionals, as in the Choosing Wisely initiative, are becoming more widely adopted.[55] Better information for patients, along with increased transparency of costs, prices, and outcomes, will also help consumers make choices. Some of the biggest questions revolve around whether current healthcare experiments will reduce costs *and* improve quality, and whether models that work in one location can be used elsewhere.

Meanwhile, some authors highlight the importance of addressing social as well as medical needs and linking healthcare systems to community resources using local innovations that may hold promise for broader geographic areas.[41] Given the prominent role of chronic conditions in healthcare spending, [12] and evidence that risk factors contributing to these conditions are amenable to both individual and population-level prevention,[58] these are logical priorities. Public health has a critical role to play in the changing healthcare delivery system and reducing the burden of preventable illness in the population by linking population-based prevention efforts to clinical care.

FOR ADDITIONAL STUDY

Henry J. Kaiser Foundation. Health Care Costs: A Primer. 2012. http://kff.org/health-costs/report/health-care-costs-a-primer/.

Gawande A. The Cost Conundrum. *The New Yorker.* 2009. http://www.newyorker.com/reporting/2009/06/01/090601fa_fact_gawande?currentPage=all.

Gawande A. The Hot Spotters. *The New Yorker.* 2011. http://www.newyorker.com/reporting/2011/01/24/110124fa_fact_gawande.

REFERENCES

1. HealthCare.gov. [website]. 2014. https://www.healthcare.gov/get-started/. Accessed May 24, 2014.
2. KFF. Summary of the Affordable Care Act. 2013. http://kff.org/health-reform/fact-sheet/summary-of-new-health-reform-law/. Accessed May 24, 2014.
3. Adamy J. Senate bill removes 'botax,' adds tanning tax. *Wall Street Journal Online.* 2009. http://blogs.wsj.com/washwire/2009/12/19/senate-bill-removes-botax-adds-tanning-tax/tab/print/. Accessed May 24, 2014.
4. Page S. *USA Today*/Pew poll: Health care law faces difficult future. *USA Today.* 2013. http://www.usatoday.com/story/news/politics/2013/09/16/usa-today-pew-poll-health-care-law-opposition/2817169/. Accessed May 24, 2014.
5. KFF. Health Reform. 2014. http://kff.org/health-reform/. Accessed October 3, 2014.
6. Murray CJ, Frenk J. Ranking 37th—measuring the performance of the U.S. health care system. *N Engl J Med.* 2010;362(2):98–99.
7. Lowrey A. Health care spending's recent surge stirs unease. *The New York Times.* 2014. http://www.nytimes.com/2014/04/19/business/economy/health-care-spendings-recent-surge-stirs-unease.html. Accessed May 24, 2014.
8. Rosenthal E. The $2.7 trillion medical bill: Colonoscopies explain why U.S. leads the world in health expenditures. *The New York Times.* 2013. http://www.nytimes.com/2013/06/02/health/colonoscopies-explain-why-us-leads-the-world-in-health-expenditures.html?pagewanted=all. Accessed May 24, 2014.
9. Kliff S. Nearly all hospitals will give you the price of parking. Barely any will give you the price of health care. *The Washington Post Wonkblog.* 2013. http://www.washingtonpost.com/blogs/wonkblog/wp/2013/12/03/nearly-all-hospitals-will-give-you-the-price-of-parking-barely-any-will-give-you-the-price-of-care/. Accessed May 24, 2014.
10. Bernstein JR, Bernstein J. Availability of consumer prices from Philadelphia area hospitals for common services: Electrocardiograms vs parking. *JAMA Intern Med.* 2014;174(2):292–293.
11. Rosenthal E. Patients' costs skyrocket; Specialists' incomes soar. *The New York Times.* 2014. http://www.nytimes.com/2014/01/19/health/patients-costs-skyrocket-specialists-incomes-soar.html. Accessed May 24, 2014.
12. Appleby J, Kaiser Health News. Seven factors driving up your health care costs. *PBS NewsHour.* 2012. http://www.pbs.org/newshour/rundown/seven-factors-driving-your-health-care-costs/. Accessed May 24, 2014.
13. *U.S. health in international perspective: Shorter lives, poorer health.* Washington, DC: The National Academies Press; 2013.
14. CMS. National health expenditures 2012 highlight. 2012. http://www.cms.gov/Research-Statistics-Data-and-Systems/Statistics-Trends-and-Reports/NationalHealthExpendData/downloads/highlights.pdf. Accessed June 4, 2014.
15. CMS. Centers for Medicare and Medicaid Services: Research, statistics, and data. 2014. http://www.cms.gov/Research-Statistics-Data-and-Systems/Statistics-Trends-and-Reports/NationalHealthExpendData/NationalHealthAccountsProjected.html. Accessed November 2, 2014.
16. Godell S, Ginsburg PB. The Synthesis Project: High and rising health care costs: demystifying U.S. health care spending. 2008. http://www.rwjf.org/en/research-publications/find-rwjf-research/2008/10/high-and-rising-health-care-costs.html. Accessed May 24, 2014.

17. Goodman L, Norbeck T. Who's to blame for our rising healthcare costs? *Forbes.com.* 2013. http://www.forbes.com/sites/realspin/2013/04/03/whos-to-blame-for-our-rising-healthcare-costs/. Accessed May 24, 2014.

18. KFF. Health care costs: A primer. 2012. http://kff.org/health-costs/report/health-care-costs-a-primer/. Accessed May 24, 2014.

19. KFF. Snapshots: Health care spending in the United States and selected OECD countries. 2011. http://kff.org/health-costs/issue-brief/snapshots-health-care-spending-in-the-united-states-selected-oecd-countries/. Accessed November 2, 2014.

20. Moses H 3rd, Matheson DH, Dorsey ER, George BP, Sadoff D, Yoshimura S. The anatomy of health care in the United States. *JAMA.* 2013;310(18):1947–1963.

21. Pasternak S. End-of-life care constitutes third rail of U.S. health care policy debate. *The Medicare Newsgroup.* 2013. http://www.medicarenewsgroup.com/context/understanding-medicare-blog/understanding-medicare-blog/2013/06/03/end-of-life-care-constitutes-third-rail-of-u.s.-health-care-policy-debate. Accessed June 4, 2014.

22. The Dartmouth Atlas of Health Care: Understanding of the efficiency and effectiveness of the health care system. 2014. http://www.dartmouthatlas.org/. Accessed June 4, 2014.

23. Goodman DC, Esty AR, Fisher ES, Chang CH. Trends and variation in end-of-life care for Medicare beneficiaries with severe chronic illness. 2011. http://www.rwjf.org/en/research-publications/find-rwjf-research/2011/04/trends-and-variation-in-end-of-life-care-for-medicare-beneficiar.html. Accessed June 4, 2014.

24. Goodman DC, Morden NE, Chang C, Fisher ES, Wennberg JE. Trends in cancer care near the end of life. *Dartmouth Atlas of Health Care Brief.* 2013. http://www.rwjf.org/content/dam/farm/reports/issue_briefs/2013/rwjf407663. Accessed June 4, 2014.

25. Rattner S. Beyond Obamacare. *The New York Times.* 2012. http://www.nytimes.com/2012/09/17/opinion/health-care-reform-beyond-obamacare.html. Accessed June 4, 2014.

26. Dowless RM. The health care cost-shifting debate: Could both sides be right? *J Health Care Fin.* 2007;34(1):64–71.

27. KFF. Health care expenditures per capita by state of residence. 2014. http://kff.org/other/state-indicator/health-spending-per-capita/#map. Accessed November 2, 2014.

28. CMS. Medicare provider utilization and payment data: Physician and other supplier. 2014; http://www.cms.gov/Research-Statistics-Data-and-Systems/Statistics-Trends-and-Reports/Medicare-Provider-Charge-Data/Physician-and-Other-Supplier.html. Accessed June 4, 2014.

29. CMS releases trove of Medicare physician billing data. *Kaiser Health News.* 2014. http://www.kaiserhealthnews.org/daily-reports/2014/april/09/medicare-billing-data.aspx. Accessed June 4, 2014.

30. Rosenthal E. Medicine's top earners are not the M.D.s. *The New York Times.* 2014. http://www.nytimes.com/2014/05/18/sunday-review/doctors-salaries-are-not-the-big-cost.html. Accessed June 4, 2014.

31. Chronic Conditions Overview. 2014. http://www.cms.gov/Research-Statistics-Data-and-Systems/Statistics-Trends-and-Reports/Chronic-Conditions/index.html. Accessed June 4, 2014.

32. Reichard J. Medicare releases trove of claims data showing regional variations. *Washington Health Policy Week in Review.* 2014. http://www.commonwealthfund.org/publications/newsletters/washington-health-policy-in-review/2014/jun/jun-9-2014/medicare-releases-trove-of-claims-data-showing-regional-variations. Accessed June 4, 2014.

33. Rosenthal JA, Lu X, Cram P. Availability of consumer prices from US hospitals for a common surgical procedure. *JAMA Intern Med.* 2013;173(6):427–432.

34. Bernstein N. How to charge $546 for six liters of saltwater. *The New York Times.* 2013. http://www.nytimes.com/2013/08/27/health/exploring-salines-secret-costs. html?emc=edit_hh_20130827&nl=health&nlid=67811076. Accessed May 24, 2014.

35. Rosenthal E. As hospital prices soar, a stitch tops $500. *The New York Times.* 2013. http://www.nytimes.com/2013/12/03/health/as-hospital-costs-soar-single-stitch-tops-500.html?_r=0. Accessed May 24, 2014.

36. KFF. Health Reform: Subsidy Calculator: Premium assistance for coverage in exchanges. 2014. http://kff.org/interactive/subsidy-calculator/. Accessed June 4, 2014.

37. CMS. Medicare.gov hospital compare. 2014. http://www.medicare.gov/hospitalcompare/search.html?AspxAutoDetectCookieSupport=1. Accessed June 4, 2014.

38. Creswell J, Abelson R. New laws and rising costs create a surge of supersizing hospitals. *The New York Times.* 2013. http://www.nytimes.com/2013/08/13/business/bigger-hospitals-may-lead-to-bigger-bills-for-patients.html?pagewanted=all. Accessed May 24, 2014.

39. Delbanco S. Medical mergers are driving up health costs. *Wall Street Journal Online.* 2014. http://online.wsj.com/articles/suzanne-f-delbanco-medical-mergers-are-driving-up-health-costs-1412119178. Accessed October 2, 2014.

40. Gawande A. The cost conundrum. *The New Yorker.* 2009. http://www.newyorker .com/ reporting/2009/06/01/090601fa_fact_gawande?currentPage=all. Accessed June 4, 2014.

41. Gawande A. The hot spotters. *The New Yorker.* 2011. http://www.newyorker.com/reporting/2011/01/24/110124fa_fact_gawande. Accessed May 24, 2014.

42. Auerbach J, Chang D, Hester JA, Magnan S. Opportunity knocks: Population health in state innovation models. 2013. http://www.iom.edu/~/media/Files/Perspectives-Files/2013/Discussion-Papers/BPH-OpportnuityKnocks.pdf. Accessed June 4, 2014.

43. Harbage Consulting for RWJF and Consumers Union. State-based approaches to health care value: Cost and quality. *Consumers Union.* 2013. http://consumersunion.org/healthcosts/StateApproaches_FINAL.pdf. Accessed May 24, 2014.

44. Rosenthal MB, Friedberg MW, Singer SJ, Eastman D, Li Z, Schneider EC. Effect of a multipayer patient-centered medical home on health care utilization and quality: The Rhode Island chronic care sustainability initiative pilot program. *JAMA Intern Med.* 2013;173(20):1907–1913.

45. CMS. Accountable care organizations (ACO). 2014. http://www.cms.gov/Medicare/Medicare-Fee-for-Service-Payment/ACO/. Accessed June 4, 2014.

46. AHRQ. The state of accountable care organizations. 2014. https://innovations.ahrq .gov/perspectives/state-accountable-care-organizations. Accessed October 2, 2014.

47. Taubman SL, Allen HL, Wright BJ, Baicker K, Finkelstein AN. Medicaid increases emergency-department use: Evidence from Oregon's health insurance experiment. *Science.* 2014;343(6168):263–268.

48. Zhang J. Maryland reins in hospital costs by setting rates: State commission aims to keep expenses lower, gain charity care in exchange for greater regulation. *Wall Street Journal Online.* 2009. http://online.wsj.com/news/articles/SB125288688445707403. Accessed May 24, 2014.

49. Porter E. Lessons in Maryland for costs at hospitals. *The New York Times.* 2013. http://www.nytimes.com/2013/08/28/business/economy/lessons-in-maryland-for-costs-at-hospitals.html. Accessed May 24, 2014.

50. Nabel EG, Ferris TG, Slavin PL. Balancing AMCs' missions and health care costs: Mission impossible? *N Engl J Med.* 2013;369(11):994–996.
51. McWilliams JM, Landon BE, Chernew ME. Changes in health care spending and quality for Medicare beneficiaries associated with a commercial ACO contract. *JAMA.* 2013;310(8):829–836.
52. Choosing Wisely: An initiative of the ABIM Foundation. 2014. http://www.choosingwisely.org/about-us/. Accessed June 4, 2014.
53. Choosing Wisely. [website]. 2013. http://consumerreports.org/cro/health/doctors-and-hospitals/choosing-wisely/index.htm. Accessed June 4, 2014.
54. Owens DK, Qaseem A, Chou R, Shekelle P, Clinical Guidelines Committee of the American College of Physicians. High-value, cost-conscious health care: Concepts for clinicians to evaluate the benefits, harms, and costs of medical interventions. *Ann Intern Med.* 2011;154(3):174–180.
55. ACP. Choosing Wisely: American College of Physicians: Five things physicians and patients should question. 2014. http://www.choosingwisely.org/doctor-patient-lists/american-college-of-physicians/. Accessed June 4, 2014.
56. Gever J. Doctors say 45 common tests 'overused'. *Medpagetoday.com.* 2012. http://www.medpagetoday.com/PublicHealthPolicy/GeneralProfessionalIssues/32028. Accessed June 4, 2014.
57. Commonwealth Fund. Confronting Costs: Stabilizing U.S. health spending while moving toward a high performance health care system. *Fund Reports.* 2013. Accessed June 4, 2014.
58. Mokdad AH, Marks JS, Stroup DF, Gerberding JL. Actual causes of death in the United States, 2000. *JAMA.* 2004;291(10):1238–1245.

CHAPTER 9

Health Reform: Improving Health

LEARNING OBJECTIVES

- Discuss the determinants of health. What role does health care play?
- Identify components of the ACA that contribute to improved individual and population health.
- Describe the relationship between clinical and community preventive services.
- Identify evidence-based strategies to improve health status during proposed changes in the healthcare delivery system in the United States.

THE CONTROVERSY

Who would have thought disease prevention was so controversial? During congressional debate and final passage of the Patient Protection and Affordable Care Act (ACA), signed into law on March 23, 2010,[1] there were myriad controversies, including new strategies to provide access to both clinical and community prevention. One section (Section 2713 of the Public Health Service Act, added by the ACA[2]) required health insurance plans to provide birth control coverage without cost sharing, sparking a huge public debate, and ultimately, a longer timeline for implementation.[3] The rule was issued in 2011, and exempted churches (religious employers) but not hospitals or educational institutions that were "affiliated" with churches.[3] However, the rule was further amended in February 2013, clarifying and broadening the definition for "religious employer exemption."[2] Despite these changes, one source noted the changes prompted more than 400,000 public comments, more than any previous government regulation,[4,5] and at least 60 legal filings.[5] Why the big fuss? One blogger, writing in the *California Healthline,* said this particular regulation hit a variety of "pressure points: politics, religion, sex, federal mandates, and federal entitlements."[5]

Also under attack is the Prevention and Public Health Fund, which supports population and community-based public health prevention programs. Initially funded at a level of $500 million in 2010, with proposed increases to $2 billion annually by fiscal year 2015,[6] it has been the target of ongoing scrutiny and cuts since ACA passage. Dubbed a "slush fund" by some critics because it lacked detailed funding priorities,[7] and viewed by others as a back-door strategy to fund health exchanges, the House Appropriations bill in January 2014 proposed cuts of $1 billion from this fund.[7] Supported by the administration as a way to enhance funding for public health infrastructure, prevention research, and prevention funding for such public health issues as HIV, obesity, tobacco, and substance abuse,[6] critics claim it is "vaguely defined" and pays for "calming techniques" offered by massage therapists, as well as Zumba and kickboxing.[8]

Why is this fund so controversial? In part because of its size, a perception that funded activities may bypass the usual appropriations process, and concerns that grant funds are inappropriately used for "lobbying" for such policy initiatives as higher tobacco taxes, price increases on sugar-sweetened beverages, or outdoor smoking bans.[8] Furthermore, in response to the administration's using $453.8 million from this fund to jump-start health insurance exchanges, one senator said, "To slash money from this fund . . . is to cannibalize the Affordable Care Act in ways that will cost both money and lives."[8] Others write that such prevention activities are "politically charged" and it remains to be seen whether or not the United States will effectively transition from a "sick care" to a "healthcare" system.[9]

BACKGROUND AND SCOPE OF THE PUBLIC HEALTH AND HEALTH POLICY ISSUE

The United States, when measured against other peer countries, spends more on health care but fares worse in population health status measures and life expectancy.[10,11] Why is this? In part, because many factors that determine health, such as population-level changes to promote health habits and behaviors, social and economic factors, and the environment (especially the built environment), may lie largely outside the realm of health professionals.[10,12] In addition, many people are still without adequate and high-quality health care.[10] Medical care's role in improving health status and reducing premature death has been estimated at about 10%.[10,13,14] Other factors, habits, and behaviors, such as tobacco use, alcohol use, poor nutrition, and sedentary behavior, contribute an estimated 40% to premature deaths in the United States, with genetics (30%) and social factors (15%) critical in determining our poorer collective health.[10]

In addition, there is a huge "spending mismatch"[15] between what factors contribute to population health status and how we allocate health spending resources: in the estimated $2.6 trillion spent in the United States on health, 90% was for medical services, 9% for programs or activities related to healthy behaviors, and 1% on "other."[15] This spending proportion stands in contrast to the estimated 6% contribution of access to health care and a 37% contribution of healthy behaviors to determining health (along with 20% from genetics, 22% from our socioeconomic and physical environment, and 15% from the interaction of these factors).[15] In addition, performance of the U.S. healthcare system ranks last in overall measures of health insurance coverage, healthcare quality, efficiency, and health status outcomes compared to 10 other countries: Australia, Canada, France, Germany, the Netherlands, New Zealand, Norway, Sweden, Switzerland, and the United Kingdom.[16] The ACA[1] improves access to health insurance for an estimated "millions of Americans" as of the end of 2013[17] and also contains provisions to strengthen other factors contributing to improvements in population health.[6]

EVIDENCE BASE FOR PREVENTION AND PRACTICE

Clinical and Community Preventive Services

For individuals, an independent panel, the U.S. Preventive Services Task Force (USPSTF) reviews scientific evidence related to a wide variety of clinical preventive healthcare services.[18] Services may include preventive screening tests, the effectiveness of prevention counseling, or other office-based strategies. The Task Force uses a systematic approach to make recommendations based on the strength of the evidence, and gives letter grades, such as "A" (strongly recommends), "B" (recommends), "C" (neither recommends for or against), "D" (recommends against), or "I" (insufficient evidence to make a recommendation).[18] Examples of topics covered include low back pain, alcohol misuse, blood pressure, breast cancer, colorectal cancer, cervical cancer, or dementia screening.[18]

For communities or populations, The Community Preventive Services Task Force uses a similar evidence-based approach for population health interventions.[19] The Task Force makes recommendations based on systematic reviews of the available scientific literature to determine the evidence for effective prevention in community settings, including costs.[19] The Task Force publishes recommendations in "The Community Guide: What Works to Promote Health" and includes such topics as adolescent health, diabetes, obesity, tobacco, vaccination, and many others.[20] For example, in the area of increasing physical activity, the Community Guide outlines recommendations in areas of behavioral and social approaches (such as school-based physical education), campaigns and informational approaches (such as community-wide campaigns), and environmental and policy approaches (such as urban design and land use policies).[21] These two groups, the USPSTF and the Community Preventive Services Task Force, both comprised of experts, make complementary recommendations from different perspectives, focusing on individuals and communities, respectively.[19]

What the ACA Includes to Improve Population Health

In the ACA, there are a variety of provisions that have potential to improve both individual and population health.[1] Insurance coverage increases, including individuals with preexisting conditions, allow many more individuals financial access to health care.[22] Dependent coverage was expanded to include children and young adults up to age 26 for all individual and group policies that went into effect 6 months after the law was passed.[23] This allows young adults, recently entering the workforce or still completing their education, to have another potential source of health insurance.

Regarding preventive services, available estimates suggest individuals in the United States get only 50% of recommended clinical preventive services.[6] One way the ACA facilitates access to preventive services is to eliminate cost sharing for qualified health plans, Medicare, states offering Medicaid-covered clinical preventive services with an "A" or "B" rating by the USPSTF (and some other nationally recognized groups).[6,23] In addition, for those aged 65 and older, Medicare covers an annual wellness visit, beginning in 2011, and a personalized prevention plan with individual risk assessment.[6,23] Although preventive services for women, specifically contraception, has been one of the most controversial provisions in the

ACA, the Kaiser Family Foundation emphasizes the ACA will enhance other preventive services not readily available, particularly for uninsured women.[24] For example, general preventive counseling for tobacco or alcohol use, depression, cholesterol screening, immunizations, or screening for breast and cervical cancer, are just some examples of services more readily available under ACA requirements to help remedy access gaps[24] (see **Figure 9–1**).

Other approaches include creating a nonprofit Patient-Centered Outcomes Research Institute to compare clinical effectiveness of different medical treatments and a national quality improvement strategy to improve health-care service delivery, health outcomes, and population health.[23] Additional reporting from the U.S. Department of Health and Human Services (HHS) Secretary is required to highlight progress in reducing health disparities; providing health care in rural and underserved populations and for individuals with disabilities; and requiring better data on sex, race, ethnicity, and primary language.[23]

To promote primary care, primary care physicians were paid higher Medicaid fees for 2013 and 2014 and a 10% Medicare bonus payment (2011 through 2015).[23] To improve patient access to primary care, funding was increased for the National Health Service Corps and community health centers, school-based health centers, and nurse-managed health clinics.[23] Other workforce strategies include a national Workforce Advisory Committee, redistributing unused Graduate Medical Education (GME) slots, emphasizing primary care and general surgery, and creating Teaching Health Centers.[23] A variety of incentives to increase primary care were included: scholarships and loans, state grants in underserved areas, mental and behavioral health support, oral health training programs, and additional strategies to help reduce the shortage of nursing professionals. Approaches to increase recruitment and retention of nursing professionals include loan repayment and grants to increase numbers of family nurse practitioners providing primary care in health centers and clinics.[23]

Grants to promote worksite wellness and Community Transformation Grants to promote health were also included in the ACA.[6,25] They include funds allocated for small employers to create worksite wellness programs.[23] Research suggests that worksite wellness programs produce a positive return on investment (ROI), in some cases saving $3.27 in medical costs for each dollar invested, and cost savings have been reported by large public and private employers.[25] The ACA also required nutritional content to be provided by chain restaurants and on vending machines to allow informed consumer choices.[23]

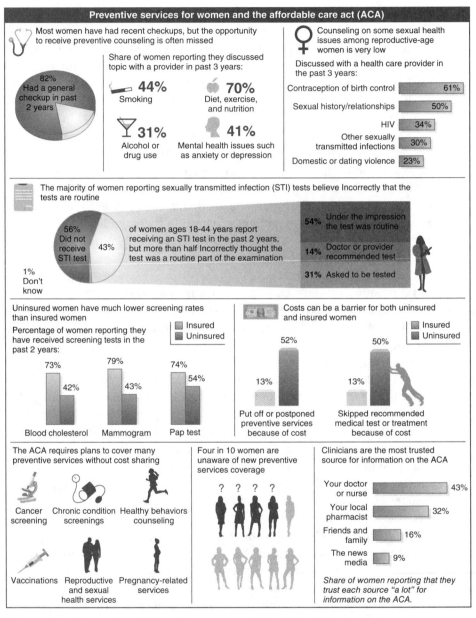

Figure 9–1 Preventive services for women and the Affordable Care Act.

Reproduced from Kaiser Family Foundation. Visualizing Health Policy: Preventive Services for Women and the Affordable Care Act. Available at http://kff.org/womens-health-policy/press-release/visualizing-health-policy-preventive-services-for-women-and-the-affordable-care-act/

ACA funding to support population-based healthcare models such as community health teams and patient-centered medical homes, allows coordinated, team-based care, especially important for patients with chronic conditions.[22] These healthcare models may detect problems earlier, help patients keep track of their medications, and facilitate access to other needed services such as nutrition or community social services.[22]

The ACA also created the National Prevention, Health Promotion, and Public Health Council to develop a comprehensive approach for the nation.[6,26] The Prevention and Public Health Fund (PPHF) provides funds for population-based prevention and is administered by HHS.[6] Funds are used for wellness, prevention research, health screenings, and immunization programs.[23] Grant programs were established to enhance evidence-based community prevention, emphasizing prevention of chronic diseases, improving rural health, and reducing health disparities.[6,23]

Laiteerapong and Huang conclude that ACA-related improvements in population health and chronic diseases, will be determined by "the size of the uninsured population, their prevalence of chronic diseases, effectiveness of chronic disease prevention and treatment, and size of the primary care workforce."[22] Other authors note the importance of the elimination of cost sharing for clinical preventive services, new funding for community preventive services, and funding for workplace wellness, as critical components to improve individual and population-based prevention.[9] Other reports emphasize the importance of using technology to connect primary care providers with their patients and using healthcare data to improve care (and measurable outcomes) of entire population of patients, termed "practice-based population health" (PBPH).[27] In 2012, the Institute of Medicine's Committee on Integrating Primary Care and Public Health published recommendations to broadly enhance collaboration to improve population health.[28]

Health Reform in Massachusetts: Changes in Mortality

Health reform and access to health insurance will result in measurable health improvements in individuals and populations by removing at least some of the financial barriers to health care, although even this basic assertion is controversial.[29] In 2014, there were huge geographic variations across the United States in how much people paid for health insurance under the ACA[30] (see **Figure 9–2**).

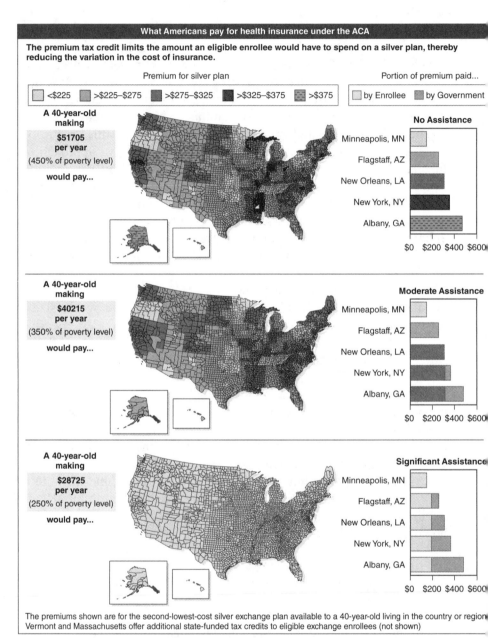

Figure 9–2 What Americans pay for health insurance under the ACA.

Reproduced from Kaiser Family Foundation: Visualizing Health Policy: What Americans Pay for Health Insurance Under the ACA. Available at http://kff.org/infographic/visualizing-health-policy-what-americans-pay-for-health-insurance-under-the-aca/

Does having a regular relationship with a primary care provider, made easier with health insurance and access to preventive care, make a difference? A 2014 study of changes in Massachusetts after their implementation of health reform provides some additional insights. Death rates in people aged 20–64 years in Massachusetts before (2001–2005) and after (2007–2010) health reform were compared with similar "control group" counties in other states in the United States.[31] Investigators studied deaths from all causes, as well as deaths from specific treatable medical conditions (such as heart disease, stroke, infections, or cancer) that might be improved with access to health care. When the researchers compared Massachusetts to control counties, they found a statistically significant decrease in deaths from all causes, as well as a significant decline in deaths in the specific diseases related to access to care.[31] Improvements were noted in insurance coverage, having a "usual source of care," and self-reported health. Comparing counties with higher and lower incomes and uninsured rates, investigators noted larger changes after reform in the geographic areas with lower incomes and higher rates of uninsured populations to start.[31]

Workforce Concerns: Do We Have Enough Health Professionals?

Comparing the United States to peer nations, in addition to examining costs and health status, also highlights the importance of a strong primary care workforce. Many authors agree that better healthcare quality, along with lower spending, is consistently seen in healthcare systems with a stronger primary care foundation.[32] Other authors make the case for dramatic primary care reform, whether from a government, patient, or provider perspective.[33] However after implementation of the ACA, one of the commonly asked questions is: Will we have enough primary care providers? The Health Resources and Services Administration (HRSA) estimates that about 20% of Americans live in geographic areas in the United States where there are not enough primary care physicians.[34] Furthermore, the Association of American Medical Colleges (AAMC) projects that the United States will need 45,000 additional primary care physicians by 2020.[34] This situation is not entirely related to physician-to-population ratios, as shortages are uneven across the United States, and some geographic areas are especially challenged. In addition, some of the health insurance expansion under the ACA is through state-based Medicaid expansions, and not all physicians (including psychiatrists) or dentists accept Medicaid insurance.[34]

Additional costs related to GME (residency training after graduating from medical school) were also a point of controversy while drafting the ACA, but rather than increase GME slots to improve physician supply, currently unused GME positions were redistributed, emphasizing primary care and general surgery.[35] The U.S. Census Bureau projects a 36% increase in numbers of Americans over age 65 in the next decade, whereas numbers of physicians will increase by only 7%.[34] Potential solutions include growing use of technology (such as telemedicine) in healthcare settings and new team-based practice models. Expanding scope of practice for nurse practitioners, physician assistants, or pharmacists is an approach used in some states, although it is often controversial.[34]

A research and projections report by the AAMC in 2010, based on increases in physician utilization, impact of the obesity epidemic, and moderate increase in productivity (due to increases in physician assistants and nurse practitioners) projected a shortage of 91,500 and 130,600 physicians in 2020 and 2025; primary care physician shortages were projected as 45,400 in 2020 and 65,800 in 2025.[36] However, some describe these acute shortages (62,900 physicians short in 2015) as an "invisible problem" that results in patients waiting longer for care or, more likely, using the emergency department because they cannot get regular primary care visits.[37]

Massachusetts, a state that implemented health reform in 2006 before the rest of the nation, provides insight into the kind of provider shortages we can expect. One published study compared per capita employment in the healthcare industry before and after health reform in Massachusetts compared to other states in the United States.[38] Since 2006, investigators found total per capita healthcare employment grew faster than the rest of the United States, increasing at a rate of 9.5%, compared to a rate of 5.5% for the rest of the United States during this same time.[38]

Surprisingly, most of the healthcare employment growth in Massachusetts was in administrative positions (18.4%), which was also statistically different from the rest of the United States (8%). Furthermore, growth was also seen in patient care support personnel (therapists, technicians, aides) who, as a group, increased by 18%. In contrast, growth in other healthcare positions—physicians and nurses—increased at a rate similar to the rest of the United States.[38] The authors concluded that, at least for Massachusetts health reform, healthcare employment grew faster in administrative positions (management, business, financial operations, or administrative support) and patient care support personnel than in healthcare professionals such as physicians and nurses,[38] potentially providing hints for what might be expected for the rest of the United States after ACA implementation.

One area of active health policy discussion centers on the role of nurses and nurse practitioners in the reformed healthcare system. A 2010 Institute of Medicine publication, "The Future of Nursing: Leading Change, Advancing Health"[39] recommends four major policy directions: "nurses should practice to the full extent of their education and training"; a renewed call for educational improvements with "seamless" academic progression; nurses should be "full partners" with physicians and other healthcare professionals; and improved data are needed.[39] In response to this report, a national initiative called the Future of Nursing: Campaign for Action and supported by the Robert Wood Johnson Foundation and AARP, with more than 80 health care, business, and other organizational partners, was established and state coalitions across the U.S. have worked to implement these recommendations.[40]

However, a national survey of 505 physicians and 467 nurse practitioners working in primary care setting showed substantial disagreement about their respective roles in primary care, reflecting ongoing controversy in some states.[41] Nearly 96% of nurse practitioners and 76% of physicians agreed that "nurse practitioners should be able to practice to the full extent of their education and training."[41] Nurse practitioners agreed they should be able to lead medical homes (82%) more often than did physicians (17%). However, despite some areas of agreement, the largest area of disagreement was in response to the statement, "physicians provide a higher quality of examination and consultation than nurse practitioners," where 66% of physicians agreed and 75% of nurse practitioners disagreed.[41] Although the study did not include other health professionals such as physician assistants, the authors (from public health, nursing, and medicine) expressed optimism that such data can be used in ongoing discussions and improvements in healthcare workforce needs.[41]

DISCUSSION QUESTIONS: TEMPLATE FOR DISCUSSION

1. Significance of this public health issue:
   a. Why is this health issue important?
   b. How many people does it impact?
   c. How serious is it?
   d. Is it preventable?
2. What is the evidence base for prevention?

3. What specific strategies should be used to achieve progress on this health issue?
   a. What evidence-based approach would you use?
   b. Where would you start if you are an individual citizen; public health professional; healthcare professional; community, state, or federal policymaker?
4. Specific questions for this topic:
   a. What features of the ACA have potential to improve individual and population health?
   b. What can we learn from Massachusetts' health reform experience from the perspectives of health outcomes and workforce planning?
5. What is the controversy?
   a. Define the controversy.
   b. Is controversy a good or bad thing? (Does it help or hinder progress?)
6. *Why* is this health issue controversial?
   a. What specific factors are involved?
   b. Do economics, government, scientific uncertainty, or politics play a role?
   c. What is the role of the media?
7. How would you respond to the controversy?

PERSPECTIVES TO CONSIDER

When you mention health, many people automatically think of health care, and more specifically, health insurance. However, international comparisons and other published literature have well documented the relationship of habits and behaviors, social and economic factors, the environment, and genetics to the health equation as well.[11] Some hold our progress in international comparisons of diseases related to healthcare access as the ultimate measure of the ACA's success.[42] — not the whole story

The ACA provides many opportunities for health improvements, both at the individual and population levels,[6,17,23] including the estimated "millions" with access to health insurance.[17] Highly respected organizations, such as the Institute of Medicine, write about the importance of integrating primary care and public health.[28] Many new models of population-based health care take steps in the right direction, such as patient-centered primary care medical homes, which link patients to community resources, dieticians, social workers, and specialists as needed. However, based on the contribution of health care to overall health status and our current patterns of spending,[10,15] it also makes sense to look at population health not through the lens of health care, but rather at health care through the lens of population health. Clinical prevention,[18] now more available through the ACA, is a huge step forward; however, evidence-based strategies to improve population health and evidence-based public health practices are also widely available, such as those found in "The Guide to Community Preventive Services,"[20] but are less well known or systematically utilized. These may rely on changes in our environment (bike paths), nutrition programs, or more controversial public health policies (such as taxes on tobacco, alcohol, or sugar-sweetened beverages).

Lessons from Massachusetts are both fascinating and compelling.[31,38] Their experiences show that ensuring access to health care can improve health (and reduce deaths) with health insurance and regular, preventive, and primary care. However, Massachusetts' experience in what numbers and types of additional personnel are *actually* needed to implement health reform contrasts with some other dire projections, raising a number of questions.[34,38] Will we actually need currently-projected numbers of physicians and nurses? More importantly, will the experience of other states and communities (especially in underserved areas) be similar or different?

And what about the funding for prevention in the ACA? Why are population-based strategies so controversial? Do they simply embody the controversy that accompanies public health more generally, especially when considering laws and policies? Despite all the clamor, current funding to support the public health infrastructure and research into "what works" is critical, because widespread use of evidence-based strategies can improve health status more broadly as we improve access to health care in the United States.

FOR ADDITIONAL STUDY

Sommers BD, Long SK, Baicker K. Changes in mortality after Massachusetts health care reform: a quasi-experimental study. *Ann Intern Med.* 2014;160(9):585–593.

Staiger DO, Auerbach DI, Buerhaus PI. Health care reform and the health care workforce—the Massachusetts experience. *N Engl J Med.* 2011;365(12):e24.

REFERENCES

1. HHS.gov/HealthCare. Read the law. 2014. http://www.hhs.gov/healthcare/rights/law/. Accessed June 20, 2014.
2. Department of Health and Human Services. Coverage of certain preventive services under the Affordable Care Act. *Federal Register.* 2013. http://www.gpo.gov/fdsys/pkg/FR-2013-02-06/pdf/2013-02420.pdf. Accessed June 20, 2014.

3. Aizenman N. Obama administration gives groups more time to comply with birth control rule. *The Washington Post.* 2012. http://www.washingtonpost.com/national/health-science/obama-administration-holds-to-birth-control-insurance-rule-but-gives-religious-groups-more-time-to-comply/2012/01/20/gIQAR84nDQ_story.html. Accessed June 20, 2014.

4. Kliff S. Here's Obamacare's most controversial regulation. *The Washington Post.* 2013. http://www.washingtonpost.com/blogs/wonkblog/wp/2013/03/25/heres-obamacares-most-controversial-provision/. Accessed June 16, 2014.

5. Diamond D. Birth control mandate: The most controversial regulation ever? *California Healthline.* 2013. http://www.californiahealthline.org/road-to-reform/2013/birth-control-mandate-the-most-controversial-regulation-ever?view=print. Accessed June 20, 2014.

6. Koh HK, Sebelius KG. Promoting prevention through the Affordable Care Act. *N Engl J Med.* 2010;363(14):1296–1299.

7. Easley J. Spending bill rolls back funding for controversial ObamaCare program. *The Hill.* 2014. http://thehill.com/policy/healthcare/195332-spending-bill-rolls-back-funding-for. Accessed June 16, 2014.

8. Taylor S. Obamacare's slush fund fuels a broader lobbying controversy. *Forbes.com.* 2013. http://www.forbes.com/sites/realspin/2013/05/30/obamacares-slush-fund-fuels-a-broader-lobbying-controversy/. Accessed June 16, 2014.

9. Preston CM, Alexander M. Prevention in the United States Affordable Care Act. *J Prev Med Pub Health.* 2010;43(6):455–458.

10. Schroeder SA. Shattuck Lecture. We can do better—improving the health of the American people. *N Engl J Med.* 2007;357(12):1221–1228.

11. *U.S. Health in International Perspective: Shorter Lives, Poorer Health.* Washington, DC: The National Academies Press; 2013.

12. Sallis JF, Floyd MF, Rodriguez DA, Saelens BE. Role of built environments in physical activity, obesity, and cardiovascular disease. *Circulation.* 2012;125(5): 729–737.

13. McGinnis JM, Foege WH. Actual causes of death in the United States. *JAMA.* 1993;270(18):2207–2212.

14. Mokdad AH, Marks JS, Stroup DF, Gerberding JL. Actual causes of death in the United States, 2000. *JAMA.* 2004;291(10):1238–1245.

15. NEHI. Healthy people/healthy economy. *Annual Report Card 2013.* 2013. http://www.nehi.net/writable/publication_files/file/hphe.final_2013_3rd_report_card.pdf. Accessed June 20, 2014.

16. Davis K, Strmikis K, Squires D, Schoen C. Mirror, mirror on the wall, 2014 Update: How the U.S. health care system compares internationally. *The Commonwealth Fund: Publications.* 2014. http://www.commonwealthfund.org/publications/fund-reports/2014/jun/mirror-mirror. Accessed June 20, 2014.

17. Pear R, Goodnough A. Millions gaining health coverage under law. *The New York Times.* 2013. http://www.nytimes.com/2014/01/01/us/politics/millions-gaining-health-coverage-under-law.html?ref=health&_r=0. Accessed May 24, 2014.

18. USPSTF. U.S. Preventive Services Task Force. 2014. http://www.uspreventiveservicestaskforce.org/. Accessed January 31, 2014.

19. The Guide to Community Preventive Services: What is the Task Force? 2014. http://www.thecommunityguide.org/about/aboutTF.html. Accessed June 20, 2014.

20. The Community Guide: What works to promote health. 2014. http://www.thecommunityguide.org/index.html. Accessed January 31, 2014.
21. The Guide to Community Preventive Services: Increasing physical activity. 2008. http://www.thecommunityguide.org/pa/index.html. Accessed September 6, 2013.
22. Laiteerapong N, Huang ES. Health care reform and chronic diseases: Anticipating the health consequences. *JAMA*. 2010;304(8):899–900.
23. KFF. Summary of the Affordable Care Act. 2013. http://kff.org/health-reform/factsheet/summary-of-new-health-reform-law/. Accessed May 24, 2014.
24. KFF. Visualizing health policy: Preventive services for women and the Affordable Care Act. 2014. http://kff.org/womens-health-policy/press-release/visualizing-health-policy-preventive-services-for-women-and-the-affordable-care-act/. Accessed October 2, 2014.
25. Anderko L, Roffenbender JS, Goetzel RZ, et al. Promoting prevention through the affordable care act: Workplace wellness. *Prev Chronic Dis*. 2012;9:E175.
26. National Prevention Council. 2014. http://www.surgeongeneral.gov/initiatives/prevention/about/. Accessed June 20, 2014.
27. Cusack C, Knudson, AD, Kronstadt, JL, Singer, RF, Brown, AL. Practice-based population health: Information technology to support transformation to proactive primary care. 2010. AHRQ Publication No. 10-0092-EF. http://pcmh.ahrq.gov/sites/default/files/attachments/Information%20Technology%20to%20Support%20Transformation%20to%20Proactive%20Primary%20Care.pdf Accessed June 20, 2014.
28. Committee on Integrating Primary Care and Public Health, Institute of Medicine. *Primary Care and Public Health: Exploring Integration to Improve Population Health*. Washington, DC: The National Academies Press; 2012.
29. Frakt A. Improving health through coverage expansion. *Ann Intern Med*. 2014;160(9):649–650.
30. KFF. Visualizing health policy: What Americans pay for health insurance under the ACA. 2014. http://kff.org/infographic/visualizing-health-policy-what-americans-pay-for-health-insurance-under-the-aca/. Accessed October 2, 2014.
31. Sommers BD, Long SK, Baicker K. Changes in mortality after Massachusetts health care reform: A quasi-experimental study. *Ann Intern Med*. 2014;160(9):585–593.
32. Dentzer S. Reinventing primary care: A task that is far 'too important to fail'. *Health Aff (Millwood)*. 2010;29(5):757.
33. Grundy P, Hagan KR, Hansen JC, Grumbach K. The multi-stakeholder movement for primary care renewal and reform. *Health Aff (Millwood)*. 2010;29(5):791–798.
34. Ollove M. Are there enough doctors for the newly insured? *Kaiser Health News*. 2014. http://www.kaiserhealthnews.org/Stories/2014/January/03/doctor-shortage-primary-care-specialist.aspx. Accessed June 20, 2014.
35. Iglehart JK. Health reform, primary care, and graduate medical education. *N Engl J Med*. 2010;363(6):584–590.
36. AAMC. The impact of health care reform on the future supply and demand for physicians updated projections through 2025. 2010. https://www.aamc.org/download/158076/data/updated_projections_through_2025.pdf. Accessed June 20, 2014.
37. Lowrey A, Pear R. Doctor shortage likely to worsen with health law. *The New York Times*. 2012. https://www.aamc.org/download/158076/data/updated_projections_through_2025.pdf. Accessed May 24, 2014.
38. Staiger DO, Auerbach DI, Buerhaus PI. Health care reform and the health care workforce—the Massachusetts experience. *N Engl J Med*. 2011;365(12):e24.

39. Committee on the Robert Wood Johnson Foundation Initiative on the Future of Nursing at the Institute of Medicine. The future of nursing: Leading change, advancing health. The National Academies Press. 2010. http://www.iom.edu/Reports/2010/the-future-of-nursing-leading-change-advancing-health.aspx. Accessed June 20, 2014.

40. Future of Nursing: Campaign for Action. 2014. http://campaignforaction.org/. Accessed June 20, 2014.

41. Donelan K, DesRoches CM, Dittus RS, Buerhaus P. Perspectives of physicians and nurse practitioners on primary care practice. *N Engl J Med.* 2013;368(20):1898–1906.

42. Buchanan L, Fairfield H, Yourish K. Rating a health law's success. *The New York Times.* 2014. http://www.nytimes.com/interactive/2014/05/19/health/rating-a-health-laws-success.html?_r=0. Accessed October 2, 2014.

CHAPTER 10

Health Care—Improving Veterans' Health

LEARNING OBJECTIVES

- Discuss the system of health care in the United States for active duty military personnel and veterans.
- Describe accountability for the veterans and Military Health Systems.
- Identify changes in the types of health needs in populations served by the VA.
- Discuss how the Patient Protection and Affordable Care Act (ACA) may impact health care for veterans and active duty military personnel, dependents, and retirees.
- Identify evidence-based strategies to improve health care for veterans.

THE CONTROVERSY

On April 23, 2014, CNN reported on claims that 40 or more U.S. veterans died while waiting for health care at the Phoenix VA Health Care System.[1] Further allegations described a "secret list" that was created to cover up lengthy delays in getting care. Even worse, CNN reported that officials at the health system were aware of the use of "official" and "unofficial" patient waiting lists, one entered into the electronic system and the other not—effectively masking delays in scheduling patient appointments.[1] CBS News reported that Americans blamed the Secretary of Veterans Affairs and local VA hospitals. Some even blamed the president.[2]

The situation in Phoenix was the latest allegation. Earlier, in January 2014, CNN reported delays in medical care at Veterans Administration (VA) hospitals had contributed to deaths in 19 U.S. veterans.[3] Attributed in part to delays in medical consultations and procedures such as colonoscopies and endoscopies (to screen for colorectal cancer or other gastrointestinal diagnoses), the problem was found to be widespread: from VA facilities in Florida, South Carolina, and Georgia to Texas and the Rocky Mountains.[3] In response, the House Committee on Veterans' Affairs, which had already been already investigating VA concerns for a year, traveled to some of the hot spots. One of the major themes from all of the investigations was the lack of accountability when mistakes were made. The congressional committee then gave the VA system a month to answer their questions.[4]

A long chronology of healthcare concerns has plagued the VA health system, as early as 1921 and escalating in the 1980s and 1990s.[5] These concerns have included such findings as: 93 VA physicians had regulatory actions taken against their licenses, some severe (1988); unnecessary surgery and delays in care in a Chicago VA hospital (1991); ethical lapses in human subjects clinical research in Los Angeles (1999); long wait times (2003); exposure to hepatitis and HIV from inadequately-disinfected medical equipment in Tennessee, Georgia, and Florida (2009); and many others.[5]

Following the Phoenix allegations, the VA Secretary answered questions about the existence of "secret waiting lists" before Congress on May 15, 2014.[6] During a contentious House committee hearing, one representative simply said, "Veterans died. Give us the answers, please."[7] And in response to hotline calls, the VA Secretary, and Chair of the House Committee on Veterans' Affairs, the Department of Veterans Affairs, Office of the Inspector General (OIG) issued an interim report on May 28, 2014 of VAs patients' scheduling and waiting times.[8] In previous years, the OIG had released 18 reports, citing scheduling problems at VA facilities, long waiting times, and adverse patient impact, all since 2005.[8] The OIG review found scheduling practices that did not follow Veterans Health Administration policy and also found waiting lists that were not the official electronic wait list (EWL).[8]

Their first interim recommendation to the VA Secretary was to immediately provide health care to the 1,700 veterans identified by the investigation but not found on any waiting list. In addition, OIG recommended all waiting lists at the Phoenix VA Health Care System be examined, so patients who most needed care could be identified. A national review of all waiting lists at VA healthcare facilities was also recommended.[8] The VA Secretary resigned May 30, 2014.[9]

BACKGROUND AND SCOPE OF THE PUBLIC HEALTH AND HEALTH POLICY ISSUE

What is Veterans' Health Care? What is Military Medical Care?

Health care for U.S. military personnel, veterans, retirees, and dependents is provided by programs in the Department of Veterans Affairs (VA) and Department of Defense (DoD), through a combination of direct healthcare services and health insurance.[10] In 2011, these two agencies provided care or insurance to an estimated 14 million people at a total cost of $104 billion.[10]

The VA, through its three major divisions, Veterans Benefits Administration, Veterans Health Administration, and National Cemetery Division, administers benefits, delivers health care and oversees national cemeteries.[11] The total VA budget for the Fiscal Year (FY) 2015 budget request, including all programs, is $163.9 billion, compared to $72.1 billion in Fiscal Year 2007; 36.4% of the total budget request is for medical programs.[12] A detailed breakdown of funds in areas of medical services, support, and facilities, was provided in a submission to Congress.[13] FY2015, the total amount requested for Medical Care was $59.1 billion, an increase of $1.8 billion from the previous year.[12] An increase of $309 million was requested from the previous year (total of $7.2 billion) specifically to increase all types of mental health care for veterans: inpatient, outpatient, and residential. Increases were also requested for women veterans (total budget $403 million), Iraq and Afghanistan veterans (total budget $4.2 billion), and for home Telehealth (total budget $567 million) to provide technology-based access to health care for some veterans[12] (see **Figure 10–1**).

Part of the Department of Veterans Affairs, the Veterans Health Administration (VHA) is a healthcare delivery system that includes about 1,700 healthcare facilities: hospitals, long-term care facilities, and outpatient healthcare clinics, all managed by the VHA.[14] Many health professionals delivering care in these settings are employees of the federal government.[14,15] In addition, the VHA is characterized as the largest healthcare system in the United States, employing about 15,000 physicians and 61,000 nurses.[15] The VHA provides health care to about 9 million veterans each year, and VHA facilities also serve as training sites for over 60,000 physicians and dentists.[14]

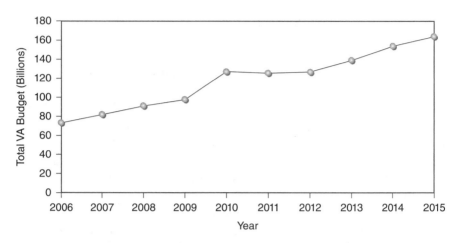

Figure 10-1 Trends in Veterans Administration budget, 2006 to 2015.

Data from VA 2015 Budget Request Fast Facts. Available at http://www.va.gov/budget/docs/summary/Fy2015-FastFactsVAsBudgetHighlights.pdf

Who Is Eligible for Veterans and Military Medical Care?

Veterans who were on active duty (and not dishonorably discharged) are eligible for VA health care. However, in recent years, the VA has not been able to meet the needs of this entire group, so eight priority groups, based on health condition, age, and income, were established in 2010 by the VHA (under direction from Congress).[14] Veterans with a service-related disability or veterans with low income receive priority for health care.[10] Not all veterans can be served, and about 1.3 million veterans did not have healthcare benefits in 2012, although some will qualify for benefits under the ACA through eligibility for health insurance subsidies or Medicaid.[15] It is estimated that 5.5 million of about 24 million living veterans receive care through the VHA on an annual basis.[10] Another program called CHAMPVA, is a health insurance program for survivors of veterans who have either died from a service-related condition or who are totally disabled; these dependents receive care in the private sector.[14]

In parallel to the healthcare system and benefits available to veterans, the DoD, through the Defense Health Agency (DHA) administers health care through hospitals and clinics of the Military Health System (MHS), using both DoD medical facilities and private healthcare providers.[16] Active duty members of the U.S. Army, Navy, Air Force, Marines, and Coast Guard receive services through 57 hospitals and nearly 400 clinics.[14,16]

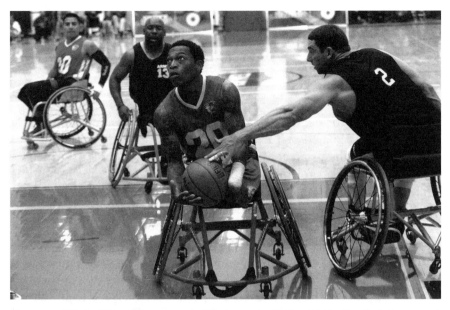

Courtesy of United States Department of Defense. Available at http://www.defense.gov/
dodcmsshare/homepagephoto/2014-10/hires_141003-D-DB155-003.jpg

The MHS also covers dependents of US military personnel on active duty, retirees and their dependents, and some reserve corps members, serving an estimated 9.7 million people through a combination of its own facilities and private sector care.[16] Also, since 1966, military dependents and retirees and their dependents have been eligible for care in the private sector through TRICARE (formerly called CHAMPUS).[16] TRICARE has several different plans, including a health maintenance organization (HMO) option, preferred provider (PPO) option, fee-for-service option (FFS), and a Medicare wrap-around option, and also includes pharmacy and dental programs.[16]

Although separate from the VHA, the MHS has had its own share of controversy. The 2010 death of a pregnant woman seeking care at an Oklahoma Army Community Hospital, which went without required investigation, resulted in a June 2014 investigative report by the *New York Times* on quality and patient safety in military hospitals.[17] This news report found that only 100 of 239 unexpected deaths were investigated from 2011 to 2013, and a review by the American College of Surgeons provided data that 50% of the largest hospitals in the MHS had "higher-than-expected" surgical complication rates.[17] In May 2014, during the same time period as the VHA crisis, the U.S. Secretary of Defense ordered a review of healthcare quality issues in the MHS, after two unexpected deaths at Army hospitals in North Carolina.[17]

Veterans' Health Issues

The demand for health care at VHA facilities has increased. As of 2011, it was estimated that more than 1.2 million soldiers, veterans of the Iraq and Afghanistan conflicts, are now eligible for VHA services.[18] Over time, the need for primary care has increased, compounding the healthcare needs of the VHA system. Aging Vietnam veterans who have both military service-related conditions and chronic conditions commonly seen in aging populations, already contribute to escalating healthcare demands on the VHA system.[6] Furthermore, prevalent conditions such as post-traumatic stress disorder (PTSD) create a need for additional services.[18]

One report notes that one-third of Iraq and Afghanistan veterans have a mental health condition, estimated at almost 730,000 men and women.[15] Only one-third of these individuals receive "evidence-based health care" for their health condition.[15] Recent veterans are more likely to experience PTSD, depression, or traumatic brain injury.[10,19] Many different reports demonstrate a high rate of PTSD and subsequent use of VHA services among Iraq and Afghanistan veterans.[18] Barriers to services for active duty personnel have been previously identified as: concerns about confidentiality and concerns about hindering career progress if they seek help.[10] Vogt, in writing a review of mental health-related beliefs, cites the importance of such beliefs in whether or not veterans and military personnel seek mental health care and recommends including mental healthcare decision making as a part of overall healthcare decision making.[20] New data systems and research, such as the Army Study to Assess Risk and Resilience in Servicemembers (Army STARRS), are now being used to better identify risks for suicide in active duty soldiers and provide better recommendations for prevention and care.[21]

In addition, there are concerns about transitioning from mental health care while on active duty (in the DoD system) to VHA services; one 2003 estimate notes that only about half of discharged individuals with a serious mental illness actually transitioned to VHA care.[10] Cost and capacity for mental health care in the VHA has resulted in new programs to integrate physical and mental health care, and provide easier access.[10] Examples include a "crisis line" for suicide prevention, and screening

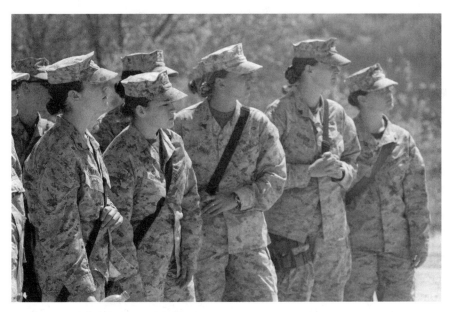

Courtesy of US Department of Defense.

veterans who seek care for other medical conditions for PTSD.[10] Recent VHA budgets have requested additional funds for all areas of mental health care for veterans.[12]

Improvements in health care for women veterans is also an urgent need. Although more than $1 billion has been spent to upgrade the healthcare services available to female veterans since 2008, nearly one-quarter of the nation's VA hospitals still do not employ a full-time gynecologist, a problem that is even worse in rural area clinics.[22] Even the basics, such as adding women's restrooms at over 1,000 VA hospitals, has been a relatively recent occurrence.[22]

In 2013, VA hospitals and clinics provided care for an estimated 390,000 female veterans, double the number of women since 2000.[22] However transitioning a largely male-veteran-oriented system to meet the needs of women has been an ongoing challenge. Women who are veterans are more likely to be on the waiting list for appointments, mammogram reports are often delayed, and healthcare providers specifically trained in women's health care are not available in nearly one-quarter of all VA hospitals, nor are they available in all rural clinics.[22] Even more worrisome was the finding that half of women veterans, often of childbearing age, were prescribed medication that could cause birth defects.[22]

Who Oversees Veterans' Health Care?

The Secretary of Veterans Affairs, a member of the president's cabinet (the president's advisory group comprised of 15 department heads), leads the Department of Veterans Affairs, and is responsible for about 235,000 employees and a budget of $90 billion.[23] The Department of Veterans Affairs has the responsibility of administering benefits, such as education, disability, pensions, medical care, and others, to veterans, families of veterans, and survivors.[23] In Congress, the House and Senate Committee on Veterans' Affairs provide oversight.[24,25] However, a variety of government departments, agencies, and offices also provide information or evaluation of the VA system, including the Department of Veterans Affairs Office of the Inspector General (OIG),[26] Government Accountability Office (GAO),[27] and even the Office of Special Counsel (OSC).[28]

The OIG, through its Office of Healthcare Inspections evaluates veterans' health care and aims to improve quality and patient outcomes.[26] According to its website, the GAO is an "independent, nonpartisan agency" that works for Congress and is often nicknamed the "congressional watchdog."[27] There are more than 1,000 reports on their website related to veterans, dating back to 1950, with more than 200 related to veterans healthcare services, since 1974.[27] GAO reports have documented concerns about long waiting times at VA facilities as early as 2000, and the OIG has scrutinized this same topic multiple times from 2005 to 2012, finding that VA scheduling policy was not being followed.[29]

In December 2012, GAO officials conducted site visits at 23 VA clinics, reviewed policies and data, and interviewed VHA personnel. They concluded that the VHA needed to make improvements in accurately measuring waiting times for medical appointments and also needed additional oversight of patient scheduling.[30] In February 2013, in a statement to the House Committee on Veterans' Affairs, GAO officials testified that "unreliable wait time measurement has resulted in a discrepancy between the positive wait time performance VA has reported and veterans' actual experiences."[31] They further recommended strategies to increase compliance with VA policies and improve access to health care through use of "best practices."[31] A May 25, 2014 report tracking progress toward the 2012 recommendations concluded, "Continued work is needed to ensure these actions are fully implemented in a timely fashion."[32] GAO further added that "Ultimately, VHA's ability to ensure and accurately monitor access to timely medical appointments is critical to ensuring quality health care to veterans, who may have medical conditions that worsen if access is delayed."[32]

The U.S. Office of Special Counsel (OSC), according to its website, is "an independent federal investigative and prosecutorial agency."[28] Some of their duties include protecting federal employees from "prohibited personnel practices;" they especially protect whistleblowers.[28] On June 23, 2014 the OSC sent a lengthy letter to the president and Congress stating "the Department of Veterans Affairs often admits to serious deficiencies in patient care, while implausibly denying any impact on veterans' health."[33] The letter detailed 10 instances, in VA facilities in Colorado, Massachusetts, Alabama, and others, where conclusions of VA investigators were in direct conflict with information found during their own investigation.[33] In response to this letter, the Chairman of the House Committee on Veterans' Affairs issued a press release stating: "In reality, the deaths of dozens of veterans across the country have been linked to delays in VA care and other severe department healthcare problems. . . . It's impossible to solve problems by whitewashing them or denying they exist."[34]

EVIDENCE BASE FOR PREVENTION AND PRACTICE

Care Redesign and Quality Measures

A much-cited 1999 Institute of Medicine (IOM) report, "To Err is Human: Building a Safer Health System," alerted the public, healthcare professionals, and public health communities that between 44,000 and 98,000 people die every year in hospitals from preventable medical mistakes.[35] These errors involved mistakes in diagnosis, treatment, prevention, communication, equipment, or system failure.[35] Subsequently, in 2001, the IOM published "Crossing the Quality Chasm: A New Health System for the 21st Century," with six aims, all with a goal to better meet the health needs of patients. According to IOM recommendations, the healthcare system should be: safe, effective, patient-centered, timely, efficient, and equitable.[36] Nationally, these two publications highlighted the changing healthcare needs of the public, emphasized "systems" aspects of health care, and propelled national momentum toward healthcare redesign in different settings and locations. The VA was no exception to the larger patient safety and healthcare quality conversations in the United States. Despite the current controversy, there is much published literature about quality measurement and improvement in the VA health system.

Kizer (former Undersecretary of Veterans Affairs) and Dudley write about the massive changes in the veterans healthcare system, which they term "extreme makeover," describing the turnaround from the mid-1990s, to an improved, redesigned system beginning in 1999, emphasizing quality, coordination of health care, information technology, and accountability.[37] Other authors echo the serious quality issues of the mid-1990s, including calls for "dismantling" the entire system, and the subsequent evidence of quality improvement, use of information technology, and shift from inpatient care to a greater emphasis on outpatient primary care.[38]

One *New England Journal of Medicine* study by Jha and colleagues compared VA healthcare quality (preventive, acute, and chronic care) in 1994 and 2000, before and after system-wide changes were implemented. Investigators also compared VA quality measures to Medicare fee-for-service care.[39] The VA had implemented a number of extensive changes to systematically measure and focus its efforts on improving healthcare quality; one important change included implementing an extensive electronic health record system across the entire system. The study used quality measures similar to those used in the private sector, and importantly, data collection was done by an independent agency.[39]

Examples of quality measures include influenza vaccination and cancer screening (preventive care), diabetes care, depression screening, hypertension control (outpatient care), and several quality measures related to the treatment of acute myocardial infarction (inpatient care). Statistically significant improvement was shown in 12 of 13 measures over multiple years of data collection. In addition, for the 11 measures that could be directly compared to Medicare, the VA health system performed significantly better.[39] Although assessment of quality outside of the specific measures chosen could not be determined, the authors concluded that the reengineering changes implemented in the VHA system were successful in improving healthcare quality.[39]

Another widely mentioned study from 2004 compared healthcare quality in 12 VHA systems and 12 communities, using 348 measures for 26 different health conditions.[40] Overall healthcare quality was significantly higher at the VHA, as was chronic disease care and preventive care, especially in those areas of health care where the VHA specifically measured quality improvement.[40] More recent studies evaluated cancer care for older men in the VHA.[41,42] When cancer care at the VHA was compared to Medicare patients, VHA patients had earlier diagnosis of colon and rectal cancer and fared better in quality measures for other cancers as well.[41] When looking at cancer deaths, VHA patients survived as often as or better than Medicare patients, in some cases due to earlier cancer diagnosis.[42]

New Directions

Following the resignation of the VA Secretary on May 30, 2014,[9] the president nominated the former CEO of Procter and Gamble rather than a career military officer to become the new VA Secretary.[43] The proposed new VA Secretary graduated from the U.S. Military Academy at West Point, NY and served in the U.S. Army.[44] Although there was support in some corners, there were also critics. *The Washington Post* called the president's pick "unorthodox" because he chose an appointee whose prior company made "detergent and toilet paper."[44] However, in July 2014, by a vote of 97 to 0, the Senate confirmed the president's choice.[45]

In September 2014, Secretary McDonald publically presented a 90-day plan with goals to "rebuild trust" and a veteran-centered approach to focus on scheduling appointments and other service delivery improvements.[46] At the same time, he reported that several federal government agencies were now in the process of investigating over 100 VHA facilities around the country and stated, "I want to personally apologize to all veterans."[47]

In addition, the new VA Secretary has traveled around the country recruiting new physicians from such medical schools as Johns Hopkins and the University of Vermont in order to try to alleviate dire shortages. The national recruitment goal is for 28,000 physicians and nurses.[48] A new proposed restructuring is designed to make it easier for veterans to understand the system and access health care.[49]

New Models of Care

Evidence is accumulating for benefits to patients and cost saving from primary care medical homes (PCMHs).[50–52] Characteristics or principles of PCMHs include emphasis on being patient-centered, comprehensive (team of providers), accessible to patients (including improved communication with patients), coordinated (includes hospital, specialty, and other support services), and using a systems approach (including health information technology) to improve quality and safety.[51,52] One 2014 review noted improvements in cost, utilization, population health measures, access to care, prevention, and patient satisfaction.[52] A 2012 CDC report summarized 58 PCMH evaluations in primary care settings, finding evidence of process measures to improve patient access and care and some evidence of cost savings, but concluded that evidence of effectiveness was not yet available.[51] Another report summarized results in a variety of different settings in the United States, showing examples of improvements in quality and cost.[50]

In April 2010, using more than $227 million, the VA began implementing patient-centered medical homes in 900 clinics over a 3-year period.[53] The VHA is using the Patient Aligned Care Team (PACT) to implement the components of the PCMH. The PACT uses different strategies to facilitate healthcare access, delivers team-based care, and aims to deliver "veteran-centered" care. Veterans have access to educational materials, an Internet site, and can use phone and secure messaging in addition to in-person visits to communicate with their healthcare team.[54] A 2013 published evaluation looking at nearly 3 years of progress noted primary care staff levels increased to support the system, phone calls and electronic communications from patients increased significantly, and numbers of patient follow-up visits after being hospitalized showed dramatic improvements.[55] Other case studies reported appointment waiting time was reduced from 90 days to appointments scheduled on the same day at one clinic site. In addition, unnecessary emergency department visits declined from 52% to 12%, and clinical improvement was seen in one-third of patients with severe diabetes.[53] One study in the VHA and VA Midwest Healthcare Network demonstrated a nearly $600 savings per patient in the PCMH chronic disease management program for patients with chronic lung disease; similar findings were noted in patients with other chronic conditions.[50]

Impact of the Patient Protection and Affordable Care Act

Some authors emphasize the complexity of the current healthcare system for veterans and other military personnel, retirees, and dependents, especially as the VHA and DoD programs relate to the rest of the healthcare delivery and insurance systems in the United States.[10] The ACA has resulted in a wide range of changes in the delivery of health care in the United States.[56] As a result of the ACA, many veterans and others served by the MHS may have options for health insurance through the healthcare exchanges, state-based Medicaid programs, as well as their current TRICARE or VHA services.[10]

Escalating healthcare costs have been an ongoing challenge in both the private and public sectors. Experiencing similar pressures as large companies, DoD officials identified a dangerous and unaffordable financial path created by rising health care and other benefits costs.[57] One report suggests that military families eligible for TRICARE, with an estimated 2014 income of $32,000, might pay similar amounts for TRICARE or getting insurance through a health exchange as part of the ACA.[10] An estimate of uninsured VHA patients further suggests that 25% have incomes that would make them Medicaid-eligible under the ACA, and 50% of uninsured veterans would qualify for healthcare subsidies to buy insurance in the exchanges.[10] These authors go a (controversial) step further, asking, ". . . does it make sense to go on operating a separate health system for veterans—especially those with no service-connected problems?"[10]

Following the president's appointment of a new VA Secretary, *The Arizona Republic* editorial board published "Advice for New VA Chief."[58] They advised the new VA Secretary, in addition to tough management and the hard task of changing the VA culture, to make the system smaller, not larger, and return to the original VA mission by caring for injuries and medical conditions that are a direct result of their service.[58] The editorial board emphasized the "strengths" of the VA system, especially in areas of biomedical research, such as developing artificial limbs, stroke rehabilitation, and new treatments for PTSD.[58] However, given the opposition to similar suggestions in the 1990s, at a time when VA health care was also in crisis,[38] it is not clear whether or not any of these ideas would be widely supported. In response to the current VA crisis, Congress added—in a show of bipartisan support and confidence in the new chief—a substantive appropriation to the VA budget to hire more physicians and nurses and to make the system more accountable.[59]

DISCUSSION QUESTIONS: TEMPLATE FOR DISCUSSION

1. Significance of this public health issue:
   a. Why is this health issue important?
   b. How many people does it impact?
   c. How serious is it?
   d. Is it preventable?
2. What is the evidence base for prevention?
3. What specific strategies should be used to achieve progress on this health issue?
   a. What evidence-based approach would you use?
   b. Where would you start if you are an individual citizen; public health professional; healthcare professional; community, state, or federal policymaker?

4. Specific questions for this topic:
   a. Why is the healthcare system for veterans and active duty military personnel so complex?
   b. Who is responsible for costs, access, and quality of veterans' health care?
   c. What changes, if any, would you propose to improve veterans' health?
5. What is the controversy?
   a. Define the controversy.
   b. Is controversy a good or bad thing? (Does it help or hinder progress?)
6. *Why* is this health issue controversial?
   a. What specific factors are involved?
   b. Do economics, government, scientific uncertainty, or politics play a role?
   c. What is the role of the media?
7. How would you respond to the controversy?

PERSPECTIVES TO CONSIDER

The healthcare system that serves veterans in the United States as well as active-duty military personnel, dependents, and retirees is huge and complicated. There are many hospitals, clinics, and insurance programs, all with different eligibility.[14] Further complicating this system is the changing needs of veterans, with aging veterans from the Vietnam War needing care, along with more recent and growing numbers of Iraq and Afghanistan veterans.[18] PTSD and mental health conditions are especially common and often untreated, for a variety of reasons.[19] Women veterans, with specific health needs, are also increasing in numbers.[22]

In addition, oversight and accountability involves a mix of executive branch departments, congressional oversight, and reports from other independent government organizations and offices. One notable feature of this oversight that garnered intense criticism in the 2014 controversy is the role of the OIG. Reports from this office originated in the same department as the one under scrutiny and other "independent" offices (OSC and GAO) were forceful in articulating their concerns about the VHA system.

In contrast, the VHA system has a track record of change in its delivery of care and achievement of quality improvement in many published reports and in priority areas for many health systems.[40] The VHA system's use of electronic health information technology to promote quality is well recognized.[37] Newer models of care delivery, specifically the PCMH models being implemented in the VA health system and widely across the country, offer optimism for targeting populations with chronic conditions and meeting the unique needs of specific patient populations by using a patient-centered and healthcare "team" approach.[52] There is substantial data already available related to improvements in care processes, quality measures, and cost savings.[53,55] More data will be available on patient outcomes over time, as many PCMHs are now being fully evaluated.

The ACA adds many new questions. The impact of the ACA on the current health care and insurance systems available to veterans, active-duty military personnel, retirees, and families, is not yet fully known. However, if history is any barometer, any proposed changes to the current system, even with potential for improvement in veterans' health, will likely be controversial.

FOR ADDITIONAL STUDY

Klein S. The Veterans Health Administration: Implementing patient-centered medical homes in the nation's largest integrated delivery system. *The Commonwealth Fund: Case Study.* 2011. http://www.qualitysolutions360.com/Assets/Commonwealth_Fund_ Veterans_Health_Administration_I.pdf.

Rosland AM, Nelson K, Sun H, et al. The patient-centered medical home in the Veterans Health Administration. *Am J Managed Care.* 2013;19(7):e263–272.

REFERENCES

1. Bronstein S, Griffin D. A fatal wait: Veterans languish and die on a VA hospital's secret list. *CNN.com.* 2014. http://www.cnn.com/2014/04/23/health/veterans-dying-health-care-delays/. Accessed June 24, 2014.
2. Who do Americans blame for the VA scandal? *CBS News.* 2014. http://www.cbsnews .com/news/who-do-americans-blame-for-the-va-scandal/. Accessed June 24, 2014.
3. Bronstein S, Black N, Griffin D. Veterans dying because of health care delays. *CNN. com.* 2014. http://www.cnn.com/2014/01/30/health/veterans-dying-health-care-delays/ index.html?iid=article_sidebar. Accessed June 24, 2014.
4. Griffin D, Black N, Bronstein S. Congress demands answers after CNN report on VA deaths. *CNN.com.* 2014. http://www.cnn.com/2014/01/07/health/congress-veterans-benefits/index.html. Accessed June 24, 2014.
5. Pearson M. The VA's troubled history. *CNN.com.* 2014. http://www.cnn.com/ 2014/05/23/politics/va-scandals-timeline/. Accessed June 24, 2014.
6. Oppel R, Jr. Veterans Affairs Secretary to face Senate questions on delayed care. *The New York Times.* 2014. http://www.nytimes.com/2014/05/15/us/politics/veterans-affairs-secretary-to-face-senate-questions-on-delayed-care.html. Accessed June 24, 2014.

7. Carter CJ. Report: 1,700 vets not on Phoenix VA wait list, at risk of being 'lost or forgotten'. *CNN.com.* 2014. http://www.cnn.com/2014/05/28/politics/phoenix-va-hospital/. Accessed June 24, 2014.

8. Office of Inspector General. Veterans Health Administration - Interim Report - Review of patient wait times, scheduling practices, and alleged patient deaths at the Phoenix Health Care System. 2014. http://www.va.gov/oig/pubs/VAOIG-14-02603-178.pdf. Accessed June 24, 2014.

9. Shear M, Oppel R, Jr. VA Chief resigns in face of furor on delayed care. *The New York Times.* 2014. http://www.nytimes.com/2014/05/31/us/politics/eric-shinseki-resigns-as-veterans-affairs-head.html. Accessed June 24, 2014.

10. The future of health care for military personnel and veterans. *Academy Health.* 2012. http://www.academyhealth.org/files/publications/AH_RIBriefMilVetsFinal.pdf. Accessed June 24, 2014.

11. Department of Veterans Affairs. 2014. http://www.allgov.com/departments/department-of-veteran-affairs?detailsDepartmentID=567. Accessed June 24, 2014.

12. VA 2015 Budget Request Fast Facts: Total VA funding has grown in 2015 by nearly 68% from 2009. *Fast Facts.* 2014. http://www.va.gov/budget/docs/summary/Fy2015-FastFactsVAsBudgetHighlights.pdf. Accessed June 24, 2014.

13. Department of Veterans Affairs: Volume II: Medical programs and information technology programs: 2015 congressional submission. 2014. http://www.va.gov/budget/docs/summary/Fy2015-VolumeII-MedicalProgramsAndInformationTechnology.pdf. Accessed June 24, 2014.

14. Rovner J. VA and military health care are separate, yet often confused. *NPR Shots.* 2014. http://www.npr.org/blogs/health/2014/05/30/317381276/va-and-military-health-care-are-separate-yet-often-confused. Accessed June 24, 2014.

15. Kliff S. Five Facts about Veterans' health care. *The Washington Post.* 2012. http://www.washingtonpost.com/blogs/wonkblog/wp/2012/11/12/five-facts-about-veterans-health-care/. Accessed June 24, 2014.

16. Jansen DJ. Miltary medical care: Questions and answers. 2014. http://fas.org/sgp/crs/misc/RL33537.pdf. Accessed June 24, 2014.

17. LaFraniere S, Lehren AW. In military care, a pattern of errors but not scrutiny. *The New York Times.* 2014. http://www.nytimes.com/2014/06/29/us/in-military-care-a-pattern-of-errors-but-not-scrutiny.html?smid=tw-bna&_r=0. Accessed June 28, 2014.

18. Shiner B. Health services use in the Department of Veterans Affairs among returning Iraq War and Afghan War veterans with PTSD. *PTSD Res Quart.* 2011;22. http://www.ptsd.va.gov/professional/newsletters/research-quarterly/v22n2.pdf. Accessed June 24, 2014.

19. Seal KH, Metzler TJ, Gima KS, Bertenthal D, Maguen S, Marmar CR. Trends and risk factors for mental health diagnoses among Iraq and Afghanistan veterans using Department of Veterans Affairs health care, 2002–2008. *Am J Public Health.* 2009; 99(9):1651–1658.

20. Vogt D. Mental health-related beliefs as a barrier to service use for military personnel and veterans: A review. *Psychiatr Serv.* 2011;62(2):135–142.

21. Schoenbaum M, Kessler RC, Gilman SE, et al. Predictors of suicide and accident death in the Army Study to Assess Risk and Resilience in Servicemembers (Army STARRS): Results from the Army Study to Assess Risk and Resilience in Servicemembers (Army STARRS). *JAMA Psychiatry.* 2014;71(5):493–503.

22. Burke G. VA falls short on medical care of servicewomen. *The Boston Globe.* 2014. http://www.bostonglobe.com/news/nation/2014/06/22/falls-short-medical-care-female-veterans/9F870XeQOFthvKyTETuO9N/story.html. Accessed June 24, 2014.

23. The Executive Branch. 2014. http://www.whitehouse.gov/our-government/executive-branch. Accessed June 24, 2014.

24. House Committee on Veterans' Affairs. 2014. http://veterans.house.gov/. Accessed October 2, 2014.

25. The United States Senate Committee on Veterans' Affairs. 2014. http://www.veterans.senate.gov/. Accessed October 2, 2014.

26. Department of Veterans Affairs Office of Inspector General: About the Office of Health Care Inspections. 2014. http://www.va.gov/oig/about/healthcare.asp. Accessed June 24, 2014.

27. GAO. About GAO. 2014. http://www.gao.gov/about/index.html. Accessed June 24, 2014.

28. U.S. Office of Special Counsel. 2014. http://www.osc.gov. Accessed June 24, 2014.

29. Hicks J. A guide to the VA health care controversy. *The Washington Post.* 2014. http://www.washingtonpost.com/blogs/federal-eye/wp/2014/05/15/a-guide-to-the-va-health-care-controversy/. Accessed June 24, 2014.

30. GAO. Reliability of reported outpatient medical appointment wait times and scheduling oversight need improvement. *GAO Highlights.* 2012. http://www.gao.gov/assets/660/651077.pdf. Accessed June 24, 2014.

31. GAO. Reported outpatient medical appointment wait times are unreliable. *GAO Statement to the Committee on Veterans' Affairs.* 2013. http://www.gao.gov/assets/660/652104.pdf. Accessed June 24, 2014.

32. GAO. VA lacks accurate information about outpatient medical appointment wait times, including specialty care consults. *GAO Highlights.* 2014. http://www.gao.gov/assets/670/663194.pdf. Accessed June 24, 2014.

33. OSC cites deficiencies in VA health care reports. 2014. https://osc.gov/News/pr14_11.pdf. Accessed June 24, 2014.

34. Cashour C. Chairman Miller statement on OSC letter to President Obama. *House Committee on Veteran's Affairs Press Release.* 2014. https://veterans.house.gov/press-release/chairman-miller-statement-on-osc-letter-to-president-obama. Accessed June 24, 2014.

35. Koln LT, Ed. *To err is human: Building a safer health system.* Institute of Medicine. Washington DC: The National Academies Press, 1999; http://www.iom.edu/Reports/1999/to-err-is-human-building-a-safer-health-system.aspx. Accessed June 28, 2014.

36. Institute of Medicine. *Crossing the quality chasm: A new health system for the 21st century.* Washington, DC: The National Academies Press, 2001; http://www.iom.edu/Reports/2001/Crossing-the-Quality-Chasm-A-New-Health-System-for-the-21st-Century.aspx. Accessed June 28, 2014.

37. Kizer KW, Dudley RA. Extreme makeover: Transformation of the Veterans Health Care System. *Annu Rev Publ Health.* 2009;30(1):313–339.

38. Longman P. The best care anywhere. *Washington Monthly.com.* 2005. http://www.washingtonmonthly.com/features/2005/0501.longman.html. Accessed June 28, 2014.

39. Jha AK, Perlin JB, Kizer KW, Dudley RA. Effect of the transformation of the Veterans Affairs Health Care System on the quality of care. *N Engl J Med.* 2003;348(22): 2218–2227.

40. Asch SM, McGlynn EA, Hogan MM, et al. Comparison of quality of care for patients in the Veterans Health Administration and patients in a national sample. *Ann Intern Med.* 2004;141(12):938–945.

41. Keating NL, Landrum MB, Lamont EB, et al. Quality of care for older patients with cancer in the Veterans Health Administration versus the private sector: A cohort study. *Ann Intern Med.* 2011;154(11):727–736.

42. Landrum MB, Keating NL, Lamont EB, et al. Survival of older patients with cancer in the Veterans Health Administration versus fee-for-service Medicare. *J Clin Oncol.* 2012;30(10):1072–1079.

43. Shear MD, Oppel R, Jr. Pick for V.A. is former corporate chief. *The New York Times.* 2014. http://www.nytimes.com/2014/06/30/us/bob-mcdonald-veterans-affairs-obama .html?_r=0. Accessed October 2, 2014.

44. Eilperin J. Bob McDonald, former P&G chief, to be Obama's nominee to lead Veterans Affairs. *The Washington Post.* 2014. http://www.washingtonpost.com/ politics/bob-mcdonald-former-pandg-chief-to-be-obamas-nominee-to-lead-veterans-affairs/2014/06/29/2fddd794-ffab-11e3-b8ff-89afd3fad6bd_story.html. Accessed October 2, 2014.

45. Kesling B. Senate confirms McDonald as VA Secretary. *Wall Street Journal Online.* 2014. http://online.wsj.com/articles/senate-confirms-robert-mcdonald-as-va-secre-tary-1406660890. Accessed October 2, 2014.

46. Druzin H. 'I'm Bob': McDonald says he will tackle VA hierarchy. *Stars and Stripes.* 2014. http://www.stripes.com/i-m-bob-mcdonald-says-he-will-tackle-va-hierar-chy-1.302048. Accessed October 2, 2014.

47. Zoroya G. VA chief: More than 100 facilities now being probed. *USA Today.* 2014. http://www.usatoday.com/story/news/nation/2014/09/08/va-mcdonald-press-confer-ence-scandal-wait-times/15272409/. Accessed October 2, 2014.

48. Oppel R, Jr. Needing to hire, chief of V.A. tries to sell doctors on change *The New York Times.* 2014. http://www.nytimes.com/2014/11/09/us/politics/needing-to-hire-chief-of-va-tries-to-sell-doctors-on-change-.html?_r=0. Accessed November 12, 2014.

49. Hicks J. VA chief unveils restructuring plan for troubled agency. *The Washington Post.* 2014. http://www.washingtonpost.com/blogs/federal-eye/wp/2014/11/10/va-chief-unveils-restructuring-plan-for-troubled-agency/. Accessed November 12, 2014.

50. Grumbach K, Grundy P. Outcomes of implementing patient centered medical home interventions: A review of the evidence from prospective evaluation studies in the United States. *Patient-Centered Primary Care Collaborative Update.* 2010. http://www.cms .org/uploads/GrumbachGrundy2010OutcomesPCPCC.pdf. Accessed June 28, 2014.

51. CDC. The patient-centered medical home: Current state of evidence. *Science-in-Brief.* 2012. http://www.cdc.gov/dhdsp/pubs/docs/science_in_brief_pcmh_evidence.pdf. Accessed June 28, 2014.

52. Nielsen M, Olayiwola JN, Grundy P, Grumback K. The patient-centered medical home's impact on cost and quality. *Patient-Centered Primary Care Collaborative Update.* 2014. http://www.milbank.org/uploads/documents/reports/Patient-Centered_ Medical_Homes_Impact_on_Cost_and_Quality.pdf. Accessed June 28, 2014.

53. Klein S. The Veterans Health Administration: Implementing patient-centered medical homes in the nation's largest integrated delivery system. *The Commonwealth Fund: Case Study.* 2011. http://www.qualitysolutions360.com/Assets/Commonwealth_Fund_Veterans_Health_Administration_I.pdf. Accessed June 28, 2014.

54. Veterans Health Administration: Patient aligned care team (PACT). 2014. http://www.va.gov/health/services/primarycare/pact/index.asp. Accessed June 28, 2014.

55. Rosland AM, Nelson K, Sun H, et al. The patient-centered medical home in the Veterans Health Administration. *Am J Man Care.* 2013;19(7):e263–272.

56. KFF. Summary of the Affordable Care Act. 2013. http://kff.org/health-reform/fact-sheet/summary-of-new-health-reform-law/. Accessed May 24, 2014.

57. Keith T. Health care costs new threat to U.S. military. *NPR.* 2011. http://www.npr.org/2011/06/07/137009416/u-s-military-has-new-threat-health-care-costs. Accessed June 28, 2014.

58. Editorial Board. *The Arizona Republic* [editorial]. Advice for new VA chief. *USA Today.* 2014. http://www.usatoday.com/story/opinion/2014/07/06/advice-va-chief-bob-mcdonald/12158427/. Accessed October 2, 2014.

59. Druzin H. At tense VA hearing, doctors link delays to patient deaths. *Stars and Stripes.* 2014. http://www.stripes.com/news/at-tense-va-hearing-doctors-link-delays-to-patient-deaths-1.303604. Accessed October 2, 2014.

CHAPTER 11

Mental Health— A Continuing Crisis

LEARNING OBJECTIVES

- Describe the public health impact of mental illness in the United States.
- Identify statistics for types of mental illness in the United States, prevalence, and state variation.
- Discuss barriers to access to care for people with mental illness.
- Identify vulnerable populations at increased risk for mental illness.
- Identify evidence-based policies that are effective in improving prevention, diagnosis, or treatment of mental illness.
- Evaluate current strategies to reduce stigma related to mental illness.
- Propose evidence-based strategies to integrate physical and behavioral health.

THE CONTROVERSY

The stories are nearly endless and always heart wrenching. A report from Connecticut describes a 30-year-old man with diagnosed autism and a history of substance abuse who lived with his mother and grandmother.[1] He was supported through high school, but struggled with access to care and support services in the many years afterwards. One counselor told his mother, "If you can't deal with him, drop him off at a (homeless) shelter."[1]

In an interview on *CBS News' 60 Minutes* entitled "Nowhere to Go: Mentally Ill Youth in Crisis," Virginia State Senator Craig Deeds told the story of his mentally ill 24-year-old son, the Senator's efforts to help him seek care, and the tragic ending. Senator Deeds said, "If he could have been hospitalized that night, they could have gotten him medicated, and I could have worked to get Gus in some sort of long-term care."[2,3] Contributing factors include huge gaps in mental healthcare resources, insurance hassles, and the way mental health diagnoses are perceived in our society.[3] One mother, when asked by *60 Minute's* Scott Pelley, "What is the difference between being the mother of a child who has mental illness and the mother of a child who might have heart disease or cancer?" answered simply, "Sympathy."[2]

Despite recent policy changes, such as the 2008 Mental Health Parity and Addiction Equity Act and also the 2010 Patient Protection and Affordable Care Act (ACA) that require mental health parity in participating insurers, a variety of obstacles remain, such as widespread shortages of mental health professionals.[4] In addition, a frequently quoted statistic that only 50% of psychiatrists accept health insurance[4] implies persistent access barriers despite improvements in insurance coverage.

Authors from South Carolina describe dramatic cuts in mental health funding, slashed numbers of state hospital beds, and longer waiting time for patients.[5] They observe that prisons are now "holding areas" for patients with psychiatric illness and "emergency rooms have become the primary source of acute treatment for many psychiatric patients,"[5] a view widely shared by others.[6] One Missouri State Representative described the state's first public mental hospital as "something out of the 1920s," continuing, "Have you ever seen 'One Flew Over the Cuckoo's Nest'? It's that, but worse."[1]

And these are not isolated state-level problems. The National Association of State Mental Health Program Directors estimates that $4.35 billion for mental health treatment services has been cut since 2010.[1,6] The National Alliance on Mental Illness (NAMI) gave the entire United States a "dismal D" based on 65 specific criteria, using data from researchers, federal agencies, healthcare, and state mental health agencies. In 2009, states across the United States varied widely, but no state received an "A," six states received a "B," and six states received a failing grade."[7] Furthermore, about 25% of all U.S. adults (61.5 million people) have mental illness each year, and 13.6 million live with a diagnosis of schizophrenia, major depression, or bipolar illness, all examples of serious mental illness.[8] Some writers argue that concerns about stigma or denial about their own illness prevents some patients from getting care when they most need it.[3] Despite progress in the broader policy arena, insurance-related barriers remain and may even create provider incentives to deliver less time-consuming care.[3] One Iowa mother of a 15-year-old adolescent who has struggled since third grade (despite psychiatrist visits) observed, "It just seems like they want to medicate rather than provide education support."[9]

BACKGROUND AND SCOPE OF THE PUBLIC HEALTH AND HEALTH POLICY ISSUE

What Is Mental Illness? What is the Public Health Impact?

Mental illness, according to the Centers for Disease Control and Prevention (CDC) includes "all diagnosable mental disorders."[10] These disorders are characterized by "sustained abnormal alterations in thinking, mood, or behavior associated with distress and impaired function."[10] Levels of impairment related to mental illness vary widely and range from minor impairment in activities of daily living, to major disruptions in all aspects of life, and even include premature death.[11] Common mental illnesses include anxiety and mood disorders.[10] It is estimated that, as of 2004, about 25% of all adults in the United States have a mental illness, and almost half of all adults in the United States will develop one or more mental illnesses.[10,11] When looking internationally, the burden of mental illness is substantial in developed countries and the largest proportion of disability of *any* category of disease can be attributed to mental illness.[10,11] Health care and societal costs are substantial in the United States, with mental health resulting in an estimated $100 billion in healthcare costs and total costs of about $300 billion annually.[11]

One frequently overlooked perspective is the adverse impact mental illness has on other health conditions. Mental illness in combination with diabetes or heart disease results in worse health outcomes for these chronic conditions, because patients may be less likely or unable to access needed health care on an ongoing basis.[11] The most common chronic heart and lung diseases seen in the U.S. population result in higher death rates in patients with serious mental illness (SMI).[12] Higher rates of risk factors such as smoking and obesity also likely contribute to development of chronic conditions. Poverty, being homeless, or struggling to live independently may create additional challenges and additional barriers to treatment.[12] Rates of tobacco use and alcohol abuse are higher in people with mental illness; rates of homicide, suicide, and motor vehicle injury are also two to six times higher.[11] A 2006 report from the National Association of State Mental Health Program Directors highlights the cumulative impact of mental health diagnoses on longevity, emphasizing that adults with SMI die an average of 25 years sooner than the general population.[12]

Data and Trends

CDC uses public health surveillance, the "ongoing and systematic collection, analysis, interpretation, and dissemination of data used to develop public health interventions that reduce morbidity and mortality and improve health," to provide useful information to health professionals, public agencies, policymakers, and the general public about mental illness in the United States.[10] In 2011, CDC summarized mental illness in the United States using a number of population-based and healthcare surveys. Data sources from population-based surveys include the Behavioral Risk Factor Surveillance System (BRFSS), National Health Interview Survey (NHIS), National Health and Nutrition Examination Survey (NHANES) and others; healthcare surveys include the National Ambulatory Medical Care Survey (NAMCS) and National Hospital Discharge Survey (NHDS), among others.[10,11] In 2012, CDC concluded there is no ongoing state or national level data gathering for anxiety disorders despite their being as common as depression and recommended this gap be addressed.[10] From surveillance data, rates of adult mental illness vary across the United States.[11] For example, rates of depression were highest in Southeastern states, with reported rates of 13.7% in both Mississippi and West Virginia, compared to 4.3% in North Dakota[10] (see **Figure 11–1**). A similar pattern was seen in adult rates of "serious psychological distress" in adults.[11]

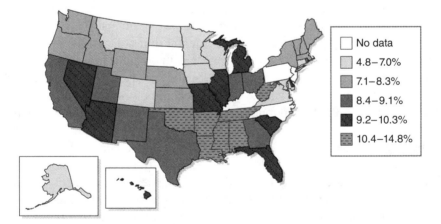

Figure 11–1 Current depression among adults—United States, 2006 and 2008.

Reproduced from Centers for Disease Control and Prevention. Current Depression Among Adults—United States, 2006 and 2008. MMWR 2010; 59(38); 1229–1235.

The National Institute of Mental Health (NIMH) also publishes statistics on prevalence, treatment and costs of mental illness in the United States.[3] Data from the 2012 National Survey on Drug Use and Health (NSDUH) showed about 9.6 million adults in the United States reported SMI in the past year (4.1% of all adults) and fewer than 60% received treatment.[13,14] In 2012, 18.6% of adults in the United States had any mental illness (about 43.7 million adults), with the highest rates reported in women (22%), those between the ages of 26 and 49 (21.2%), and individuals reporting themselves as white (19.2%) and American Indian/Alaska Native (28.3%).[13]

For depression, 6.9% of adults in the United States reported depression in the past year, higher in women (8.4%) and in individuals age 18 to 25 (8.9%). For adolescents (ages 12 to 17), 9.1% (about 2.2 million) experienced major depression in the past year, with rates higher in females (13.7%) and Hispanic (10.5%) individuals.[13] The Substance Abuse and Mental Health Services Administration (SAMHSA) publishes similar data using DSM-IV (fourth edition of the *Diagnostic and Statistical Manual of Mental Disorders*) criteria to publish state-by-state estimates.[14] Nationally, rates of any mental illness in the past year in the United States was lowest in Maryland (17.2%) and highest in Rhode Island (24.0%).[14] Rates of SMI also varied across the country with no clear regional distribution. The lowest rate of 3.5% was noted in South Dakota to the highest rate of 7.0% in Rhode Island.[14]

Suicide

According to CDC, there were 38,364 suicides in the United States, an average of 105 each day in 2010, and suicide was the 10th leading cause of death for all ages.[15] Firearms are the most common method of suicide (51%), followed by suffocation (25%), and poisoning (17%). However, for every suicide death there were 25 suicide attempts, and in 2011, there were 487,700 emergency department visits for self-inflicted injuries in the United States.[16] In adults aged 15 to 24 years, there are between 100 and 200 suicide attempts for every death from suicide.[15]

Suicide rates vary by age, gender, and geographic location. CDC mapped suicide rates in U.S. counties from 2000 to 2006, to highlight the variation seen across the United States (see **Figure 11–2**). Suicide rates were higher in western states and counties, including Alaska, some Appalachian counties of Kentucky and West Virginia, southern Oklahoma, and northern Florida.[17]

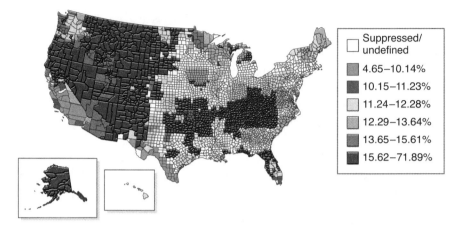

Figure 11–2 Age-adjusted suicide rates per 100,000 population, by county, United States, 2000–2006.

Reproduced from the Centers for Disease Control and Prevention. Web-based Injury Statistics Query and Reporting System (WISQARS). Fatal Injury Maps 2000–2006. Atlanta, GA: National Center for Injury Prevention and Control. Last accessed 2012 March 09. Available at http://www.cdc.gov/violenceprevention/suicide/statistics/aag.html#2

In the United States, the highest suicide rates in 2010 were in people aged 45 to 64 and those older than 85, with rates about 4 times higher in men.[18] Despite the fact that the higher rates are seen in middle-aged people, suicide is the third leading cause of death among young people age 15 to 24, accounting for 20% of all deaths in this age group.[15] Among American Indian/Alaska Native individuals in the United States aged 15–34 years, suicide rates are 2.5 times higher the national average, representing the second leading cause of death.[15]

Globally, the World Health Organization (WHO) notes there are about 800,000 suicides each year, about three-quarters of suicides are in low- and middle-income countries, and suicide represents the second leading cause of death in people aged 15 to 29 years old.[19] Hanging, using firearms, and eating pesticides represent the most common means.[19] Globally, age-standardized suicide rates vary dramatically across continents and by country[20] (see **Figure 11–3**).

Risk and Protective Factors

Research studies have identified both risk and protective factors related to suicide.[16] Risk factors include family history of suicide, history of depression or other mental illness, history of alcohol or drug abuse, previous

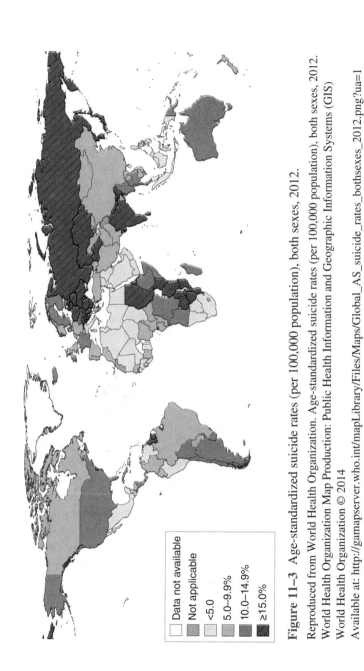

Figure 11–3 Age-standardized suicide rates (per 100,000 population), both sexes, 2012.

Reproduced from World Health Organization. Age-standardized suicide rates (per 100,000 population), both sexes, 2012. World Health Organization Map Production: Public Health Information and Geographic Information Systems (GIS) World Health Organization © 2014

Available at: http://gamapserver.who.int/mapLibrary/Files/Maps/Global_AS_suicide_rates_bothsexes_2012.png?ua=1 suicide attempt, recent loss, and access to lethal means. CDC also includes "exposure to the suicidal behavior of others" in the list of risk factors.[16] In contrast, family, community, health care, and mental health support; access to clinical care for physical and mental health disorders; cultural beliefs that include the importance of seeking help; and skills in resolving conflicts are all factors that may protect people from suicide.[16] Although suicide is still associated with both stigma and poor public understanding, research into risk factors, partnerships with national organizations,[18] and widespread public education about resources to help people at risk (such as the National Suicide Prevention Lifeline[21]) all contribute in a positive way to public health efforts to prevent suicide.[16]

Insights from Research—Genetics and Studies of Parental Age

Scientific studies suggest genetic mutations related to psychiatric illness may be partially attributed to the increase in genetic mutations in sperm in older fathers; however, there is scientific controversy related to methods used in these studies.[22] Two studies from 2014 further contributed to the complex scientific literature about the question of parental age and psychiatric disorders.[22,23]

One cohort study in Sweden from 1973 to 2001 of 2,615,081 births analyzed the association between older paternal age and psychiatric diagnoses or low educational attainment in children.[22] Conditions studied included ADHD, autism, psychosis, bipolar disorder, attempted suicide, and substance abuse. The authors found that older age of fathers was associated with increased risks for autism, psychosis, and bipolar disorder, but lower risks for others.[22] However, when they compared children born to older fathers to siblings born years earlier to the same father, children born to fathers aged 45 and older had statistically increased risks for the entire list of psychiatric illnesses studied, as well as for lower educational attainment, compared to children (siblings) born to their fathers when younger (aged 20–24).[22] This study provided additional evidence supporting the hypotheses that new genetic mutations in sperm of older fathers is related to increased risk for mental illnesses.[22]

Another comprehensive population-level study in Denmark, linking birth records and data from the Danish Psychiatric Central Research Register was used to study the association between both maternal and paternal age and psychiatric disorders.[23] In their study of 2,894,688 births, the authors noted increased risks for psychiatric disorders for children of both younger and older parents compared to those born to parents aged 25–29 years.[23] However, the types of mental health disorders seen in children of younger and older parents differed, with children born to older fathers having increased risks for schizophrenia, mental retardation, and autism spectrum disorders. In contrast, children born to younger mothers and fathers were more likely to have substance abuse and mental retardation.[23]

The Role of Stigma

Worldwide, as many as three-quarters of people with diagnosed mental illness do not receive needed treatment.[24,25] In addition to lack of services in many areas, contributing factors also include a widespread lack of public information about the signs and symptoms of mental illness and how to access available care in communities.[24] Stigma can be a barrier to treatment, and can include "social" or "public" stigma, the negative perceptions against people with mental health disorders solely as a result of their condition. There may also be "perceived stigma" or "self-stigma" which are these same feelings in the person with mental illness.[26,27]

One author of a 2014 review analyzing 144 studies on this topic said, "we now have clear evidence that stigma has a toxic effect by preventing people seeking help for mental health problems."[28] In this large review article, Clement and colleagues from the United Kingdom analyzed studies involving 90,189 participants, concluding that stigma was a substantive negative factor in patients' decisions to access help.[29] In this study, of 10 identified barriers, stigma was ranked fourth, and especially posed a barrier to care for young people, men, ethnic minority populations, and people in military and health professions.[29]

Challenges in Access to Care—Financing and Insurance

The history of the mental health system in the United States spans decades. Available psychiatric beds dropped from about 500,000 to less than 100,000 since the 1960s, because scientific views favored the benefits of treatment in local communities.[2] During this time, many large mental institutions closed. However, local community capacity never expanded sufficiently to meet the demand, leaving widespread gaps in care and treatment.[2]

The National Association of State Mental Health Program Directors and the National Association of State Alcohol and Drug Abuse Directors together reported to the U.S. Congress on state budget reductions and the huge unmet needs for mental health treatment in the United States.[6] The state directors noted reductions from 2009 to 2012 in state funding for public mental health totaling about $4.35 billion, rivaling the magnitudes of budget cuts following deinstitutionalization of mental health patients, all despite a 10% increase in demand for services.[6] In their report to Congress they stated, "We are spending money in all the wrong places— prisons, emergency departments, and homeless shelters when the illness become more serious," estimating that one of every eight emergency department visits in 2007 in the United States involved a mental health or substance abuse diagnosis.[6] One sheriff in Montana, in response to increased calls for police responders to psychiatric emergencies lamented, "People in psychiatric crisis need to receive community-based mental health services staffed by licensed professionals—not in the back of a patrol car."[6]

A "Primer on Mental Health Financing" from the Kaiser Commission on Medicaid and the Uninsured, details the many funding sources for U.S. systems to provide mental health and substance abuse services (together called the *behavioral health system*) which make it difficult to implement systematic improvements for patients.[30] Funding sources include the federal–state Medicaid program, federal Medicare program, individual states and counties, private insurance plans, out-of-pocket payments by individual consumers, and other programs.[30] Most treatment for mental health and substance abuse is provided in outpatient rather than in hospital settings and includes pharmacological treatment (medications), psychological counseling, or both.[30] Despite progress in providing needed behavioral health services, more than 60% of adults and 70% of children do *not* receive needed mental health treatment; this figure approaches 90% for both children and adults with substance abuse disorders.[30]

Total spending for behavioral health services in the United States was estimated at $135 billion in 2005. Changes since 1986 include a higher proportion of total spending on prescription medications (from 7% to 27%) and decreased spending on inpatient treatment (42% to 19%).[30] Of total national expenditure for mental health, the largest shares are paid by Medicaid (28%), private insurance (27%), and other state and local sources (18%), whereas the use of state and local funds are the largest sources of funding (36%) for substance abuse services.[30]

Financing of behavioral health services differs from physical health services, with 61% of payments for behavioral health services coming from public financing sources, compared to 46% for other healthcare services.[30] Other public financing sources include the Community Mental Health Services Block Grant (MHBG) providing state grants for patients with SMI. Although private health insurance covers the most people, it represents only 25% of the spending, due to limitations on allowed services. Charitable sources represent only 4% of overall behavioral health financing.[30] Out-of-pocket payments by individual consumers represents 11% of behavioral health spending and is higher for those with private insurance.[30]

Challenges in Access to Care—Health Professionals

Despite new national funding to train mental health professionals in local communities and state-based approaches to link young people at high risk to mental health services,[31] access to mental health professionals, such as psychiatrists (physicians specializing in the prevention, diagnosis, and treatment of mental illness, who are able to prescribe medications) continues to be challenging in many areas of the United States. A 2014 study by Bishop and colleagues looked the question of whether acceptance of health insurance by psychiatrists was an important barrier to care.[32] Using the National Ambulatory Medical Care Survey (NAMCS), a national survey from CDC's National Center for Health Statistics, investigators compared psychiatrists' acceptance of health insurance (compared to other physician specialties), looking specifically at whether physicians were accepting new patients with private insurance, Medicare, or Medicaid.[32]

The investigators found that psychiatrists were statistically less likely to accept all types of insurance than were other medical specialties, with lower acceptance rates seen for private insurance (55.3% vs. 88.7%), Medicare (54.8% vs. 86.1%), and Medicaid (43.1% vs. 73%) in 2009–2010.[32] Rates of psychiatrists' acceptance of private insurance and Medicare had declined since 2005–2006. Whether or not psychiatrists accepted insurance also varied geographically. Psychiatrists in the Midwest were statistically more likely to accept private insurance (85.1%) than psychiatrists practicing in the West, South, or Northeast.[32] Longer patient visit times needed for psychiatry compared to other healthcare specialties was cited as a potential contributing factor. The authors also found that psychiatrists practicing in a group practice were more likely to accept insurance, which may be relevant as new team-based practice models (such as patient-centered medical homes) become more common.[32]

Special Population Needs—The U.S. Military

In addition to challenges with access to mental health services, provider shortages, stigma, and other barriers to mental health care, questions remain about the needs of specific populations, such as the U.S. military. In 2014, the largest study of the U.S. military and risks for mental illness was reported in a series of research articles[33–35] that reported rates of some types of mental illness were higher in U.S. soldiers than in civilian populations.[36] The U.S. Army and the NIMH together used data from nearly 5,500 military members, called the Study to Assess Risk and Resilience in Servicemembers (STARRS).[36]

Kessler and colleagues, using the STARRS database, studied the frequency of DSM-IV diagnoses in the past month in a group of 5,428 soldiers.[34] Investigators included major depressive disorders, bipolar disorder, anxiety, panic, and post-traumatic stress, ADHD, explosive disorders, and alcohol and substance abuse in their study.[34] One-quarter of survey respondents (25.1%) met criteria for one of these diagnoses, and based on age calculations, more than three-quarters of these (76.6%) occurred before enlistment.[34]

A study using the STARRS database by Schoenbaum and colleagues measured suicide or accident deaths during active Army service. Suicide rates (from 2004 and 2009) increased both among Army soldiers who were never deployed and also in currently and previously deployed soldiers.[35] Demographic, occupational, and deployment factors associated with increased suicide risk included being a man (or women during deployment), white race/ethnicity, junior enlisted rank, recent demotion, current or previous deployment.[35] The authors argued that factors related to combat did not totally explain the increased risk, because an increased suicide risk was also reported in never-deployed U.S. Army soldiers.[35]

In another study using this database, Nock and colleagues studied lifetime risk and predictors of suicide in nondeployed US Army soldiers.[33] Suicide attempts after Army enlistment were associated with being a woman, lower rank, and previously deployment. Military members who had certain specific conditions prior to enlistment (such as post-traumatic stress disorder) and after enlistment (such as depression) had a greater risk of a suicide attempt after enlisting in the Army.[33] Surprisingly, investigators found that about one-third of suicide attempts after Army enlistment were related to mental disorders that were present *before* enlistment.[33]

An accompanying editorial by Friedman noted the importance of these studies, which were designed similarly to the famous Framingham Heart Study.[37] This editorial highlighted the surprising findings about increased suicide rates in nondeployed soldiers and the importance of mental disorders that were present *before* Army enlistment.[37] These studies have tremendous potential to better identify personal and environmental factors amenable to prevention, as well as improve screening and treatment for people enlisting in the U.S. Army.[37]

EVIDENCE BASE FOR PREVENTION AND PRACTICE

Reducing Stigma

Research about stigma suggests population-level and individual strategies that have potential to reduce the adverse consequences of stigma related to mental illness.[24] A variety of countries have initiated social marketing campaigns aimed at improving knowledge and attitudes toward mental illness. The "Time to Change" social marketing campaign began in England in 2009. Campaigns in New Zealand called "Like Minds Like Mine," "Opening Minds" in Canada, "One of Us" in Denmark, and "Beyondblue" in Australia are all examples.[24] The major challenge in evaluating these campaigns it the lack of a control group, but the "Time to Change" program in England instead used questions from an ongoing national mental health survey for this purpose. Researchers generally noted "mental health knowledge" predicted two positive outcomes, whether someone intended to get help and whether they wanted to tell family and friends about their illness.[24] In the same study, the study of attitudes toward mental illness was more complicated, but positive attitudes of "tolerance and support for community care" were associated with individuals' intentions to get help for a mental health problem.[24] One specific aspect of the "Time to Change" campaign was to strive for better quality news media coverage of mental health. One study reported a significant increase in "anti-stigmatizing" mental health articles from 2008 to 2011 in local and national newspapers in England.[38]

Other studies in the United States have reported that personal contact or experience with mental illness (including a history of psychiatric hospitalizations in themselves, their family, or their friends) is associated with more positive attitudes (less stigma) towards strangers with mental illness.[39] Boyd and colleagues note that these individuals are a substantial group of people who could help in reducing stigma among the general public.[39]

To determine how public knowledge and attitudes about mental illness were related to "self-stigma" in patients, Evans-Lacko and colleagues studied the association between public perception of mental illness and the presence of "self-stigma" in 1,835 patients with mental health conditions in 14 European countries.[40] Generally, lower rates of self-stigma in people with mental illness were found in countries with better treatment access, available mental health information, and less public stigma.[40] Their findings suggested that efforts to reduce public stigma (such as through public campaigns) may also help in reducing self-stigma in patients with mental illness but must include a comprehensive approach.[40]

Policy Initiatives and Promising Models

The ACA, the 2008 Mental Health Parity Act, and 2014 funding for mental health professional training and state-based initiatives are all examples of recent policy changes to improve access to mental health services.[30,31] The goal of the Wellstone and Domenici Mental Health Parity and Addiction Equity Act of 2008 is to eliminate differences between insurance coverage of physical health care and behavioral health services.[30] The ACA expands Medicaid nationally for people up to 133% of the federal poverty level. In addition, people with incomes as high as 400% of the federal poverty level may receive financial assistance to help them buy insurance through health insurance "exchanges."[30] Other ACA changes prohibiting insurance companies from denying insurance because of "pre-existing" health conditions, including behavioral health in required "essential health benefits" and new grants for educational training, may also contribute positively.[12,30]

However, the multiple funding sources for behavioral health services and the separation of physical health services from behavioral health services creates challenges in shaping policies and developing new models of care to benefit patients.[12,30] Massachusetts's experience with health insurance expansion (that predated the ACA) showed improvements in the percentage of insured young adults. In addition, there were small decreases in inpatient hospital admission rates for any behavioral health diagnosis and also for depression.[41]

In 2014, the Kaiser Commission on Medicaid and the Uninsured reported on "promising Medicaid models" integrating physical and behavioral health care.[12] Five general approaches that were implemented in a variety of different U.S. locations were described: universal screening, use of navigators, co-location, health homes, and system-level integration of care. These different approaches reflect a continuum of health care that ranges from coordination to co-location to totally integrated care.[12] The concept of universal screening means having primary care providers screen for behavioral health disorders using evidence-based approaches and behavioral health providers screening for commonly co-occurring chronic conditions such as high blood pressure, obesity, or pulmonary disorders. The California Institute of Mental Health has adopted this approach, screening patients for chronic disease risks in public behavioral health centers.[12]

"Navigators" are nurses, social workers, or trained professionals that help patients on Medicaid connect to needed services or advocate on their behalf. "Wellness Recovery Teams" in Montgomery County, PA use this approach, identifying patients with SMI and chronic medical conditions and using a team-based approach for behavioral and medical care. In their first 6 months, they noted an 11% decrease in emergency department visits for medical care.[12]

Co-location refers to eliminating the physical separation between physical and behavioral health services such as in Community Health Centers. Golden Valley Health Centers in California is cited as an example of co-located medical and behavioral health services.[12] "Health homes" provide comprehensive services and may be located in community mental health centers for Medicaid patients with SMI; they are eligible for short-term federal financial incentives. Missouri has utilized health homes for nearly 19,000 Medicaid patients with behavioral health diagnoses and noted a 27% decrease in hospitalizations in a 1-year period. Other states, such as Ohio, Iowa, Maryland, and Rhode Island are also currently implementing this approach.[12]

System-level care integration includes financial accountability for the entire range of physical and behavioral health services delivered in a setting or to a defined population.[12] A Medicaid managed care program in Maricopa County, AZ is an example of this model where physical health and behavioral health services for patients with SMI are managed by one entity.[12]

New York State (NYS) is systematically integrating behavioral health care (beginning with patients diagnosed with depression) into primary care settings in some academic medical centers and includes primary care residency training sites.[42] In this project, the NYS Department of Health, in collaboration with the NYS Office of Mental Health is funding academic medical centers who meet specified requirements for patient-centered medical homes. Although early, the NYS Collaborative Care Initiative (CCI) aims to implement evidence-based and fully integrated behavioral and physical health care for Medicaid patients, first starting with patients with depression. In addition, because the sites chosen are also primary care residency training sites, this model of care will become more familiar to physicians in training for primary care specialties.[42] In all of these examples, efforts to systematically integrate mental health, substance abuse, and physical health services are being tested in order to develop successful models that can be used in a variety of settings and geographic locations, all to improve patient outcomes.

DISCUSSION QUESTIONS: TEMPLATE FOR DISCUSSION

1. Significance of this public health issue:
   a. Why is this health issue important?
   b. How many people does it impact?
   c. How serious is it?
   d. Is it preventable?
2. What is the evidence base for prevention?
3. What specific strategies should be used to achieve progress on this health issue?
   a. What evidence-based approach would you use?
   b. Where would you start if you are an individual citizen; public health professional; healthcare professional; community, state, or federal policymaker?
4. Specific questions for this topic:
   a. Why is stigma about mental illness still present in the United States?
   b. What barriers prevent people from receiving treatment for mental illness?
   c. What is the role of surveillance data and public education about mental illness in overall public health strategies?
5. What is the controversy?
   a. Define the controversy.
   b. Is controversy a good or bad thing? (Does it help or hinder progress?)

6. *Why* is this health issue controversial?
   a. What specific factors are involved?
   b. Do economics, government, scientific uncertainty, or politics play a role?
   c. What is the role of the media?
7. How would you respond to the controversy?

PERSPECTIVES TO CONSIDER

Mental health, as a public health issue, has a long history. In 2009, in the United States, more than 60% of people with *any* mental illness did not receive treatment.[43] Even worse, the fact that 40% of patients with SMI do not access treatment, despite scientific advances, underscores the complexity of this problem and the many barriers to progress.[13]

Mental health and physical health continue to be viewed differently, and many areas of stigma remain. Barriers include financial ones (despite recent policy changes) and shortages of mental health professionals, especially psychiatrists.[32] Financing for behavioral health services is an amalgam of public, private, and other funding sources, making system-wide changes complex.[30] Large recent reductions in state mental health budgets exacerbate the problems and result in emergency departments becoming a source of care for many patients.[6] Chronic health conditions pose an especially large risk for people with SMI, who die years earlier than people in the general population with these same conditions.[12] Suicide remains a public health crisis among many age groups in the United States and on a global scale.[15,19]

What promising approaches are on the horizon? Challenges to health provider shortages may be ameliorated in part by new models of care that utilize a patient-centered and team-based approach, including nurse practitioners, social workers, and other healthcare professionals.[12] New pilot models to integrate mental health and physical health services in the United States are promising, and if successful, can be expanded to other locations. These models range from examples of universal screening, use of navigators, health homes, and co-location, to system-level integration of care, and some include teaching these concepts in the training of physicians.[12] Importantly, campaigns in England, New Zealand, Canada, Denmark, and Australia[24,38,40] may provide insights into strategies to reduce stigma, a longstanding barrier to mental health care at the level of the patient, community, and society as a whole.

For Additional Study

Nardone M, Snyder S, Paradise J. Integrating physical and behavioral health care: Promising Medicaid models. 2014. http://kff.org/medicaid/issue-brief/integrating-physical-and behavioral-healthcare-promisingmedicaid-models/.

References

1. Horowitz A. U.S. mental healthcare system failing patients, advocates say. *Huffington Post.* 2013. http://www.huffingtonpost.com/2012/12/26/us-mental-healthcaresystem_n_2353319.html. Accessed March 7, 2014.
2. CBS News: 60 Minutes. Nowhere to go: Mentally ill youth in crisis. Pelley S, ed. 2014.
3. Jain S. Understanding lack of access to mental healthcare in the US: 3 lessons from the Gus Deeds story. *PLOS Blogs.* http://blogs.plos.org/mindthebrain/2014/02/06/understanding-lack-access-mental-healthcare-3-lessons-gus-deeds-story/ 2014. Accessed March 7, 2014.
4. Kennedy K. Health law may not broaden access to mental treatment. *USA Today.* 2013. http://www.usatoday.com/story/news/politics/2013/12/29/only-half-of-mental-health-docs-take-insurance/4206239/. Accessed March 7, 2014.
5. Epright MC, Sade RM. Conundrums and controversies in mental health and illness. *J Law Med Eth.* 2010;38(4):722–726.
6. Glover RW. Proceedings on the state budget crisis and the behavioral health treatment gap: The impact on public substance abuse and mental health treatment systems. 2012. http://www.nasmhpd.org/docs/Summary-Congressional%20Briefing_March%2022_Website.pdf. Accessed March 7, 2014.
7. NAMI. Grading the states 2009: A report on America's health care system for adults with serious mental illness. 2009. https://www.nami.org/gtsTemplate09.cfm?Section=Grading_the_States_2009. Accessed March 7, 2014.
8. NAMI. Mental illness: Facts and numbers. 2013. http://www.nami.org/factsheets/mentalillness_factsheet.pdf. Accessed March 7, 2014.
9. Kennedy K. Controversy plagues school mental health screening. *USA Today.* 2014. http://www.usatoday.com/story/news/nation/2014/01/13/school-mental-health-screening/4454223/. Accessed March 7, 2014.
10. CDC. Fact Sheet: Mental illness surveillance among U.S. adults. 2011. http://www.cdc.gov/mentalhealthsurveillance/documents/MentalIllnessSurveillance_FactSheet.pdf. Accessed March 7, 2014.
11. CDC. Mental illness surveillance among adults in the United States. *MMWR.* 2011. Accessed March 7, 2014.
12. Nardone M, Snyder S, Paradise J. Integrating physical and behavioral health care: Promising Medicaid models. 2014. http://kff.org/medicaid/issue-brief/integrating-physical-and-behavioral-health-care-promising-medicaid-models/. Accessed March 7, 2014.
13. NIMH. National Institute of Mental Health: Statistics 2012. http://www.nimh.nih.gov/Statistics/index.shtml. Accessed March 7, 2014.
14. SAMSHA. State estimates of adult mental illness. *The NSDUH Report.* 2012. http://www.samhsa.gov/data/2k11/WEB_SR_078/SR110StateSMIAMI2012.htm. Accessed March 7, 2014.

15. CDC. Suicide: Facts at a glance. 2012. http://www.cdc.gov/violenceprevention/pdf/Suicide-DataSheet-a.pdf. Accessed March 7, 2014.

16. CDC. CDC Features: Preventing suicide. 2013. http://www.cdc.gov/features/PreventingSuicide/. Accessed March 7, 2014.

17. CDC. Suicide prevention. 2013. http://www.cdc.gov/ViolencePrevention/suicide/index.html. Accessed March 7, 2014.

18. American Foundation for Suicide Prevention: Facts and figures. 2014. http://www.afsp.org/understanding-suicide/facts-and-figures. Accessed March 7, 2014.

19. WHO. Suicide 2014. http://www.who.int/mediacentre/factsheets/fs398/en/. Accessed October 2, 2014.

20. WHO. Age-standardized suicide rates (per 100,000) population, both sexes, 2012. 2014. http://gamapserver.who.int/mapLibrary/Files/Maps/Global_AS_suicide_rates_bothsexes_2012.png?ua=1. Accessed October 2, 2014.

21. National Suicide Prevention Lifeline. 2014. http://www.suicidepreventionlifeline.org/. Accessed March 7, 2014.

22. D'Onofrio BM, Rickert ME, Frans E, et al. Paternal age at childbearing and offspring psychiatric and academic morbidity. *JAMA Psychiatry*. 2014;71(4):432–438.

23. McGrath JJ, Petersen L, Agerbo E, Mors O, Mortensen PB, Pedersen CB. A comprehensive assessment of parental age and psychiatric disorders. *JAMA Psychiatry*. Jan 22 2014;71(3):301–309.

24. Henderson C, Evans-Lacko S, Thornicroft G. Mental illness stigma, help seeking, and public health programs. *Am J Public Health*. 2013;103(5):777–780.

25. Mientka M. Mental health illness stigma is a consistent barrier to accessing treatment, even outside the US. *Medical Daily*. 2014. http://www.medicaldaily.com/mental-health-illness-stigma-consistent-barrier-accessing-treatment-even-outside-us-270098. Accessed March 7, 2014.

26. Corrigan PW, Rao D. On the self-stigma of mental illness: stages, disclosure, and strategies for change. *Can J Psych*. 2012;57(8):464–469.

27. Davey GCL. Mental health and stigma. *Psychology Today Blog*. August 20, 2013. https://www.psychologytoday.com/blog/why-we-worry/201308/mental-health-stigma Accessed March 7, 2014.

28. Stigma 'key deterrent' in accessing mental health care. *Kings College London News*. 2014. https://www.kcl.ac.uk/iop/news/records/2014/February/Stigma-key-deterrent-in-accessing-mental-health-care.aspx. Accessed March 7, 2014.

29. Clement S, Schauman O, Graham T, et al. What is the impact of mental health-related stigma on help-seeking? A systematic review of quantitative and qualitative studies. *Psych Med*. 2014:1–17.

30. Garfield RL. Mental health financing in the United States: A primer. 2011. http://kaiserfamilyfoundation.files.wordpress.com/2013/01/8182.pdf. Accessed March 7, 2014.

31. Feldman S. New funding to increase access to mental health services and new protections under the health care law. *The White House Blog*. February 18, 2014. http://www.whitehouse.gov/blog/2014/02/18/new-funding-increase-access-mental-health-services-and-new-protections-under-health- Accessed March 7, 2014.

32. Bishop TF, Press MJ, Keyhani S, Pincus HA. Acceptance of insurance by psychiatrists and the implications for access to mental health care. *JAMA Psychiatry*. 2014;71(2): 176–181.

33. Nock MK, Stein MB, Heeringa SG, et al. Prevalence and correlates of suicidal behavior among soldiers: Results from the Army Study to Assess Risk and Resilience in Servicemembers (Army STARRS). *JAMA Psychiatry.* 2014;71(5):514–522.

34. Kessler RC, Heeringa SG, Stein MB, et al. Thirty-day prevalence of DSM-IV mental disorders among nondeployed soldiers in the US Army: Results from the Army Study to Assess Risk and Resilience in Servicemembers (Army STARRS). *JAMA Psychiatry.* 2014;71(5):504–513.

35. Schoenbaum M, Kessler RC, Gilman SE, et al. Predictors of suicide and accident death in the Army Study to Assess Risk and Resilience in Servicemembers (Army STARRS): Results From the Army Study to Assess Risk and Resilience in Servicemembers (Army STARRS). *JAMA Psychiatry.* 2014;71(5):493–503.

36. Willingham V. Study: Rates of many mental disorders much higher in soldiers than in civilians. *CNN.com.* 2014. http://www.cnn.com/2014/03/03/health/jama-military-mental-health/. Accessed March 7 2914.

37. Friedman MJ. Suicide risk among soldiers: Early findings from Army Study to Assess Risk and Resilience in Servicemembers (Army STARRS). *JAMA Psychiatry.* 2014;71(5):487–489.

38. Thornicroft A, Goulden R, Shefer G, et al. Newspaper coverage of mental illness in England 2008–2011. *Brit J Psych.* 2013;55:s64–69.

39. Boyd JE, Katz EP, Link BG, Phelan JC. The relationship of multiple aspects of stigma and personal contact with someone hospitalized for mental illness, in a nationally representative sample. *Soc Psych Psych Epid.* 2010;45(11):1063–1070.

40. Evans-Lacko S, Brohan E, Mojtabai R, Thornicroft G. Association between public views of mental illness and self-stigma among individuals with mental illness in 14 European countries. *Psych Med.* 2012;42(8):1741–1752.

41. Meara E, Golberstein E, Zaha R, Greenfield SF, Beardslee WR, Busch SH. Use of hospital-based services among young adults with behavioral health diagnoses before and after health insurance expansions. *JAMA Psychiatry.* 2014;71(4):404–411.

42. Sederer LI. What does it take for primary care practices to truly deliver behavioral health care? *JAMA Psychiatry.* 2014;71(5):485–486.

43. SAMSHA. Mental Health, United States, 2010. 2010. http://www.samhsa.gov/data/2k12/MHUS2010/MHUS-2010.pdf. Accessed October 2, 2014.

CHAPTER 12

Immunizations—Parent Choice vs. Public Health

LEARNING OBJECTIVES

- Explain the public health impact of vaccines on vaccine-preventable diseases in the United States.
- Describe trends in immunization rates and identify population(s) at risk.
- Describe changes in the epidemiology of vaccine-preventable diseases.
- Evaluate the role of the Internet and social media in parent decisions about vaccines.
- Discuss the role of health professionals in parent decisions about vaccines.
- Identify evidence-based strategies to improve immunization rates in children and adolescents in the United States.

THE CONTROVERSY

In 2014, the Centers for Disease Control and Prevention reported 288 cases of measles between January 1 and May 23, 2014 (including an outbreak in progress in Ohio), the highest total in 20 years.[1] The vast majority of patients were unvaccinated (nearly 70%) or their vaccination status was not known (20%).[1] One major outbreak was in an Ohio Amish community where four unvaccinated community members had traveled to the Philippines (where measles is an epidemic) on a service mission and returned with the infection.[2,3] In six Ohio counties, 164 measles cases were reported and more than 8,000 Amish people willingly came to free vaccination clinics offered by the Ohio Department of Health.[2,3] In 2013, a Texas megachurch experienced 21 measles cases, mostly among its unvaccinated members, after a person traveling to Indonesia contracted the infection and visited the church.[4]

Measles (rubeola) is a highly contagious viral infection. Before 1963, when measles vaccine was first introduced, it was responsible for 30% of all deaths from vaccine-preventable diseases. Additionally, 1 in 1,000 children developed encephalitis, a swelling of the brain.[5,6] Each year in the United States in the 1950s and early 1960s, there were 3 to 4 million measles infections, 400 to 500 deaths, 48,000 hospitalizations, and 1,000 people disabled for life as a result of measles encephalitis.[6] In 2000, CDC reported measles elimination in the United States, but measles cases imported from other areas of the world continue and outbreaks in the United States are most often in people who are not vaccinated.[1]

In 1998, Dr. Wakefield and colleagues' paper in *The Lancet* entitled "Ileal-lymphoid-nodular hyperplasia, non-specific colitis, and pervasive developmental disorder in children," concluded, "We identified associated gastrointestinal disease and developmental regression in a group of previously normal children, which was generally associated in time with possible environmental triggers."[7] The paper, which suggested a link between MMR (measles, mumps, rubella) vaccine and autism ignited concerns among parents about vaccine safety that was critical to subsequently organized anti-vaccination efforts.[8] In a 2004 *Lancet* article, 10 of the 12 original authors retracted the interpretation of their data, stating "no causal link was established between MMR vaccine and autism as the data were insufficient."[9] A statement by *The Lancet* editors in the same issue of the 2004 journal published six allegations of research misconduct, including questions about ethics, selection of research subjects, potential conflicts of interest, and the authors' responses.[10] The editors wrote, "we have decided to pursue a course of full disclosure and transparency concerning these allegations, the authors' responses, the institution's judgment, and our evaluation."[10]

But the damage had already been done. MMR vaccination rates plummeted in the United Kingdom, from more than 90% before 1998 to less than 80% in 2004.[11] Ultimately, following the conclusions of the United Kingdom General Medical Council's Fitness to Practise Panel, the editors of *The Lancet* retracted Wakefield's 1998 paper.[12]

This was not the only controversy regarding vaccines and links to autism. From 1999 to 2000, thimerosal (a mercury-containing preservative) was removed from nearly all vaccines despite the fact there were no scientific studies supporting harmful effects.[13] "Green Our Vaccines," a celebrity-supported and highly visible campaign to remove "toxins" from vaccines was also launched. Earlier, DTP (diphtheria, tetanus, and pertussis) vaccine was the subject of a 1982 documentary, "DPT Vaccination Roulette," and a 1991 book, *A Shot in the Dark*, detailed claims of health risks from the vaccine.[13] The President of the National Vaccine Information Center (NVIC) at the 2008 "Rally for Conscientious Exemption to Vaccination" said, "No American should be legally forced to play vaccine roulette with a child's life . . ."[14]

A 2010 California pertussis (whooping cough) outbreak responsible for 9,120 cases and 10 deaths was at least partially attributed to groups of people (called *exemption clusters*) who refused vaccination.[15,16] And in 2014, *USA Today* wrote the "Anti-vaccine movement is giving diseases a second life," highlighting the vulnerability of infants, who are too young to be vaccinated.[17] In 2014, the American Academy of Arts and Sciences recommended more research about how parents make vaccine decisions.[18]

BACKGROUND AND SCOPE OF THE PUBLIC HEALTH AND HEALTH POLICY ISSUE

Vaccines and their role in disease prevention have been cited by the Centers for Disease Control and Prevention (CDC) as one of the "Ten Great Public Health Achievements."[19] As of 2011, 17 diseases were the focus of prevention efforts using both new and older vaccines, immunization programs, and policies.[19] For example, from 2000 to 2008, pneumococcal conjugate vaccine prevented more than 200,000 infections and 13,000 deaths.[19] In the 20th century, between 95% and 100% reductions in deaths and illness have been documented in nine vaccine-preventable diseases: smallpox, diphtheria, pertussis, tetanus, paralytic poliomyelitis, measles, mumps, rubella, and *Haemophilus influenza* type b (Hib) infections.[20,21]

Haemophilus influenza bacteria (including Hib), in addition to ear infections, can cause serious bacterial diseases, called "invasive disease," including such epiglottitis, arthritis, blood infections, skin infections, pneumonia, and meningitis.[22,23] The development and widespread use of Hib vaccine has resulted in a 99% reduction in invasive Hib disease.[23] In contrast, before the vaccine was available, young children in the United States experienced an estimated 20,000 serious Hib infections

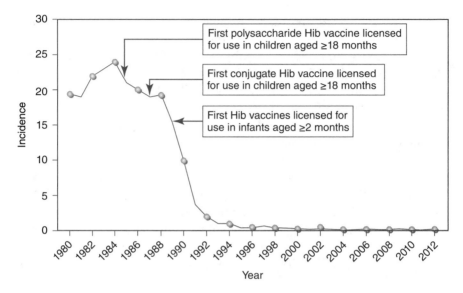

Figure 12–1 Estimated annual incidence of invasive *Haemophilus influenzae* type b (Hib) disease in children aged <5 years—United States, 1980–2012.

Reproduced from Centers for Disease Control and Prevention. Briere EC RL, Moro PL, Cohn A, Clark T, Messonnier N. Prevention and Control of Haemophilus influenzae Type b Disease: Recommendations of the Advisory Committee on Immunization Practices (ACIP). *MMWR*. 2014. Available at http://www.cdc.gov/mmwr/preview/ mmwrhtml/rr6301a1.htm

each year, with 3–6% dying from them. Furthermore, before the vaccine, Hib infection was the most common cause of bacterial meningitis in young children.[22-24] Following the introduction and use of the Hib vaccine, during 1989 to 2000, rates of invasive Hib infections in young children dropped by 99%, and remained at a low level from 2000 to 2012.[23] (see **Figure 12–1**).

Overall, the adverse public health impact of most vaccine-preventable diseases has been greatly reduced or eliminated altogether in the last 50 years.[25] However during the period from 2000 to 2010, despite dramatic declines in rates of most vaccine-preventable diseases, changes occurred in patterns of some diseases that prompted further improvements in vaccines or vaccination policy. For example, waning immunity from pertussis vaccine (to prevent whooping cough) resulted in a development of a new vaccine that could be used in older children, adolescents, and adults.[25] Successful immunity to varicella (chicken pox) was determined to require two shots, and recommendations were changed.[25] Measles cases doubled in 2008, concentrated in intentionally unvaccinated children, as rates of vaccination exemptions as a result of personal beliefs increased.[25] In addition, experts cite potential benefits of the Patient Protection and Affordable Care Act (ACA) for improving immunization rates in both children and adults through improved access to preventive health care.[25]

Information about U.S. vaccination rates and policies can be found on the CDC website.[24] The CDC website contains information for health professionals and the public about the rationale for immunization, vaccine safety and side-effects, vaccine-preventable diseases, immunization rates, immunization schedules, and requirements and laws.[24] The site also contains information for the public and health professionals about the Vaccine Adverse Event Reporting System (VAERS), a national safety monitoring system of both CDC and Food and Drug Administration (FDA), that collects information about adverse events or possible side effects that occur after someone has received a vaccine. Data are used to identify risks, track additional side effects, and if needed, to make changes to national vaccine recommendations.[24]

Project Tycho, published in 2013 (and also made publically available), compiled digitized weekly CDC *Morbidity and Mortality Weekly Reports* (MMWR) of nationally notifiable diseases in all U.S. cities and states from 1888 to 2011.[26] A total of 87,950,807 individual reports of diseases with location and time (week) were presented. In addition, the investigators chose seven vaccine-preventable diseases for additional analysis (polio, measles, rubella, mumps, hepatitis A, diphtheria, and pertussis), and used the year that vaccines against these diseases were licensed, to determine the extent of disease prevention due to vaccine use.[26] The authors estimated that 103.1 million cases of these infectious diseases had been prevented since 1924 due to vaccines, with an estimated 25% (26 million cases) prevented in the last 10 years.[26] Furthermore, about 40 million diphtheria cases were prevented (since 1924), followed by 35 million cases of measles (since 1963).[26] The authors concluded that vaccination programs contributed to dramatic declines in these diseases.[26]

Trends in Immunization Rates

CDC publishes immunization schedules for infants and children (birth through age 6), preteens and teens (age 7 through 18), and adults (age 19 and older).[24] The Advisory Committee on Immunization Practices

(ACIP) is a group of 15 experts (14 from medicine, nursing, public health, or scientific experts, and 1 consumer representative) who make recommendations about vaccines in the United States.[24] For example, currently, MMR vaccine is recommended at age 12–15 months and a second dose at 4–6 years of age.[24]

CDC (through the MMWR) reports rates of immunizations among very young children, aged 19–35 months, using information from the National Immunization Survey (NIS), a telephone survey.[27] Across the United States in 2012, immunization rates were near or above the goal of 90% for MMR, poliovirus vaccine, hepatitis B vaccine, and varicella vaccine.[27] However, vaccination rates vary by state, and when looking at combined vaccination recommendations for this age group in 2013, Alaska (59.5%) has the lowest coverage rate and Hawaii (80.2%) the highest.[27] In addition to geographic differences, rates of immunization against many vaccine-preventable diseases were lower for children and families living below the poverty level.[27]

Vaccination rates for school-aged children and adolescents also vary geographically.[28,29] CDC regularly publishes vaccination rates for children entering school in the United States using a sample or census of children in public and private school kindergartens but not home-schooled children.[28] Children are considered "up-to-date" on their vaccinations if they have received all required immunizations for school entry, which may vary in different geographic locations. Information on immunization exemptions is also collected including medical, religious, or philosophical.[28]

For the 2012–2013 school year, among 48 states and the District of Columbia, who reported vaccination rates in their kindergarten populations, examples of vaccination rates for the recommended two doses of MMR vaccine was 94.5% overall, varying from a low of 85.7% in Colorado to a high of more than 99.9% in Mississippi.[28] Rates for DTP vaccine were 95.1% overall, with a low of 82.9% in Colorado to more than 99.9% in Mississippi.[28]

For vaccine exemptions, of a total population of 4,242,558 children in kindergarten, there were approximately 91,453 exemptions, ranging from less than 0.1% in Mississippi to 6.5% in Oregon, with an average of 1.8% exemptions overall.[28] CDC notes that even though overall immunization rates may be high, they may mask local "clusters" of unvaccinated children that may put children at risk for vaccine-preventable diseases.[28,30] Regarding exemptions, CDC emphasizes that children

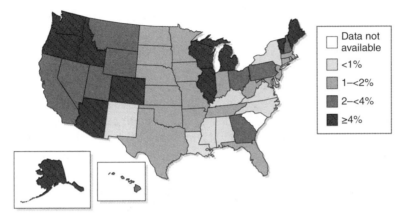

Figure 12–2 Estimated percentage of children enrolled in kindergarten who have been exempted from receiving one or more vaccines—United States, 2012–2013 school year.

Reproduced from Centers for Disease Control and Prevention. CDC. Vaccination Coverage Among Children in Kindergarten—United States, 2012–13 School Year. MMWR. 2013. Available at http://www.cdc.gov/mmwr/preview/mmwrhtml/mm6230a3.htm.

with exemptions may still receive one or more vaccines, and more exemptions are typically found in areas where gaining exemptions is easier[28] (see **Figure 12–2**).

Vaccination Policy and Trends in Exemptions

State laws requiring immunizations for school entry have been cited as a critical factor in assuring high rates of childhood immunization.[31] All states allow medical exemptions, such as for children with severe allergies or weakened immune systems, 48 states allow religious exemptions, and 20 states allow philosophical or personal belief exemptions, as of January 2014.[24]

A 2006 study examined whether or not nonmedical exemptions for required immunizations were increasing in the United States, especially in states where the exemptions are easier to obtain. The investigators also studied whether increases in pertussis were related to exemption rates.[32] They found vaccination exemption rates were higher in states that allowed "personal belief" exemptions and in states that granted them easily.[32] In states that allowed personal belief exemptions, exemption rates increased from less than 1% in 1991 to 2.54% in 2004, and increased from 1.26% in 1991 to 2.51% in 2004 in states that easily granted them.[32] Exemption rates and ease of obtaining exemptions were also related to increases in pertussis.[32] A later study from 2005 to 2011 affirmed these findings. This study assessed changes in nonmedical (philosophical or personal belief) exemptions, as well as whether the impact of administrative ease or difficulty in getting a nonmedical exemption ultimately influenced the number of exemptions.[33] Rates of nonmedical exemptions increased: nonmedical exemptions were 2.5 times higher in states that allowed philosophical exemptions than in states allowing only religious exemptions. In addition, the ease of getting an exemption also influenced exemption rates: exemptions were 2.3 times higher in states with easier rather than more difficult administrative exemption requirements.[33]

How do these research studies relate to current efforts to change vaccination policy? Using data from the Immunization Action Coalition (IAC), a nonprofit organization working closely with CDC to educate health professionals about vaccine recommendations,[34] Omer and colleagues studied state legislation introduced between 2009 and 2012 proposing personal belief exemptions and the difficulty or ease of their administrative requirements.[31] During this time, 18 states introduced legislation related to immunization exemptions. Proposed legislation varied in terms of how easy or difficult it was to gain an exemption. Administrative requirements included such steps as using a health department form, requirements for education or signature from a healthcare professional, notarization, time limits on the exemption, or others.[31] Of the 36 total bills introduced in these states, 14 (39%) had 3 to 5 administrative requirements, 7 (19%) had 1 or 2 administrative requirements, and 15 (42%) had no administrative requirements at all.[31] The website of the National Conference of State Legislatures (NCSL) summed up the challenges of state legislators, as "They are asked to balance the need to protect the public's health against the difficulties presented by funding the recommended vaccines and addressing concerns of citizens who may object to mandatory immunization recommendations."[35]

Information about Vaccines—the Role of the Internet

Internet usage, including searching for health-related information, is increasingly common. One estimate of the prevalence of general use of the Internet is 74% for Americans and 72% for Canadians, with up to 80% of people looking for online health information and nearly three-quarters of them using what they found to help make health decisions.[36] In one interesting study, investigators Google-searched for immunization Internet sites and evaluated themes found on sites opposing childhood vaccination.[36] Researchers found more anti-vaccination websites for the United States. If the term "immunization" was used, 100% of the sites were supportive or "pro-vaccination," whereas use of the term "vaccine" produced 25% "anti-vaccination" sites and the word "vaccination" resulted in 71% anti-vaccination sites.[36] Common themes on the anti-vaccination sites included: safety and effectiveness, conspiracies, alternative medicine, ideology, and civil liberties. Website designs commonly included emotional appeals, personal stories, and graphic visuals; inaccurate information was common.[36]

Another extensive study explained strategies, tactics, and "tropes" used by individuals and groups opposing childhood vaccinations.[37] For example, categories such as "skewing the science" (rejecting current scientific evidence) and "shifting hypotheses" (suggesting new theories) were commonly noted on anti-vaccination sites, as well as "attacking the opposition." "Tropes" or common phrases, arguments, or mottos included such statements as "I'm an expert on my own child," "vaccines are toxic," "vaccines are unnatural," "choosing between diseases and vaccine injuries," and "you can't prove vaccines are safe."[37]

Some Internet sites questioning or opposing childhood vaccinations are clear in their position: the Vermont Coalition for Vaccine Choice website promotes, "It's a human right" and characterizes vaccines as "injectable, for-profit pharmaceutical products."[38] Vactruth.com states, "Discover what your doctor injects into your child."[39] Another site claims, "Kids given vaccines have 22 times the rate of ear infections.[40] The National Vaccine Information Center (NVIC), founded in 1982, states its mission is "dedicated to the prevention of vaccine injuries and deaths through public education and to defending the informed consent ethic in medicine."[41] Their site says they are not advocating for or against vaccines, but for "the right of consumers to make educated, voluntary healthcare choices," and their title includes "Your Health. Your Family. Your Choice."[41]

A study of parents in 2002 and 2003 found that younger parents with more education and who opposed school requirements for childhood vaccination were more likely to use the Internet for health information about vaccines.[42] Internet vaccine information seekers were also less likely to believe vaccines were safe and effective, and their children more often had nonmedical vaccine exemptions.[42] Other authors note that Web 2.0 applications, such as social media, provide challenges of scientific misinformation "virally" spreading, but these applications also afford opportunities for public health professionals to provide education and engage parents.[43]

Price as a Barrier to Childhood Immunizations

An article in *The New York Times* highlights the impact of rising vaccine prices as a barrier to immunizations for some children and families.[44] An example from San Antonio, TX details the challenges of some physicians being able to purchase and keep vaccines in their practices due to the rising prices.[44] In a national survey, as many as 44% of family physicians sent children and adolescent patients elsewhere for some vaccines.[45] One physician noted that "Those (vaccines) in the refrigerator recently cost $70,000 more than I paid for 4 years of medical school."[44] This situation makes it challenging for some families in some locations to easily find immunizations for their children.[44] According to CDC, improvements in older vaccines and the development of new ones, have resulted in increased costs (from $100 to $2,192) to vaccinate a child with private insurance to age 18, since the mid-1980s.[44]

EVIDENCE BASE FOR PREVENTION AND PRACTICE

How Do Parents Make Decisions about Immunizations?

A review of reasons for parental "vaccine hesitancy" identified factors potentially contributing to parental concerns about childhood immunizations.[46] For example, concerns about the role of pharmaceutical companies, interest in "natural" treatments, perceptions of the likelihood of risk for side effects, and ease of finding both accurate and inaccurate information on the Internet were all cited.[46] In addition, parents' changing and more active role in healthcare decision making is likely important.[46]

A national telephone survey of 1,600 parents with young children, published in 2000, found that most respondents supported the importance of childhood immunization in children's health.[47] However, a substantial number of respondents (25%) felt that too many immunizations actually weakened a child's immune system and nearly a quarter (23%) also believed children receive too many vaccines.[47] An online survey published in 2010 tried to determine how parents' concerns about vaccines ultimately influenced their decisions to immunize their children.[48] In this survey, although 90% of respondents agreed that vaccines were "a good way to protect my children from disease," 54% of responding parents were concerned about "serious adverse effects of vaccines," 25% agreed that "some vaccines cause autism in healthy children," and 11% agreed that children don't need vaccines for diseases that are no longer frequently seen.[48] Overall, 11.5% had ever refused a vaccine for their child, with highest refusal rates seen for MMR, varicella, meningococcal conjugate, or HPV vaccines.[48]

In another large study of 11,206 parents whose children were between the ages of 2 and 3 during the 2009 National Immunization Survey interview, researchers evaluated the impact of the beliefs of parents who either delayed or refused specific vaccines for their children.[49] In this study, 25.8% of parents delayed some vaccines, 8% refused some vaccines, and about 6% did both. Three important beliefs associated with children's vaccine status included whether or not parents believed "vaccines are necessary to protect the health of children," "if I do not vaccinate my child he/she may get a disease," or whether "vaccines are safe."[49] Compared to parents whose children were up-to-date for all recommended vaccines (60% of parents in the survey), parents who refused or delayed vaccines were significantly *less* likely to believe these three statements, and vaccination rates were significantly lower for all 10 childhood vaccines in their children.[49]

A 2013 study in North Carolina of 1,847 children up to age 18 found that 12% of parents refused or delayed a vaccine. Safety concerns (34%) were the most common reason for nonvaccination and a substantial percentage of parents (18%) did not believe the vaccine was needed.[50] In addition, investigators noted that parents in higher socioeconomic groups and those very focused on other areas of their children's health, specifically nutrition, were also more likely to refuse vaccines.[50] In Washington State, refusing vaccines was also associated with refusing topical fluoride in dental clinics.[51]

In Oregon, researchers surveyed nearly 3,000 parents of children who were elementary school aged in 2004–2005 to identify factors related to parents' decisions to exempt their children from vaccines.[52] Parents who exempted children from vaccines were significantly more likely to have vaccine concerns, not trust physicians, and use chiropractic health care for their children.[52] In addition, in a geographic analysis, the level of exemptions in a community, or "community norms," were found to influence vaccination decisions.[52]

Because narratives (stories) are so commonly found on the Internet, a novel study of German university students investigated the impact of reading online narratives on vaccine perceptions and intention to vaccinate.[53] Using an online bulletin board to portray both statistical information about risk and narratives that described adverse events from vaccines, the researchers conducted a series of experiments. Narratives were important in how study participants perceived vaccine risks. Narratives that were more emotional had a bigger impact.[53] In addition, the numbers of narratives describing negative effects were related to the intention to vaccinate, with greater numbers of these narratives associated with less intention to vaccinate.[53] Other investigators describing the limitations of this experiment conducted on university students called for more research using actual decision makers for children and simulating realistic online interactions.[54]

Disease Outbreaks

A 2010 outbreak of pertussis was attributed in part to clusters of children with nonmedical exemptions (NMEs) to vaccination, as clusters of children with NMEs were statistically associated with clusters of pertussis.[16] In addition, children with pertussis were less likely to have received all five recommended doses of pertussis vaccine or it had been a long time since their fifth dose.[55] Pertussis is challenging and experts note that pertussis immunization or even the disease itself does not produce lifelong immunity.[56] The current acellular pertussis vaccine (DTaP) is less "potent" than the prior DTP.[56] In addition, some authors suggest the potential for genetic changes in the bacteria that cause pertussis as another contributing factor.[56,57]

The Ohio measles outbreak in 2014 was the largest in the United States since 1996.[58] CDC reported a 2013 measles outbreak in Brooklyn, NY in members of a religious community beginning after a 17-year-old intentionally unvaccinated adolescent returned to NY from London infected with measles.[59] Fifty-eight people were infected with measles including unvaccinated family members and children whose vaccination was delayed.[59] Another 2013 outbreak of measles that infected 23 people began in unvaccinated travelers to India, where they contracted the disease. Most of the people infected were part of a rural North Carolina religious community in which many people were unvaccinated.[60]

In 2008, the largest measles outbreak since 1991 impacted San Diego, CA originating from an unvaccinated child returning from Switzerland, where he acquired the infection.[61] Researchers mapped geographic areas where children were intentionally unvaccinated to determine whether clusters of unvaccinated children were important in this outbreak. Twelve people developed measles and more than 800 people were exposed.[61]

Nine individuals with measles were intentionally unvaccinated; 48 cases were in children too young to be vaccinated. Using mapping, clusters of individuals refusing vaccines can be seen in specific geographic areas, as well as in private or public charter schools, and represent people, families, or entire communities at risk for infection.[61]

CDC's analysis of measles in the United States in the first half of 2014 showed that of the 288 cases, 97% were imported from 18 countries, with about half of the infections contracted in the Philippines.[1] Nearly 70% of infected people were unvaccinated, and an additional 20% had unknown vaccination status.[1] Among the 165 unvaccinated people with measles, 85% were not vaccinated because of personal objections, religious reasons, or philosophical reasons, and some were too young to be vaccinated.[1] Other areas in the United States have demonstrated increased risks in areas of geographic clusters of unvaccinated individuals, such as pertussis in Michigan and Colorado and measles in Washington State.[62]

Conversely, in response to a pertussis outbreak in England that included illness and deaths in young infants, a vaccination program for pregnant women began in the fall of 2012.[63] In evaluating the program, researchers compared pertussis cases and hospitalizations in 2013 to the same time period in 2012. They found the largest drop in pertussis cases, as well as hospitalizations, occurred in very young infants, and attributed to effectiveness of the vaccine and the program.[63] Vaccinating pregnant women, in this study, conferred about 90% protection to infants, representing the first documentation of the effectiveness of this approach on a national level.[63]

Health Professionals and Parent Decision Making

Healthcare providers are the most frequent source of information about vaccinations, as noted by parents of both vaccinated and unvaccinated children.[62] There is not much scientific literature about health professionals or health professional students and their knowledge, attitudes, and beliefs about immunizations or what impact these factors may have on immunization rates. However, one systematic review from 2013 summarized studies about healthcare workers' intention to vaccinate and their knowledge, beliefs, and attitudes in developed countries.[64] Fifteen studies met the author's criteria for inclusion. In all studies, beliefs that fit with available scientific evidence and showed positive attitudes about vaccination were associated with higher rates of intention to vaccinate by the health professionals. However, the limitations of these studies was their cross-sectional design, making it impossible to establish cause and effect.[64]

In a study of healthcare professionals, 551 primary care providers in Colorado, Massachusetts, Missouri, and Washington returned mail surveys asking about their knowledge and attitudes toward vaccines (84.3% response rate). The researchers compared results in providers where children were vaccinated and providers of children whose parents exempted them from vaccination.[65] Providers of children exempt from vaccinations had significantly more concerns about vaccine safety, and were also more likely to believe multiple vaccines adversely affected children's immune systems, immunity from the disease was superior to vaccine-induced immunity, and vaccine side effects are underreported.[65]

A large study of the parents of 7,695 children aged 19–35 months sampled from the National Immunization Survey in 2001 and 2002 looked at the influence of healthcare providers on parents' vaccination decisions.[66] According to parents, 21.5% reported that healthcare providers did not influence their vaccination decisions. In this study, health providers had an important role in parents' decisions to vaccinate their children, even in parents who did not believe vaccines were safe. Of parents who reported that vaccination decisions were influenced by a healthcare provider, immunization rates for their children were 24.1% higher than in children whose parents made decisions independently from healthcare providers.[66] These studies and others that report focus-group discussions between parents and healthcare providers emphasize the importance of clinicians in facilitating discussions about the importance of immunizations and concerns about vaccine risks and safety.[62]

Reduction in the Burden of Vaccine-Preventable Diseases

CDC reminds us of the impact of immunization on vaccine-preventable diseases, especially looking longitudinally. For example, in 1950 there were 5,796 cases of diphtheria and 410 deaths; none have been reported in the United States since 2003.[67] From the Tycho project at the University of Pittsburgh, more than 100 million cases of contagious diseases have been prevented since 1924 by childhood vaccination.[26,68] But, in an article in *Time* magazine called "4 Diseases Making a Comeback Thanks to Anti-Vaxxers," an interactive map of the globe shows in graphic detail—better than statistics and words—the resurgence of vaccine-preventable diseases.[69]

DISCUSSION QUESTIONS: TEMPLATE FOR DISCUSSION

1. Significance of this public health issue:
   a. Why is this health issue important?
   b. How many people does it impact?
   c. How serious is it?
   d. Is it preventable?
2. What is the evidence base for prevention?
3. What specific strategies should be used to achieve progress on this health issue?
   a. What evidence-based approach would you use?
   b. Where would you start if you are an individual citizen; public health professional; healthcare professional; community, state, or federal policymaker?
4. Specific questions for this topic:
   a. How important is the Internet in parental vaccination decisions?
   b. What are the primary concerns of parents who exempt their children from vaccination?
   c. What is the role of health professionals in achieving high population vaccination levels?
5. What is the controversy?
   a. Define the controversy.
   b. Is controversy a good or bad thing? (Does it help or hinder progress?)
6. *Why* is this health issue controversial?
   a. What specific factors are involved?
   b. Do economics, government, scientific uncertainty, or politics play a role?
   c. What is the role of the media?
7. How would you respond to the controversy?

PERSPECTIVES TO CONSIDER

Immunizations against vaccine-preventable diseases are one of public health's greatest achievements, but in recent years vaccines have become increasingly controversial. Dramatic disease declines make it seem that risks for infection are low, even though progress is due to years of systematic prevention and vaccination efforts.[25] There are many contributing factors to the resurgence of vaccine-preventable diseases. These include an organized movement against required vaccines, widespread use of the Internet, and the pace at which information, both accurate and not, spreads through Web-based resources and social media.[36,37,46] State legislatures are struggling with conflicting requests of constituents and public health recommendations and requirements, and the boom in exemptions parallels these state-based discussions.[35] Unfortunately, so does the increase in outbreaks of vaccine-preventable diseases (especially measles) and the risk of clusters of intentionally unvaccinated individuals even with otherwise high overall state vaccination rates.[1,16,61]

Parent concerns span issues of civil liberties, concerns about vaccine safety, beliefs that vaccines are no longer needed, and may even be fueled by celebrity attention.[13] But are decisions about vaccines best approached on the Internet? There is far too little research about conversations between parents and physicians, nurses, and other health professionals. However published studies[66] shed light on the important influence of healthcare professionals in these decisions in educating, and ensuring accurate evidence-based information for parents and families, and in credibly answering questions and concerns.

For Additional Study

van Panhuis WG, Grefenstette J, Jung SY, et al. Contagious diseases in the United States from 1888 to the present. *N Engl J Med.* 2013;369(22):2152–2158.

Siddiqui M, Salmon DA, Omer SB. Epidemiology of vaccine hesitancy in the United States. *Hum Vaccin Immunother.* 2013;9(12):2643–2648.

Kata A. Anti-vaccine activists, Web 2.0, and the postmodern paradigm—an overview of tactics and tropes used online by the anti-vaccination movement. *Vaccine.* May 28 2012;30(25):3778–3789.

References

1. Gastanaduy PA, Redd SB, Fiebelkorn AP, et al. Measles—United States, January 1–May 23, 2014. *MMWR Morb Mortal Wkly Rep.* 2014;63(22):496–499.
2. Harris R. Measles hits Amish communities, and U.S. cases reach 20-year high. *NPR.* 2014. http://www.npr.org/blogs/health/2014/05/29/317045500/measles-hits-amish-communities-and-u-s-cases-reach-20-year-high. Accessed July 1, 2014.
3. Aleccia J. Measles cases in U.S. spike to highest level in 20 years. *NBC News.* 2014. http://www.nbcnews.com/health/health-news/measles-cases-u-s-spike-highest-level-20-years-n117561. Accessed July 1, 2014.
4. Silverman L. Texas megachurch at center of measles outbreak. *NPR.* 2013. http://www.npr.org/2013/09/01/217746942/texas-megachurch-at-center-of-measles-outbreak. Accessed July 1, 2014.

5. Bronfin DR. Childhood immunization controversies: What are parents asking? *Ochsner Journ.* 2008;8(3):151–156.

6. CDC. Measles (rubeola): Measles vaccination. 2014. http://www.cdc.gov/measles/vaccination.html. Accessed July 2, 2014.

7. Wakefield AJ, Murch SH, Anthony A, et al. Ileal-lymphoid-nodular hyperplasia, non-specific colitis, and pervasive developmental disorder in children. *Lancet.* 1998;351(9103):637–641.

8. Olpinski M. Anti-vaccination movement and parental refusals of immunization of children in USA. *Pediatric Polska.* 2012;87(4):381–385.

9. Murch SH, Anthony A, Casson DH, et al. Retraction of an interpretation. *Lancet.* 2004;363(9411):750.

10. Horton R. A statement by the editors of *The Lancet. Lancet.* 2004;363(9411):820–821.

11. Katz SL. Has the measles-mumps-rubella vaccine been fully exonerated? *Pediatrics.* 2006;118(4):1744–1745.

12. Retraction—Ileal-lymphoid-nodular hyperplasia, non-specific colitis, and pervasive developmental disorder in children. *Lancet.* 2010;375(9713):445.

13. History of anti-vaccination movements. 2014. http://www.historyofvaccines.org/content/articles/history-anti-vaccination-movements. Accessed July 1, 2014.

14. Vaccines pros and cons: Should any vaccines be required for children? 2014. http://vaccines.procon.org/view.answers.php?questionID=001606. Accessed July 1, 2014.

15. Healy M. Vaccine refusal linked to California pertussis outbreak. *USA Today.* 2013. http://www.usatoday.com/story/news/nation/2013/09/30/whooping-cough-california/2877343/. Accessed July 1, 2014.

16. Atwell JE, Van Otterloo J, Zipprich J, et al. Nonmedical vaccine exemptions and pertussis in California, 2010. *Pediatrics.* 2013;132(4):624–630.

17. Alcindor Y. Anti-vaccine movement is giving diseases a 2nd life. *USA Today.* 2014. http://www.usatoday.com/story/news/nation/2014/04/06/anti-vaccine-movement-is-giving-diseases-a-2nd-life/7007955/. Accessed July 1, 2014.

18. American Academy report calls for more research on parental decision-making on childhood vaccines. [press release]. *American Academy of Arts & Sciences.* 2014. http://www.amacad.org/content/news/pressReleases.aspx?pr=218. Accessed July 1, 2014.

19. CDC. Ten great public health achievements—United States, 2001–2010. *MMWR.* 2011. http://www.cdc.gov/mmwr/preview/mmwrhtml/mm6019a5.htm. Accessed July 2, 2014.

20. CDC. Ten great public health achievements in the 20th century. 2013. http://www.cdc.gov/about/history/tengpha.htm. Accessed January 31, 2014.

21. CDC. Impact of vaccines in the 20th and 21st centuries. 2011. http://www.cdc.gov/vaccines/pubs/pinkbook/downloads/appendices/G/impact-of-vaccines.pdf. Accessed July 1, 2014.

22. CDC. *Haemophilus influenzae* disease (including Hib): Types of infecions *Haemophilus influenzae* can cause. 2014. http://www.cdc.gov/hi-disease/about/types-infection.html. Accessed October 2, 2014.

23. Briere EC, Rubin L, Moro PL, Cohn A, Clark T, Messonnier N. Prevention and control of *Haemophilus influenzae* Type b disease: Recommendations of the advisory committee on immunization practices (ACIP). *MMWR.* 2014. http://www.cdc.gov/mmwr/preview/mmwrhtml/rr6301a1.htm. Accessed July 2, 2014.

24. CDC. Vaccines and immunizations. 2012. http://www.cdc.gov/vaccines/default.htm. Accessed July 1, 2014.

25. Hinman AR, Orenstein WA, Schuchat A. Vaccine-preventable diseases, immunizations, and MMWR—1961–2011. *MMWR.* 2011. http://www.cdc.gov/mmwr/preview/ mmwrhtml/su6004a9.htm. Accessed July 2, 2014.

26. van Panhuis WG, Grefenstette J, Jung SY, et al. Contagious diseases in the United States from 1888 to the present. *N Engl J Med.* 2013;369(22):2152–2158.

27. CDC. National, state, and local area vaccination coverage among children aged 19–35 months—United States, 2012. *MMWR.* 2013. http://www.cdc.gov/mmwr/ preview/mmwrhtml/mm6236a1.htm. Accessed July 2, 2014.

28. CDC. Vaccination coverage among children in kindergarten—United States, 2012–13 school year. *MMRW.* 2013. http://www.cdc.gov/mmwr/preview/mmwrhtml/ mm6230a3.htm. Accessed July 2, 2014.

29. CDC. National and state vaccination coverage among adolescents aged 13–17 years— United States, 2012. *MMWR.* 2013. http://www.cdc.gov/mmwr/preview/mmwrhtml/ mm6234a1.htm. Accessed July 1, 2014.

30. Omer SB, Enger KS, Moulton LH, Halsey NA, Stokley S, Salmon DA. Geographic clustering of nonmedical exemptions to school immunization requirements and associations with geographic clustering of pertussis. *Am J Epid.* 2008;168(12): 1389–1396.

31. Omer SB, Peterson D, Curran EA, Hinman A, Orenstein WA. Legislative challenges to school immunization mandates, 2009–2012. *JAMA.* 2014;311(6):620–621.

32. Omer SB, Pan WK, Halsey NA, et al. Nonmedical exemptions to school immunization requirements: Secular trends and association of state policies with pertussis incidence. *JAMA.* 2006;296(14):1757–1763.

33. Omer SB, Richards JL, Ward M, Bednarczyk RA. Vaccination policies and rates of exemption from immunization, 2005–2011. *N Engl J Med.* 2012;367(12): 1170–1171.

34. About us: The Immunization Action Coalition. 2014. http://www.immunize.org/ aboutus/. Accessed July 2, 2014.

35. NCSL. Immunizations policy issues overview. 2011. http://www.ncsl.org/research/ health/immunizations-policy-issues-overview.aspx. Accessed July 2, 2014.

36. Kata A. A postmodern Pandora's box: Anti-vaccination misinformation on the Internet. *Vaccine.* 2010;28(7):1709–1716.

37. Kata A. Anti-vaccine activists, Web 2.0, and the postmodern paradigm—an overview of tactics and tropes used online by the anti-vaccination movement. *Vaccine.* 2012;30(25): 3778–3789.

38. Vermont Coalition for Vaccine Choice. Vermont Coalition for Vaccine Choice: It's a human right, 2014. http://www.vaxchoicevt.com/. Accessed July 2, 2014.

39. Vactruth.com. Your child. your choice. 2014. http://vactruth.com/. Accessed July 2, 2014.

40. Vaccines articles. 2014. http://vaccines.mercola.com/. Accessed July 2, 2014.

41. National Vaccine Information Center. 2014. http://www.nvic.org/. Accessed July 2, 2014.

42. Jones AM, Omer SB, Bednarczyk RA, Halsey NA, Moulton LH, Salmon DA. Parents' source of vaccine information and impact on vaccine attitudes, beliefs, and nonmedical exemptions. *Ad Prev Med.* 2012;2012:1–8.

43. Betsch C, Brewer NT, Brocard P, et al. Opportunities and challenges of Web 2.0 for vaccination decisions. *Vaccine.* 2012;30(25):3727–3733.

44. Rosenthal E. The price of prevention: Vaccine costs are soaring. *The New York Times.* 2014. http://www.nytimes.com/2014/07/03/health/Vaccine-Costs-Soaring-Paying-Till-It-Hurts.html?_r=0. Accessed July 2, 2014.

45. Campos-Outcalt D, Jeffcott-Pera M, Carter-Smith P, Schoof BK, Young HF. Vaccines provided by family physicians. *Ann Fam Med.* 2010;8(6):507–510.

46. Siddiqui M, Salmon DA, Omer SB. Epidemiology of vaccine hesitancy in the United States. *Hum Vaccin Immunotherapeut.* Dec 2013;9(12):2643–2648.

47. Gellin BG, Maibach EW, Marcuse EK. Do parents understand immunizations? A national telephone survey. *Pediatrics.* 2000;106(5):1097–1102.

48. Freed GL, Clark SJ, Butchart AT, Singer DC, Davis MM. Parental vaccine safety concerns in 2009. *Pediatrics.* 2010;125(4):654–659.

49. Smith PJ, Humiston SG, Marcuse EK, et al. Parental delay or refusal of vaccine doses, childhood vaccination coverage at 24 months of age, and the Health Belief Model. *Public Health Rep* 2011;126(Suppl 2):135–146.

50. Gilkey MB, McRee AL, Brewer NT. Forgone vaccination during childhood and adolescence: Findings of a statewide survey of parents. *Prev Med.* 2013;56(3-4):202–206.

51. Chi DL. Caregivers who refuse preventive care for their children: The relationship between immunization and topical fluoride refusal. *Am J Public Health.* 2014;104(7):1327–1333.

52. Gaudino JA, Robison S. Risk factors associated with parents claiming personal-belief exemptions to school immunization requirements: community and other influences on more skeptical parents in Oregon, 2006. *Vaccine.* 2012;30(6):1132–1142.

53. Betsch C, Ulshofer C, Renkewitz F, Betsch T. The influence of narrative v. statistical information on perceiving vaccination risks. *Med Decis Making.* 2011;31(5):742–753.

54. Brown K, Sevdalis N. Lay vaccination narratives on the web: Are they worth worrying about? *Med Decis Making.* 2011;31(5):707–709.

55. Misegades LK, Winter K, Harriman K, et al. Association of childhood pertussis with receipt of 5 doses of pertussis vaccine by time since last vaccine dose, California, 2010. *JAMA.* 2012;308(20):2126–2132.

56. Cherry JD. Epidemic pertussis in 2012—the resurgence of a vaccine-preventable disease. *N Engl J Med.* 2012;367(9):785–787.

57. Cherry JD. Why do pertussis vaccines fail? *Pediatrics.* 2012;129(5):968–970.

58. Aleccia J. Ohio measles outbreak is biggest in U.S. since 1996. *NBC News.* 2014. http://www.nbcnews.com/health/health-news/ohio-measles-outbreak-biggest-u-s-1996-n103581. Accessed July 1, 2014.

59. Notes from the field: Measles outbreak among members of a religious community—Brooklyn, New York, March–June 2013. *MMWR.* 2013. http://www.cdc.gov/mmwr/preview/mmwrhtml/mm6236a5.htm. Accessed July 2, 2014.

60. Notes from the field: Measles outbreak associated with a traveler returning from India—North Carolina, April–May 2013. *MMWR.* 2013. http://www.cdc.gov/mmwr/preview/mmwrhtml/mm6236a6.htm. Accessed July 2, 2014.

61. Sugerman DE, Barskey AE, Delea MG, et al. Measles outbreak in a highly vaccinated population, San Diego, 2008: Role of the intentionally undervaccinated. *Pediatrics.* 2010;125(4):747–755.

62. Omer SB, Salmon DA, Orenstein WA, deHart MP, Halsey N. Vaccine refusal, mandatory immunization, and the risks of vaccine-preventable diseases. *N Engl J Med.* 2009;360(19):1981–1988.

63. Amirthalingam G, Andrews N, Campbell H, et al. Effectiveness of maternal pertussis vaccination in England: An observational study. *Lancet.* 2014; 384(9953):1521–1528.

64. Herzog R, Alvarez-Pasquin MJ, Diaz C, Del Barrio JL, Estrada JM, Gil A. Are healthcare workers' intentions to vaccinate related to their knowledge, beliefs and attitudes? A systematic review. *BMC Public Health.* 2013;13:154.

65. Salmon DA, Pan WK, Omer SB, et al. Vaccine knowledge and practices of primary care providers of exempt vs. vaccinated children. *Hum Vaccin.* 2008;4(4):286–291.

66. Smith PJ, Kennedy AM, Wooten K, Gust DA, Pickering LK. Association between health care providers' influence on parents who have concerns about vaccine safety and vaccination coverage. *Pediatrics.* 2006;118(5):e1287–1292.

67. CDC. Reported cases and deaths from vaccine preventable diseases, United States, 1950–2011. 2011. http://www.cdc.gov/vaccines/pubs/pinkbook/downloads/appendices/G/cases-deaths.pdf. Accessed July 2, 2014.

68. Lohr S. The vaccination effect: 100 million cases of contagious disease prevented. *The New York Times.* 2013. http://bits.blogs.nytimes.com/2013/11/27/the-vaccination-effect-100-million-cases-of-contagious-disease-prevented/. Accessed July 1, 2014.

69. Sifferlin A. 4 Diseases making a comeback thanks to anti-vaxxers. *Time.com.* 2014. http://time.com/27308/4-diseases-making-a-comeback-thanks-to-anti-vaxxers/. Accessed July 1, 2014.

CHAPTER 13

Prescription Drug Abuse

THE CONTROVERSY

The U.S. Centers for Disease Control and Prevention (CDC) has called prescription drug abuse an "epidemic" and identified it as one of five top national "health threats" for 2014.[1] Overdose deaths from opioid and narcotic painkillers exceed those from heroin and cocaine.[2] Furthermore, CDC says, "Enough prescription painkillers were prescribed in 2010 to medicate every American adult for a month."[3,4] Some people think the trend may have started when a 1986 article published in the journal *Pain* described long-term use of opioid painkillers in 38 patients without cancer.[5] Portenoy and Foley found that managing pain medication was challenging only in two patients who had previously abused drugs.[5] Based on their study, they concluded that long-term opioid pain medications, "can be a safe, salutary and more humane alternative to the options of surgery or no treatment in those patients with intractable non-malignant pain and no history of drug abuse."[5]

Estimated numbers of patients with chronic conditions whose pain was not adequately treated was staggering—between 37 and 46% of arthritis patients, 50% of cancer patients, and nearly three-quarters of patients having a painful condition for which they sought medical attention.[6] In response to a growing cry for better pain treatment for patients, whether the pain was related to cancer, surgery, or other medical causes, The Joint Commission (the organization accrediting or certifying more than 20,000 U.S. healthcare organizations[7]) implemented pain management standards on January 1, 2001.[8,9] The standards were developed with the University of Wisconsin Medical School and funded by the Robert Wood Johnson Foundation. They included a broadly configured expert panel on the issue.[8] The Joint Commission estimated there were more than 76 million pain-sufferers in the United States and their new standard required screening for pain (asking patients about pain), providing appropriate treatment for pain, and educating patients and families about pain. In addition, the standard emphasized these new requirements were "patient rights."[8]

Pain became the "fifth vital sign," a term coined by the American Pain Society in 1995,[10] and along with measuring pulse, respirations, temperature, and blood pressure, it became part of the critical initial assessment of all patients, especially those using emergency care. In 2001, the American College of Physicians, one of the largest medical organizations in the United States, published stories of near-miraculous changes in patients when their pain was appropriately treated—whether untreated cancer pain or from other chronic conditions such as arthritis, fibromyalgia, or migraine headaches.[6]

Around 2000, a shift also occurred in the education of physicians and attitudes of state licensing boards and regulatory organizations. This shift was in response to the widely recognized need to better treat patients' pain with medications and nondrug approaches such as acupuncture, nutrition, and mind/body approaches.[6] However, even at that time, not all health professionals agreed, with one physician predicting in 2000 that, "Encouraging the use of opiates for treating chronic nonmalignant pain in a large vulnerable population can be expected to significantly increase the number of drug abusers and addicts."[11]

In 2014, the standard remains, with The Joint Commission emphasizing that patients are encouraged to "speak up" about their pain."[8] Meanwhile, CDC reports that deaths from prescription painkiller overdoses have skyrocketed.[12] Overdose deaths are the tip of the iceberg—for every one overdose death from prescription pain medications, there are 10 hospitalizations, 32 emergency room visits, 130 people abusing prescription painkillers, and 825 people using pain medications for nonmedical reasons.[12] With an estimated 18 women dying daily from overdoses of prescription painkillers[13] and what many view as a public health crisis, some *JAMA* writers are calling on healthcare professionals and regulatory agencies to "rethink opioid prescribing."[14] One medical blogger wondered if The Joint Commission's 2001 pain standard actually ignited the current epidemic, asking is it "coincidence or regulatory unintentional consequences?"[15] An emergency department physician clearly describes the conflicting nature of the current environment: "We err on the side of treating pain and it is a huge potential for abuse."[16] In a 2012 *Wall Street Journal* article entitled, "Pain-Drug Champion Has Second Thoughts," Dr. Portenoy, lead author of the critical 1986 study says, "We didn't know then what we know now."[17]

BACKGROUND AND SCOPE OF THE PUBLIC HEALTH AND HEALTH POLICY ISSUE

Pharm 101—What Drugs Are the Problem? How Do They Work?

Categories of commonly abused prescription medications include opioids, central nervous system depressants, and stimulants.[18] The National Institute on Drug Abuse (NIDA) reported that 7 million people in the United States intentionally used prescription medications for nonmedical reasons in 2010.[19] Painkillers ranked highest (with an estimated 5.1 million people using them for nonmedical reasons), followed by tranquilizers (2.2 million people), stimulants (1.1 million), and sedatives (0.4 million).[19]

Opioid Pain Medications

Opioids are used to treat pain. Once taken, they enter the body and bind to proteins called "opioid receptors," which results in a person perceiving less pain. Because the opioid receptors are located in organs such as the brain and gastrointestinal tract, they may cause sleepiness, decrease respirations, and cause nausea or constipation.[18] These other effects are important and potentially serious when too much of the medication is taken or when taken in a way that rapidly delivers increased drug levels, such as through injection or inhalation.[18] Examples of these medications include hydrocodone (e.g., Vicodin), oxycodone (e.g., OxyContin, Percocet), morphine (e.g., Kadian, Avinza), and codeine.[18]

Central Nervous System (CNS) Depressants

These medications may be used in the treatment of difficulty sleeping or anxiety and may commonly be called *sedatives* or *tranquilizers*.[18] Their mechanism of action is through increasing the neurotransmitter GABA (gamma-amino-butyric acid), which decreases brain activity.[18] Examples of medications include benzodiazepines (diazepam [Valium], alprazolam [Xanax], triazolam [Halcion], estazolam [ProSom]); non-benzodiazepine sleep medications (zolpidem [Ambien], eszopiclone [Lunesta], zalepon [Sonata]); and barbiturates (mephobarbital [Mebaral], phenobarbital [Luminal Sodium], pentobarbital sodium [Nembutal]).[18] These medications have varying levels of risk for abuse, dependence, tolerance, and addiction and are especially risky if used in combination with pain medications, some over-the-counter medications, and especially when used in combination with alcohol.[18]

Stimulants

These prescription medications are used to treat conditions such as ADHD (attention deficit hyperactivity disorder), and their mechanism of action is to increase the effects of the neurotransmitters norepinephrine and dopamine.[18] Used appropriately, they may improve attention and alertness, but as their name implies, they cause in increases in heart rate and blood pressure, and may create "euphoria" because of their effect on the neurotransmitter dopamine. Examples include dextroamphetamine (Dexedrine, Adderall) and methylphenidate (Ritalin, Concerta).[18]

What Is Prescription Drug Abuse? How Serious Is It?

According to the NIDA, prescription drug abuse is defined as "the use of a medication without a prescription, in a way other than as prescribed, or for the experience or feelings elicited."[18] Data from the 2010 National Survey on Drug Use and Health (NSDUH) suggests that 2.4 million people in the United States used a prescription medication for nonmedical purposes within the past year.[18] Young people, girls, and women are especially at risk: of the 6,600 people who begin to use prescription medications each day for nonmedical reasons, one-third were aged 12–17 years and more than half were female.[18] Young adults, aged 18–25 years have the highest rates of prescription drug abuse, with nearly 6% of this age group reporting prescription drug abuse in the past month, and except for ages 12–17, prescription drug abuse is seen more often in males than females.[18]

One of the most commonly cited surveys, NIDA's Monitoring the Future (MTF) Survey, shows the types of prescription medications commonly used for nonmedical reasons by high school students.[20] In 2012, high school seniors reported use of the following prescription medications for nonmedical reasons: Adderall (7.6%), Vicodin (7.5%), cough medicine (5.6%), tranquilizers (5.3%), OxyContin (4.3%) as examples.[20] Use of *any* prescription medication for nonmedical reasons was reported by 15.0% of U.S. high school seniors in 2013.[21] Where are high school students getting these prescription medications? In the MTF 2011 survey, 70% of high school seniors got them from a friend or relative, with sparse attempts to get them over the Internet.[19]

In addition to the effects from abuse of these medications themselves, data from a variety of national surveys shows that young people using prescription medications also have higher rates of binge drinking, marijuana, cocaine, and other illegal drug use.[18,19] In addition, there is much concern that abuse of prescription opioid painkillers may be a first step to heroin abuse. Several studies have reported that 50% of young adults injecting heroin previously abused prescription painkillers but used heroin because of easier access and lower price.[20,22] Another 2014 article places risk even higher: Cicero and colleagues report that 75% of the heroin users in their study first used prescription painkillers.[23]

Data from the U.S. Department of Defense suggests that active duty personnel aged 18–25 years use illegal drugs at rates much lower than the general population.[24] However, abuse of prescription drugs is increasing, with 11% of service members reporting nonmedical use of prescription medications in 2008 with opioid painkillers being the medications most commonly used.[24]

The World Health Organization (WHO) characterizes prescription drug misuse (PDM) as a global problem, and despite the fact that this is well recognized in the United States it is also an international public health issue.[25] Lack of knowledge or even indifference in both the general public and trained health professionals may contribute. For example, in New Zealand, where it is geographically challenging to import heroin, prescription medications comprise most opioid abuse.[25] On a global level, the WHO cites a variety of contributing factors, as established programs for addiction to illegal drugs may not be acceptable to either patients or health professionals for treatment of prescription drug abuse.[25] Further, policies required to prevent abuse of prescription medications while still ensuring treatment for patients' pain is a difficult balance.[25]

Health Consequences: Abuse vs. Dependence vs. Addiction vs. Overdose

Abuse is defined as using prescription medications for reasons other than why they were prescribed, and in most cases, use by others who were not prescribed the medication.[18,26] It may also include taking larger doses than prescribed, taking the medication to "get high" or taking the medication by a different route, such as by injecting or inhaling crushed pills.[26] NIDA reminds us that "physical dependence" is very different from addiction and is a result of the body's normal physiological reaction to long-term medication use. This dependence may also include "tolerance," which means that the individual needs to take higher medication doses, over time, to achieve the same medical effect.[18] Prescription opioid painkillers can be extremely addictive as they interact with the same receptors as heroin, made easier when people inhale or inject crushed pills.[19] Addiction may include dependence but also includes negative behaviors such as "compulsive drug seeking" or continued use without regard for negative consequences such as legal consequences of drug seeking or use.[18] Experts characterize addiction as a "brain disease," and over time, actual changes in the brain may be seen.[27] As a result, addiction can be challenging to treat, chronic, and characterized by relapses, especially when drug abuse begins at young ages.[27]

Prescription opioid overdose may be caused by combining medications with alcohol or other prescription medications, increasing medication doses, or using different routes of administration, such as inhaling or injecting the medications that are prescribed in pill form—all potentially contributing to serious or lethal depression of respirations.[19] Methadone, due to its potential for accumulation in the body and narrow window between the effective dose and potential overdose, is especially dangerous.[28] HIV risk may be increased through injecting crushed medications with nonsterile needles or sharing such equipment.[19] Risks of abuse of CNS depressants include addiction as well as potentially life-threatening withdrawal symptoms (for example, seizures) when these medications are discontinued abruptly and without medical supervision.[19] Adverse effects from stimulants include addiction, as well as seizures, psychosis, and cardiac effects.[19] Irregular heart rhythms, heart failure, and hazardous increases in body temperature have all be reported.[20]

Deaths from Prescription Drug Abuse—Data and Trends

CDC reports prescription medication overdose deaths as "epidemic."[2] In 2010, 12 million Americans aged 12 or older had used prescription pain medications for nonmedical reasons in the previous year.[2]

In the United States in 2009, prescription painkillers resulted in 500,000 emergency room visits and overdoses caused 15,500 deaths,[28] a dramatic increase from the 4,000 deaths reported in 1999.[2] In addition, misuse of prescription painkillers has resulted in $72.5 billion in additional health-care costs each year.[2] Higher risks for prescription painkiller overdoses are seen in men, middle-aged adults, non-Hispanic white, American Indian, or Alaska Native individuals, and people living in rural areas.[2]

The Trust for America's Health, a Washington nonprofit organization, reports that between 1999 and 2010, deaths from drug overdoses have doubled (or more) in 29 states and are higher than combined deaths from heroin and cocaine.[3,29] Deaths from drug overdoses are now greater than those from motor vehicle crashes in some states, and prescription drug overdoses are highest in Appalachia and the Southwestern United States.[29] Overdose deaths in West Virginia for example, have increased 605% since 1999, with overdose death rates of nearly 29 deaths per 100,000 people. High rates are also reported in New Mexico, Kentucky, Nevada, and Oklahoma.[29] Scientific studies note a relationship between sales of opioid pain medications and overdose deaths,[30] and CDC says that states with the highest average per capita painkiller sales and abuse rates also experience more deaths[2,4] (see **Figure 13–1**). The Drug Abuse Warning Network (DAWN),

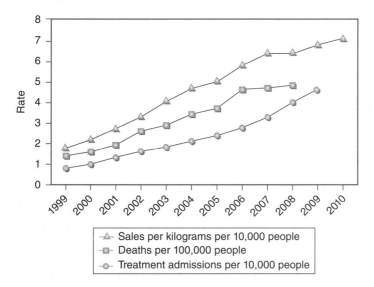

Figure 13–1 Rates of prescription painkiller sales, deaths, and substance abuse treatment admissions (1999–2010).

Reproduced from Centers for Disease Control and Prevention. Prescription painkiller overdoses in the US infographic. Available at http://www.cdc.gov/vitalsigns/painkilleroverdoses/infographic.html

which reports on emergency department (ED) visits from prescription drug misuse or abuse, reported almost 4.6 million drug-related ED visits in 2009, with ED visits for misuse or abuse of prescription medications exceeding those for illegal drugs.[31]

Women

In the United States, although men are more likely to die from overdoses than women, overdoses in women from prescription painkillers are increasing, with an estimated 6,600 deaths in 2010, which translates to 18 women dying daily[13] (see **Figure 13–2**). Highest death risks are seen in women aged 45–54 years and 70% of deaths involve painkillers, as women are more often prescribed these medications and in higher dosages than men.[13] In addition, risks are highest among non-Hispanic white and American Indian or Alaska native women. CDC estimates that, "Every 3 minutes, a woman goes to the emergency department for prescription painkiller misuse or abuse."[13]

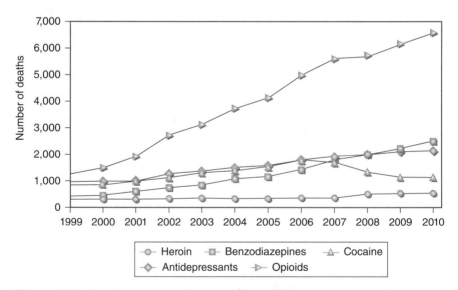

Figure 13–2 Prescription painkiller overdose deaths–A growing problem among women.

Reproduced from Centers for Disease Control and Prevention. Prescription Painkiller Overdoses: A growing epidemic, especially among women. CDC Vital Signs. 2013. Available at http://www.cdc.gov/vitalsigns/prescriptionpainkilleroverdoses/index.html

Methadone

Increases in methadone overdoses have been especially worrisome, because although methadone represents only 2% of all pain medication prescriptions, it is responsible for nearly one-third of all overdose deaths from prescription painkillers.[28] Further, this is a six-fold increase in deaths in just 10 years.[28] Methadone is sometimes prescribed for chronic pain and has a low-cost available generic formulation. More than 4 million prescriptions for methadone were written in 2009.[28] Some of the risk may be due to the characteristics of methadone and the way it is metabolized in the body, with a small difference between the optimal therapeutic dose and harmful or lethal dose.[28]

Place Matters

Per capita sales of pain medication and overdose deaths are related,[2,4] and prescribing practices for painkillers varies geographically[32] (see **Figure 13–3**). CDC reminds us that numbers of prescriptions for painkillers per person is twice as high in the United States as Canada, and within the United States prescribing varies markedly.[32] For example, southern states have the highest prescribing rates per person for

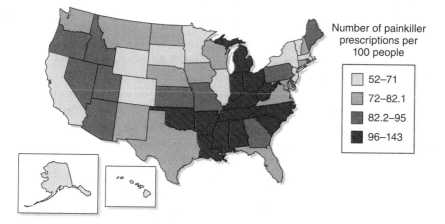

Figure 13–3 Opioid painkiller prescribing in the United States.

Reproduced from Centers for Disease Control and Prevention: Opioid Painkiller Prescribing Infographic. Available at http://www.cdc.gov/vitalsigns/opioid-prescribing/infographic.html#map

pain medications. The specific type of painkillers prescribed may also vary geographically, such as the use of long-acting pain medications in Maine and New Hampshire.[32]

Why is this Happening?

A number of factors may contribute to the current crisis. A *New York Times* article from 1999 noted a transition in how chronic pain was treated in the United States, noting the expanding number of states passing laws to protect doctors when they prescribed medications to adequately treat pain in their patients.[33] In addition, around that time model guidelines were written by the Federation of State Medical Boards to guide and protect physicians prescribing narcotic painkillers for pain.[33]

This shift and the 2001 Joint Commission standard[8] followed many studies that documented unmet pain-control needs of patients and fears of physicians. In the 1995 study to understand prognoses and preferences for outcome and risks of treatments (SUPPORT) trial, 9,105 hospitalized adults with serious and advanced chronic conditions were studied.[34] One of the key findings was that one-half of patients dying in the hospital who were awake and aware often had moderate to severe pain much of the time.[34] A 1999 *JAMA* study of 13,625 older cancer patients in nursing homes in five states found between 24–38% of older patients reported daily pain.[35] Furthermore, more than one-quarter of patients (26%) with daily pain received *no* pain medication and this percentage was higher in older and minority patients.[35]

Several well-publicized cases of physician prosecution had a dramatic dampening effect on painkiller prescribing; however, physicians' fear of causing addiction in patients and the fear of prosecution or license sanctions eased during the late 1990s.[33] The Joint Commission president said, "We believe patients have an explicit right to effective assessment and management of existing pain," and Joint Commission pain management standards went into effect January 1, 2001.[8,33]

Numbers of pain medication prescriptions have increased dramatically since the early 1990s and some authors feel increased medication availability is a contributing factor.[18,19] Data from NIDA confirms that from 1991 to 2010 the number of prescriptions for opioid painkillers increased from 75.5 million to 209.5 million, and stimulant prescriptions increased from 5 million to about 45 million.[19] CDC notes that some states struggle with healthcare "pill mills" and finding ways of managing individuals' seeking additional (but medically unneeded) prescriptions for painkillers.[4] In addition, there may be a false sense of security about the safety of prescription medications because they are regulated and prescribed by healthcare professionals.[19] In addition, some authors describe a "taking a pill for what ails you" mindset, which relies on medications in lieu of other effective treatments.[18] Reasons for taking prescription medications for nonmedical reasons range from "getting high" to relieving anxiety, improving sleep, or improving mental acuity.[19]

EVIDENCE BASE FOR PREVENTION AND PRACTICE

CDC recommends policies and practices to reduce the public health impact of prescription pain medication abuse and deaths. In general, four strategies are promoted: improving tracking (surveillance) systems to track prescriptions, evaluating and promoting programs and policies that are effective (i.e., what works), increased focus on healthcare prescribing by using evidence-based guidelines, and education for health professionals, the public, and policymakers.[12,32] Systems that allow prescription tracking are a key public health strategy. Many states have systems, called prescription drug monitoring programs (PDMP), that use electronic surveillance or tracking systems to monitor painkiller prescriptions.[4] CDC notes the need to improve these systems by linking them to state Medicaid programs, workers' compensation data, and electronic health records.[2,4] Recommendations for healthcare professionals emphasize educating patients about safekeeping and disposal of prescription medications and increasing access to nondrug pain treatments such as physical therapy.[4,32]

States can ensure access to treatment for prescription medication abuse,[2,32] and this is especially important for adolescents and young adults who underutilize substance abuse treatment.[36,37] Only 16–17% of adolescents used treatment for opioid use or dependence,[37,38] despite its effectiveness, with a variety of barriers documented in this age group.[37] In addition, for methadone, CDC recommends that health insurers rethink including methadone on preferred drug lists because of trends in overdose deaths specifically related to this pain medication.[28]

Policy Approaches

The White House published "Epidemic: Responding to America's Prescription Drug Abuse Crisis" in 2011, which called for increased education, tracking and monitoring, proper medication disposal, enforcement, and setting prescription drug abuse improvement goals.[39] In response to overdose deaths and increasing crime, New York City took a bold approach in 2013 and restricted use of narcotic painkillers in the city's 11 public hospitals, with 3-day limits for some prescribed narcotics, strict policies for lost prescriptions, and eliminating use of some painkillers altogether.[40] This step preempted guidelines from health professional societies and was criticized by some physicians as "legislative medicine."[40] In October 2013, describing the current situation as reaching a "tipping point," the U.S. Food and Drug Administration (FDA) announced new recommendations with stricter controls on how healthcare providers prescribe narcotic pain medications that included limits on numbers of refills, total medication prescribed without a new prescription, and in-person pharmacy pickup requirements.[41]

The U.S. Drug Enforcement Administration (DEA) uses five categories to regulate prescription drugs (also chemicals to make drugs) based on their medical use and how likely they are to cause drug dependence or abuse.[42] For example, Schedule III drugs have a "moderate to low potential for physical and psychological dependence," whereas Schedule II drugs have a "high potential for abuse."[42] One of the most dramatic changes recommended by the FDA advised the DEA reclassify some mediations, including oxycodone prescribed for pain and medications prescribed for ADHD, into the Schedule II category.[41] In August, 2014 the DEA proposed its final regulation that rescheduled hydrocodone combination products (HCPs) from Schedule III to Schedule II.[43]

CDC has published "Policy Impact Guide for Prescription Painkiller Overdoses" to highlight the epidemiology, trends, differences among states and populations at highest risk.[44] As a resource for state health departments and policymakers, CDC has also studied and published a summary of seven types of state laws addressing prescription drug overdose, including laws regulating pain clinics, requiring physical examination prior to prescribing, requiring tamper-proof prescription forms, prescription drug limits, patient identification in pharmacies, regulating pain clinics, and others.[45]

Future Directions

The Trust for America's Health reports that the majority of states in the United States are not yet using evidence-based or best practices to reduce prescription drug abuse.[3] On their report card, only Vermont and New Mexico scored 10 out of 10 possible strategies, whereas Washington, DC and 28 other states scored 6 or less, with Missouri and

Nebraska scoring 3 and South Dakota scoring only 2 out of 10.[3] This report emphasizes the need for public education, responsible prescribing, proper medication disposal, improved tracking systems (PDMPs), and adequate treatment services for those abusing prescription medications, similar to policy recommendations made by CDC.[3,44] NIDA notes the continuing challenge of balancing appropriate pain treatment while preventing prescription drug misuse. They cite the critical need to develop of new painkillers that remain effective but are nonaddicting.[18]

NIDA emphasizes the importance of healthcare professionals using evidence-based guidelines for prescribing.[18] However, developing high-quality guidelines is challenging. The American College of Physicians (ACP), one of the largest physician organizations in the United States, reported that high-quality guidelines for opioid prescribing are not readily available.[46] However, there were a few highly-rated and evidence-based guidelines found, such as those developed by the American Pain Society, the American Academy of Pain Medicine,[47] and the Canadian National Opioid Use Guideline Group.[46,48] Organizations such as the ACP provide current and evidence-based physician education for prescribing opioids.[49] An updated Cochrane Review from 2014, another important source of evidence-based information, emphasized the lack of evidence for "effectiveness and safety" of lengthy treatment with opioid pain medications for chronic low back pain.[50] In addition to professional guidelines, innovative approaches such as vaccines for oxycodone and hydrocodone have demonstrated "early proof-of-efficacy" in rats and represent a promising direction for future research.[51,52]

DISCUSSION QUESTIONS: TEMPLATE FOR DISCUSSION

1. Significance of this public health issue:
   a. Why is this health issue important?
   b. How many people does it impact?
   c. How serious is it?
   d. Is it preventable?
2. What is the evidence base for prevention?
3. What specific strategies should be used to achieve progress on this health issue?
   a. What evidence-based approach would you use?
   b. Where would you start if you are an individual citizen; public health professional; healthcare professional; community, state, or federal policymaker?

4. Specific questions for this topic:
   a. What specific, evidence-based policies, if systematically applied, could result in reductions in prescription drug misuse?
   b. What approaches might be better used to balance the needs for effective pain treatment and prevention of prescription drug abuse and overdose?
5. What is the controversy?
   a. Define the controversy.
   b. Is controversy a good or bad thing? (Does it help or hinder progress?)
6. *Why* is this health issue controversial?
   a. What specific factors are involved?
   b. Do economics, government, scientific uncertainty, or politics play a role?
   c. What is the role of the media?
7. How would you respond to the controversy?

PERSPECTIVES TO CONSIDER

In the year 2000, the treatment of chronic pain was framed by The Joint Commission as a "patients' rights" issue. State regulatory restrictions were relaxed and prescribing of opioid pain medications increased.[4,33] Some questioned the effectiveness of pain as the fifth vital sign and a study of a general outpatient medicine clinic suggested that pain management was unimproved.[53] Others raised questions about funding and relationships with the pharmaceutical industry and the depth of the original data used to draw conclusions about the safety of long-term opioid treatment.[14,17] Other critics wondered whether cheaper costs of treating pain with pills, rather than physical therapy and other nonpharmacologic approaches, has also contributed.[54]

Emergency department physicians complain of patients coming in with pain and the challenges of managing the appropriate treatment of pain in the current environment.[16] Others are more direct, calling for health professionals to "rethink" opioid prescribing to better protect the public's health.[14] Scientific evidence that looks at both risks and benefits of opioid treatment is missing for many nonmalignant chronic conditions, and use of opioids for treatment of chronic back pain, for example, lacks scientific backing.[14]

Many are not surprised by the current epidemic, with prescription drug abuse and the risk to public health a result of trends in increased prescribing.[3,4,13,28,32] Most telling is a 2012 *Wall Street Journal* interview with the original principle investigator of the 1986 study of 38 patients that concluded "opioid maintenance therapy can be a safe, salutary and more humane alternative..."[5] The interview and article described a shift in thinking, policy, and practice, and potential relationships between industry, professional and regulatory organizations, were all the topic of a Senate Finance Committee investigation in 2012.[17,55,56]

How do we regain that delicate balance with what we now know? The reason this trend started was because so many patients suffered and died in pain,[34,35] and we now have both skills and treatments to effectively treat pain for many, if not all, patients. No one suggests a return to that era. But the dramatic increase in prescribing opioid pain medications has also (as an unintended consequence) contributed to prescription drug abuse and an epidemic of overdose deaths. Experts recommend that increased public awareness, professional education, practice guidelines, new policies, better tracking, research, and even new laws may be needed.[3,44] However the Joint Commission 2001 standard remains,[8] and some might wonder if pain really *is* the fifth vital sign or if we should go back to the original four.

FOR ADDITIONAL STUDY

Levi J, Segal LM, Miller, AF. Prescription drug abuse: Strategies to stop the epidemic. *Trust for America's Health: Reports.* 2013. http://healthyamericans.org/reports/drugabuse2013/.

Alexander GC, Kruszewski SP, Webster DW. Rethinking opioid prescribing to protect patient safety and public health. *JAMA.* 2012;308(18):1865–1866.

REFERENCES

1. CDC. CDC's top ten: 5 health achievements in 2013 and 5 health threats in 2014. 2014. http://blogs.cdc.gov/cdcworksforyou24-7/2013/12/cdc%e2%80%99s-top-ten-5-health-achievements-in-2013-and-5-health-threats-in-2014/. Accessed January 29, 2014.
2. CDC. CDC Features: Prescription painkiller overdoses in the U.S. 2011. http://www.cdc.gov/Features/Vitalsigns/PainkillerOverdoses/. Accessed February 2, 2014.
3. Levi J, Segal LM, Miller, AF. Prescription drug abuse: Strategies to stop the epidemic. *Trust for America's Health: Reports* 2013. http://healthyamericans.org/reports/drugabuse2013/. Accessed February 2, 2014.
4. CDC. Prescription painkiller overdoses in the US. *CDC Vital Signs.* 2011. http://www.cdc.gov/vitalsigns/pdf/2011-11-vitalsigns.pdf. Accessed February 2, 2014.
5. Portenoy RK, Foley KM. Chronic use of opioid analgesics in non-malignant pain: Report of 38 cases. *Pain.* 1986;25(2):171–186.

6. Kelly C. Managing the fifth vital sign: Your patients' pain. *ACP Internist.* 2001. http://www.acpinternist.org/archives/2001/04/managepain.htm. Accessed February 7, 2014.

7. The Joint Commission: About the Joint Commission. 2014. http://www.jointcommission.org/about_us/about_the_joint_commission_main.aspx. Accessed February 8, 2014.

8. The Joint Commission: Facts about pain mangement. 2014. http://www.jointcommission.org/pain_management/. Accessed February 8, 2014.

9. Phillips DM. JCAHO pain management standards are unveiled. Joint Commission on Accreditation of Healthcare Organizations. *JAMA.* 2000;284(4):428–429.

10. Lafleur K. Taking the fifth (vital sign). *Modernmedicine.com.* 2004. http://www.modernmedicine.com/modern-medicine/news/taking-fifth-vital-sign. Accessed February 2, 2014.

11. Hansen G. Assessment and management of pain. *JAMA.* 2000;284(18): 2317–2318.

12. CDC. Preventing prescription painkiller overdoses: Fact sheet. 2012. http://www.cdc.gov/injury/pdfs/NCIPC_Overview_FactSheet_PPO-a.pdf. Accessed February 2, 2014.

13. CDC. Prescription painkiller overdoses: A growing epidemic, especially among women. *CDC Vital Signs.* 2013. http://www.cdc.gov/vitalsigns/prescriptionpainkilleroverdoses/index.html. Accessed February 2, 2014.

14. Alexander GC, Kruszewski SP, Webster DW. Rethinking opioid prescribing to protect patient safety and public health. *JAMA.* 2012;308(18):1865–1866.

15. Cato A. How pain as a vital sign contributed to prescription pill mills. *KevinMD.com.* November 12, 2011. Accessed February 2, 2014.

16. Saint Louis C. E.R. doctors face quandary on painkillers. *The New York Times.* 2012. http://www.nytimes.com/2012/05/01/health/emergency-room-doctors-dental-patients-and-drugs.html. Accessed February 2, 2014.

17. Catan T, Perez E. A pain-drug champion has second throughts. *Wall Street Journal Online.* 2012. http://online.wsj.com/news/articles/SB10001424127887324478304578173342657044604. Accessed February 2, 2014.

18. NIDA. Research report series: Prescription drugs: Abuse and addiction. 2011. http://www.drugabuse.gov/sites/default/files/rrprescription.pdf. Accessed February 2, 2014.

19. NIDA. Prescription drug abuse. 2011. http://www.drugabuse.gov/sites/default/files/prescription_1.pdf. Accessed February 2, 2014.

20. NIDA. DrugFacts: Prescription and over-the-counter medications. 2013. http://www.drugabuse.gov/sites/default/files/drugfacts_rx_otc_5_2_13_ew2_0.pdf. Accessed February 2, 2014.

21. NIDA. DrugFacts: High school and youth trends. 2014. http://www.drugabuse.gov/sites/default/files/drugfactsmtf2013.pdf. Accessed February 2, 2014.

22. NIDA. DrugFacts: Heroin. 2013. http://www.drugabuse.gov/publications/drugfacts/heroin. Accessed October 2, 2014.

23. Cicero TJ, Ellis MS, Surratt HL, Kurtz SP. The changing face of heroin use in the United States: A retrospective analysis of the past 50 years. *JAMA Psychiatry.* 2014;71(7):821–826.

24. NIDA. DrugFacts: Substance abuse in the military. 2013. http://www.drugabuse.gov/publications/drugfacts/substance-abuse-in-military. Accessed Feburary 8, 2014.

25. WHO. Prescription drug misuse: Issues for primary care: Report of findings. 2008. http://apps.who.int/medicinedocs/en/d/Js19984en/. Accessed February 2, 2014.

26. MedlinePlus: Prescription drug abuse. 2013. http://www.nlm.nih.gov/medlineplus/prescriptiondrugabuse.html. Accessed February 2, 2014.

27. Prescription drug abuse 2012. http://www.webmd.com/mental-health/abuse-of-prescription-drugs. Accessed February 2, 2014.

28. CDC. CDC Vital signs: Prescription painkiller overdoses: Methadone. 2012. http://www.cdc.gov/Features/VitalSigns/MethadoneOverdoses/. Accessed February 2, 2014.

29. Brinkerhoff N. More U.S. deaths from prescription drug abuse than from heroin and cocaine combined. *ALLGOV.* 2013. http://www.allgov.com/news/controversies/more-us-deaths-from-prescription-drug-abuse-than-from-heroin-and-cocaine-combined-131011?news=851366. Accessed February 2, 2014.

30. Paulozzi LJ, Ryan GW. Opioid analgesics and rates of fatal drug poisoning in the United States. *Am J Prev Med.* 2006;31(6):506–511.

31. Highlights of the 2009 Drug Abuse Warning Network (DAWN) findings on drug-related emergency department visits. *The DAWN Report.* 2010. http://oas.samhsa.gov/2k10/dawn034/edhighlights.htm. Accessed February 2, 2014.

32. CDC. Opioid painkiller prescribing: Where you live makes a difference. *CDC Vital Signs.* 2014. http://www.cdc.gov/vitalsigns/opioid-prescribing/index.html. Accessed October 2, 2014.

33. Noble HB. A shift in the treatment of chronic pain. *The New York Times.* 1999. http://www.nytimes.com/1999/08/09/us/a-shift-in-the-treatment-of-chronic-pain.html?pagewanted=print. Accessed February 8, 2014.

34. A controlled trial to improve care for seriously ill hospitalized patients. The study to understand prognoses and preferences for outcomes and risks of treatments (SUPPORT). The SUPPORT Principal Investigators. *JAMA.* 1995;274(20):1591–1598.

35. Bernabei R, Gambassi G, Lapane K, et al. Management of pain in elderly patients with cancer. SAGE Study Group. Systematic assessment of geriatric drug use via epidemiology. *JAMA.* 1998;279(23):1877–1882.

36. Ilgen MA, Schulenberg J, Kloska DD, Czyz E, Johnston L, O'Malley P. Prevalence and characteristics of substance abuse treatment utilization by U.S. adolescents: National data from 1987 to 2008. *Addict Behav.* 2011;36(12):1349–1352.

37. Wu LT, Blazer DG, Li TK, Woody GE. Treatment use and barriers among adolescents with prescription opioid use disorders. *Addict Behav.* 2011;36(12):1233–1239.

38. NIDA. Few teens with prescription opioid use disorders receive treatment. 2012. http://www.drugabuse.gov/news-events/nida-notes/2012/07/few-teens-prescription-opioid-use-disorders-receive-treatment. Accessed February 2, 2014.

39. Epidemic: Responding to America's prescription drug abuse crisis. 2011. http://www.whitehouse.gov/sites/default/files/ondcp/issues-content/prescription-drugs/rx_abuse_plan_0.pdf. Accessed February 2, 2014.

40. Hartocollis A. New York City to restrict prescription painkillers in public hospitals' emergency rooms. *The New York Times.* 2013. http://www.nytimes.com/2013/01/11/nyregion/new-york-city-to-restrict-powerful-prescription-drugs-in-public-hospitals-emergency-rooms.html?emc=tnt&tntemail0=y&_r=1&&pagewanted=print. Accessed February 4, 2014.

41. Meier B. FDA urging a tighter rein on painkillers. *The New York Times.* 2013. http://www.nytimes.com/2013/10/25/business/fda-seeks-tighter-control-on-prescriptions-for-class-of-painkillers.html?_r=0. Accessed February 8, 2014.

42. DEA US. Drug Scheduling 2014. http://www.justice.gov/dea/druginfo/ds.shtml. Accessed October 2, 2014.

43. DEA US. Schedules of controlled substances: Rescheduling of hydrocodone combination products from schedule III to schedule II. 2014. https://www.federalregister .gov/articles/2014/08/22/2014-19922/schedules-of-controlled-substances-rescheduling-of-hydrocodone-combination-products-from-schedule. Accessed October 2, 2014.

44. CDC. Policy impact: Prescription painkiller overdoses. 2011. http://www.cdc.gov/ homeandrecreationalsafety/rxbrief/. Accessed February 2, 2014.

45. CDC. Prescription drug overdose: State laws. 2012. http://www.cdc.gov/ HomeandRecreationalSafety/Poisoning/laws/index.html. Accessed February 2, 2014.

46. ACP. Few high-quality guidelines exist for prescribing opioids. *ACPHOSPITALIST.* 2013. http://www.acphospitalist.org/weekly/archives/2013/11/13/index.html. Accessed February 8, 2014.

47. Chou R, Fanciullo GJ, Fine PG, et al. Clinical guidelines for the use of chronic opioid therapy in chronic noncancer pain. *J Pain.* 2009;10(2):113–130.

48. Nuckols TK, Anderson L, Popescu I, et al. Opioid prescribing: A systematic review and critical appraisal of guidelines for chronic pain. *Ann Intern Med.* 2014; 160(1): 38–47.

49. ACP. Education program for prescribing opioids now available. 2014. http://www .acponline.org/education_recertification/cme/safe_opioid_prescribing.htm. Accessed February 8, 2014.

50. Chaparro LE, Furlan AD, Deshpande A, Mailis-Gagnon A, Atlas S, Turk DC. Opioids compared with placebo or other treatments for chronic low back pain: An update of the Cochrane Review. *Spine.* 2014;39(7):556–563.

51. Pravetoni M, Le Naour M, Tucker AM, et al. Reduced antinociception of opioids in rats and mice by vaccination with immunogens containing oxycodone and hydrocodone haptens. *J Med Chem.* 2013;56(3):915–923.

52. NIDA. Oxycodone vaccine passes early tests. *NIDA Notes.* 2013. http://www .drugabuse.gov/news-events/nida-notes/2013/05/oxycodone-vaccine-passes-early-tests. Accessed February 2, 2014.

53. Mularski RA, White-Chu F, Overbay D, Miller L, Asch SM, Ganzini L. Measuring pain as the 5th vital sign does not improve quality of pain management. *J Gen Intern Med.* 2006;21(6):607–612.

54. Meier B. Profiting from pain. *The New York Times.* 2013. http://www.nytimes. com/2013/06/23/sunday-review/profiting-from-pain.html. Accessed February 8, 2014.

55. Meier B. Senate inquiry into painkiller makers' ties. *The New York Times.* 2012. http://www.nytimes.com/2012/05/09/health/senate-panel-to-examine-narcotic-drug-makers-financial-ties.html. Accessed Feburary 8, 2014.

56. Baucus, Grassley seek answers about opioid manufacturers' ties to medical groups. *The United States Senate Committee on Finance.* 2012. http://www.finance.senate.gov/ newsroom/chairman/release/?id=021c94cd-b93e-4e4e-bcf4-7f4b9fae0047. Accessed Feburary 8, 2014.

CHAPTER 14

Infectious Diseases: Climate Change and Public Health

LEARNING OBJECTIVES

- Discuss the public health effects of climate change related to infectious diseases.
- Describe the factors contributing to uncertainty about climate change, public health, and infectious diseases.
- Critically assess evidence for effective strategies to prevent the public health impact of climate change and infectious diseases.
- Predict the impact of rising temperatures, changing rainfall patterns, and "extreme" weather on infectious diseases and public health.
- Discuss examples of climate-sensitive diseases.
- Identify evidence-based policies and practices that can reduce the public health impact of climate change.
- Propose evidence-based strategies to reduce the public health impact on vulnerable populations.

THE CONTROVERSY

The U.S. Centers for Disease Control and Prevention (CDC) reported an infection in a 12-year-old girl with the brain-eating amoeba *Naegleria fowleri*.[1] This organism thrives in warm freshwater bodies, usually enters through the nose after swimming or diving, and causes primary amebic meningoencephalitis (PAM), a serious and often-fatal brain infection.[1,2] Investigators suspected a water park in Arkansas as the potential infection source.[1] *N. fowleri* infections are usually reported in southern states during warmer summer months, especially after prolonged heat spells resulting in lower water levels and warmer water.[2,3]

A CDC official noted that from 2003 to 2012, 31 infections had been reported in the entire United States, with half reported in Texas and Florida.[1] Although the infection is not common, it is nearly always (97%) fatal: from 1962 to 2013, of 132 infected individuals, only three have survived.[2] In the summer of 2013, three of four children reported with the infection died.[3] A *N. fowleri* infection reported in Minnesota in 2012 was a new finding. In answer to the question about whether climate change could be causing the infection to spread to new locations, one CDC epidemiologist said, "We don't have data right now to show that the infections are increasing, but just by the virtue of the fact that it's a thermophilic organism and we're seeing warmer temperatures, I think put those two together."[3] Another CDC spokesperson noted, "It may not be that there are more infections . . . but it could be that infections occur in places where they have previously not occurred, such as Minnesota, Kansas, places we've seen recent infections."[3]

To help answer the question about whether climate change is causing more or different patterns of disease, *Science* published an entire issue in 2013 highlighting the complex research questions surrounding connections between climate change and infectious diseases.[4] The Harvard School of Public Health says infections such as malaria and dengue fever are "climate sensitive," because mosquito vectors that transmit these diseases do not live and spread disease if weather is cooler.[5] A blogger for *The Huffington Post* writing about climate change and public health asks, "Will dengue fever mosquitos touch down someday soon in Chicago? Will the *Anopheles* family, better known as the Malaria Mob, buzz the rooftops of Miami in the not too distant future?"[6]

BACKGROUND AND SCOPE OF THE PUBLIC HEALTH AND HEALTH POLICY ISSUE

Health Effects and Trends

Weather and climate have dramatic effects on public health, including infectious diseases.[7] Information about climate norms and variation is available from the National Oceanic and Atmospheric Administration (NOAA) National Climatic Data Center.[8] The Global Change Research Act of 1990 requires a U.S. National Climate Assessment, every 4 years, to provide data to the public, the private sector, and policymakers.[9] The results of the third national climate assessment reported 12 key findings, including impacts of climate change on air quality, water quality, and infectious

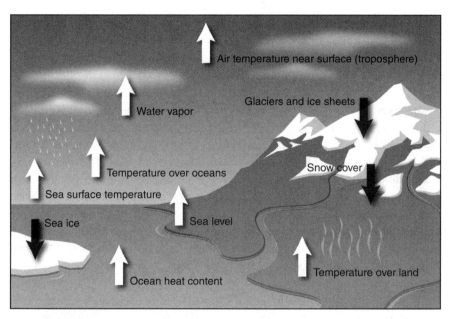

Figure 14–1 Ten indicators of a warming world.

Reproduced from NOAA NCDC based on data updated from Kennedy et al. 2010.
Available at http://www.ncdc.noaa.gov/sites/default/files/Ten-Indicators-of-a-Warming-
World-third-National-Climate-Assessment.png

diseases. Disruptions to ecosystems and agriculture, and other adverse effects are projected to worsen throughout this century[9] (see **Figure 14–1**).

CDC emphasizes a range of potential health effects that may occur worldwide in different locations and populations, from climate changes such as higher temperatures to weather conditions such as hurricanes, floods, droughts, and air pollution.[10] These health effects may include acute health issues and injuries, infectious diseases, and exacerbation of chronic conditions. For example, elevated temperatures, causing "heat waves" may cause heat stress and increased deaths in very young and older populations and people with underlying cardiovascular and respiratory diseases.[10] Injuries and drowning may result from hurricanes and floods. Air pollution, including increased ozone and allergens, may particularly impact young children, older adults, and those with pre-existing respiratory conditions.[10] Severe storms may cause injuries, homelessness, and prolonged stress in families and communities and increase the need for both mental health and healthcare services.[10] In addition to health effects from prolonged heat and severe weather, increased temperatures, droughts, and floods may precipitate increases in infectious diseases, whether food-borne, waterborne, or related to disease vectors such as mosquitos and ticks.[10] The Lancet Commission agrees that climate changes may impact health though "extreme" weather, water (floods and droughts), food and nutrition, housing, changes in population, and changes in the distribution of diseases.[11]

Globally, an estimated 150,000 deaths each year are attributed to the health effects of climate changes such as increased temperatures and rainfall, with impacts not evenly distributed. Temperate latitudes, areas near the Pacific and Indian oceans, sub-Saharan Africa, and large urban areas are felt to be at increased risk.[12] The Lancet Commission reported that 5.5 million disability adjusted life years (DALYs) lost can be attributed to climate change worldwide in the year 2000.[11] Furthermore, they predict people in lower income countries, urban settings, the very old and very young, and populations living in coastal regions will experience a greater proportion of the negative health impacts.[11]

CDC described the public health impacts of climate change and related weather events on vector-borne and zoonotic diseases, waterborne diseases, foodborne diseases, and nutrition.[13] For vector-borne diseases, potential changes in a variety of weather-related factors makes it hard to predict with certainty the exact impact on human health. For example, changes in local habitats of insects and animals and how temperature and humidity influence reproductive and life cycle of disease pathogens, may all have an influence on vector-borne and zoonotic diseases.[13] In addition, human-related behaviors such as travel, population migration, and land use may also contribute to changes in disease incidence.[13]

Potential impacts of climate change on infectious diseases includes recurrence of diseases previously seen, the introduction of new diseases, such as West Nile virus, or changes in the geographic distribution of currently reported diseases, such as Lyme disease and hantavirus.[13] Waterborne diseases, such as cholera, may be influenced by floods, droughts, or changes in water temperature related to changing climates.[13] Rises in sea levels or changes in pH or salinity of ocean ecosystems may also contribute to changes in incidence of waterborne diseases.[13] Changes in surface temperatures in the ocean may result in more *Vibrio* bacteria, including *Vibrio vulnificus* and *Vibrio parahaemolyticus,* causative agents in seafood-related illness.[13] Other authors note that malaria, dengue, and viral encephalitis, all related to mosquito vectors, are especially climate-sensitive diseases.[14]

Other factors such as transportation and travel, nutritional status, presence of antibiotic resistance, quality of housing, and urban or rural setting may also impact the incidence of infectious diseases.[15] In addition, potential mitigating factors such as the presence of preventive measures, public education, public health infrastructure, and access to health care, may also vary in different geographic regions. Ultimately, this may influence whether or not adverse health impacts are actually *seen* in human populations.[13]

The World Health Organization (WHO) describes the relationship between climate change, waterborne diseases, and public health, on a global scale.[7] Eight out of ten deaths (of an estimated 2 million annual deaths) worldwide from diarrheal diseases such as cholera are children under the age of 5.[7] Factors related to "extreme weather" such as droughts, floods, hurricanes, and severe storms include water contamination and threats to sanitation and result in increased risks for infectious diseases.[7] Developing countries, which are less likely to have systems to ensure safe drinking water and modern sanitation systems, may have the greatest increasing population risks from diseases such as cholera, a situation already seen in certain areas of Africa and Asia.[7]

Some scientists characterize discussion of the long-term impact of climate change on rates of infectious disease as a "polarizing debate," with arguments centering on the variable effects climate change has on local ecosystems and how mitigating factors and human behaviors might impact the development and spread of a variety of climate-sensitive diseases.[16] For example, there is no consensus about the impact of climate change on vector-borne diseases, such as malaria. Some scientists suggest, in contrast to predictions of huge increases in infectious disease incidence in many geographic areas, that we may instead observe changes in geographic distribution of infectious diseases without large total increases because of the variety of ecologic factors at play.[17] Other scientists from the University of Georgia describe global variation in factors that may help countries reduce health impacts of climate changes, including available resources and access to health care, and that "the climate signal, in many cases, is hard to tease apart from other factors like vector control and vaccine and drug availability."[18] Another scientist from the University of Calgary says, "The Arctic is like a 'canary in the global coal mine,'" arguing that because of the relative speed of temperature changes seen in the Arctic, increased growth and development of some parasites is already happening.[18]

Other examples are found in Caribbean coral reefs, where rising water temperatures have resulted in disease-causing bacteria and fungi.[16,18] Other scientists emphasize the importance of biodiversity loss in infectious diseases, for example, in Lyme disease and West Nile virus.[18] These same scientists point out the many gaps in current research, call for improved surveillance systems especially at local levels, and the need to test predictive models in real-world situations.[16,18] Also needed are better ways to predict where vulnerable locations and populations might be at increased risk, to drive "practical solutions" that better protect both animal and human health.[16]

Examples of Climate-Sensitive Diseases

Malaria

Humans are infected with the malaria parasite from the bite of female *Anopheles* mosquitos.[19] About 30 to 40 *Anopheles* species can transmit malaria.[19] *Plasmodium vivax* and *Plasmodium falciparum* (spread by mosquitos) represent the most important malaria-causing parasites worldwide.[7] WHO estimates range from 200 to 500 million malaria cases annually that result in an estimated 1 million deaths each year. Eighty percent of all malaria cases worldwide and 90% of deaths from malaria are found in 35 countries in central Africa and are related to their rural environments, lack of public health and healthcare resources, and an abundance of mosquito species and malaria parasites that cause more serious disease.[7] In addition to the strength of control measures, temperature, humidity, and rainfall all impact malaria incidence in a region because of the impact of these climate factors on both mosquito populations and how well the malaria parasite thrives.[7] Because of rising global temperatures, one model predicts between 260 and 320 million additional people will develop malaria by 2080 because of the spread of mosquito populations to new locations.[11]

Dengue

Nearly 400 million people are infected worldwide by one of the four viruses causing dengue, which may cause high fever, headache, muscle and bone pain, rash, and sometimes bleeding.[20] Dengue is spread by *Aedes* mosquitos and there is currently no vaccine to prevent the disease. Public health efforts focus on mosquito control and preventing mosquito bites.[20] The Natural Resources Defense Council reports that between 1995 and 2005, approximately 4,000 cases of dengue fever were reported in the United States; reports from Florida in 2009 and 2010 showed the first outbreak of dengue in decades.[21] According to the WHO, dengue causes about 15,000 deaths each year from infections occurring in about 100 tropical and subtropical countries.[7] Both climate and socioeconomic factors are felt to play important roles in creating environments where infections can occur. Climate changes, especially heavy rainfall and elevated temperatures can increase the numbers of mosquitos and rising temperatures can also speed virus development.[7] In addition to the impact of climate, with dengue showing seasonal fluctuation in many areas, factors such as travel, population density, and mosquito prevention and control activities can all impact the extent of disease in a given geographic area.[7]

Meningitis

Meningitis is an inflammation of the covering of the brain and spinal cord, often from infection of the surrounding fluid with bacteria, viruses, parasites, or fungi.[22] One cause of severe bacterial meningitis is *Neisseria meningitidis*.[22] In Africa, most meningitis is seen in a part of sub-Saharan Africa called the "Meningitis Belt." Meningitis epidemics regularly occur during the dry season that runs from December to May and has resulted in more than 250,000 cases and 25,000 deaths in the past decade.[7] Although the exact cause of this seasonal pattern is not known, one theory is that the prolonged dry air causes drying of the mucous membranes in the nose, enabling the bacteria to more easily enter the body and cause infection.[7]

Eastern Equine Encephalitis (EEE)

Spread by the bite of infected mosquitos, EEE is an uncommon viral infection. It usually occurs in the Eastern United States, causing potentially fatal brain swelling (encephalitis).[23] In 1933, there was a large EEE animal outbreak (epizootic) in horses in mid-Atlantic states, and an outbreak of 34 human cases (25 deaths) was reported in Massachusetts as early as 1938.[24,25] A New Jersey outbreak was reported in 1959 with 32 human cases, and an outbreak was reported in New Hampshire in 2005.[24,25] In subsequent years, infections have been reported in the Northeast in New York,

Rhode Island, Vermont, Connecticut, Maine, and as far north as Canada, places where this often-fatal infection was rarely or never seen.[24,25] Some authors are calling EEE an "Old Enemy, New Threat,"[25] as this resurgence has coincided with climate changes. There is currently no vaccine or specific treatment, and case-fatality rates are estimated to range between 35–75%, with many survivors experiencing long-lasting brain damage.[23,25]

Scientists attribute outbreaks to changes in the environment that allow virus growth and subsequent horse or human infections.[25] Although changes in population density and land-use may also be contributing factors, rainfall and warmer winters may directly affect the size of mosquito populations and the speed of EEE virus reproduction and potential human risks for infection. Public health surveillance programs, public education, and mosquito control are recommended population-level prevention strategies.[25]

Lyme Disease

Lyme disease, transmitted by the bite of an infected tick, is caused by the bacterium *Borrelia burgdorferi* and causes a red rash, called *erythema migrans*, fever, head and muscle aches, and other generalized symptoms.[26] Six out of ten people who have Lyme disease that is not diagnosed and treated may later develop arthritis, especially in their knees; a smaller percentage (about 5%) may develop symptoms in their nervous system months to years later.[26] Humans become infected by a bite from a black-legged tick infected with the causative bacteria. In some eastern and central parts of the United States the blacklegged tick, also called the deer tick (*Ixodes scapularis*), transmits the disease to humans and in western states the western blacklegged tick (*Ixodes pacificus*) is the responsible disease vector.[26]

Confirmed cases of Lyme disease in the United States have increased since 2001, when there were 17,029 confirmed Lyme disease cases reported to CDC.[26] By 2013, Lyme disease was the sixth most common disease reported in the United States as part of CDC's list of nationally notifiable diseases and there were 27,203 confirmed cases reported (see **Figures 14–2 and 14–3**). In addition, according to CDC, 95% of all reported cases of Lyme disease were from 14 states, predominantly in the northeast and parts of the Midwest (see Figure 14–3).[26]

Scientists and public health officials have tracked the progression of Lyme disease, and its relation to changing climate, observing that both temperature and moisture may impact the specific ticks that transmit

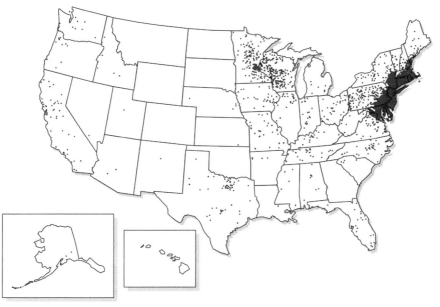

1 dot placed randomly within county of residence for each reported case

Figure 14–2 Reported cases of Lyme disease–United States, 2001.

Reproduced from Centers for Disease Control and Prevention, Lyme Disease, Interactive Lyme Disease Map. Available at http://www.cdc.gov/lyme/stats/maps/interactiveMaps.html

B. burgdorferi.[27] Other scientists have studied the relationship between oak trees, white-footed mice, Lyme disease, and climate changes. An abundance of acorns in a given year will also result in more mice; researchers found that high acorn yields in 2010 resulted in an explosion of mice in 2011.[27] Why are mice important in the spread of Lyme disease? Along with deer, mice carry the *B. burgdorferi* bacterium; mice are accessible hosts to this infectious process because they don't become ill from the infection and are easily bitten by ticks.[27] Ticks generally have a 2-year life span that is comprised of three stages: larva, nymph, and adult and they drink blood at each of these stages in their development.[28] Humans may be later infected from a tick bite.[27] Scientists from Canada have recently observed more ticks along their U.S. border, discovered that "ticks move faster" when temperatures are warmer, and Canada is now experiencing an increase in Lyme disease cases.[27]

Other scientists have studied the mechanism of climate change's impact on the overall transmission and severity of Lyme disease.[28] According

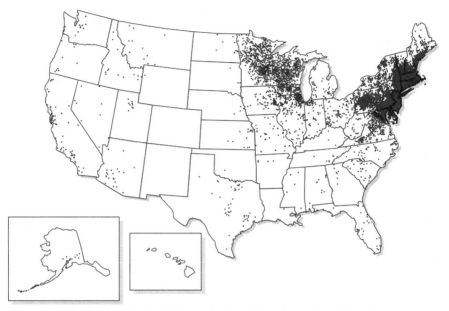

1 dot placed randomly within county of residence for each confirmed case

Figure 14–3 Reported cases of Lyme disease–United States, 2013.

Reproduced from Centers for Disease Control and Prevention, Lyme Disease, Interactive Lyme Disease Map. Available at http://www.cdc.gov/lyme/stats/maps/interactiveMaps.html

to Yale University scientists, climate changes directly impact feeding patterns of deer ticks. They studied both the blacklegged tick and *B. burgdorferi* in 30 different geographic locations in the Northeastern and Midwestern United States.[29] They observed that the timing of tick feeding at each life stage in more moderate climates caused a longer interval between each of the three feedings and resulted in human infections from hardier bacteria that were able to survive longer.[29] Their observations in the Northeast and Midwest paralleled the numbers of reported cases observed in these regions, suggesting that climate predicted the distribution of blacklegged ticks and different strains of *B. burgdorferi*, both with implications for the distribution of human infections.[28,29] Yale scientists also developed an environmental and climate model to predict distribution of the tick *I. scapularis* and future risk for Lyme disease.[30] Their model predicted the current distribution of this Lyme disease vector with nearly 90% accuracy. It predicts more than a doubling of the Canadian tick population by 2080 and increased risk for Lyme disease in Canada and also predicts tick migration into the central part of the United States.[30]

EVIDENCE BASE FOR PREVENTION AND PRACTICE

Public Health and Meteorology

The WHO assembled an "Atlas of Health and Climate," in partnership with the World Meteorological Organization, noting that "climate affects the geographical and temporal distribution of large burdens of disease and poses important threats to health security, on time scales from hours to centuries."[7] In addition to climate, the authors suggest that poverty, human behavior, and the availability of health services are additional determinants for the manifestations of infectious diseases in human populations.[7] Available research from a variety of disciplines, including meteorological data, is currently used globally to protect public health, especially through public health preparedness.[7]

One Health

The concept of "One Health" is not a new one, beginning in the 1800s when Virchow, a German pathologist, used the term "zoonosis" to describe infections passed between animals and humans.[31] However, the term One Health is more recent and is often attributed to Calvin Schwabe, who in 1984[32] emphasized a more holistic and interdisciplinary approach relating human health to both animal health and the environment.[31] This approach is especially important as new diseases or patterns of diseases are noted.[31] Zoonotic diseases may include viruses, bacteria, or other pathogens that spread from animals to humans through a variety of routes.[31] Many authors have written about the complexity of factors related to global climate change and human health, especially zoonotic and vector-borne diseases, emphasizing the need for a strong research agenda.[33–35]

Coker reminds us that a huge proportion (about two-thirds) of all human pathogens are zoonotic and that this is increasing. It is estimated that about 75% of new (emerging) infections and reemerging infectious diseases are zoonotic, necessitating a framework for One Health policy on a global level.[36] Experts hypothesize a variety of ways that climate change can ultimately impact human health, such as changes in habitats, vector populations, and changes in diseases that occur in animals and plants.[37] The complex interplay between climate, changes in the environment, and the impact on animal and human health requires a broad range of expertise to understand how diseases develop and spread in a changing environment.[37] Veterinarians, physicians and other healthcare professionals, public health experts, and environmental scientists are just some of the professions involved in adopting this "one health" approach. A summary of the American Veterinary Medical Association's (AVMA) One Health Initiative Task Force, articulates the benefits of this approach.[32] A One Health approach is both holistic and collaborative and has potential to improve animal and human health globally, anticipate new health threats, develop areas and centers of excellence, and through research, contribute to the creation of new health programs.[32]

Future Needs

The Natural Resources Defense Council reports that 11 U.S. states, from Alaska to New York to New Hampshire, have developed preparedness approaches for climate change and public health, which include better infectious disease and vector monitoring.[21] Early warning systems have been successfully used in Southern Africa to reduce the impact of malaria. Climate forecasts, developed in partnership with weather organizations such as the National Meteorological and Hydrological Services (NMHS) have been used by health ministries to prepare for likely malaria epidemics several months in advance.[7] Similar surveillance systems are being tested in several South American countries.[7]

Mapping techniques that superimpose weather conditions such as heavy precipitation and flooding on maps of disease incidence, may help indicate high-risk areas of developing waterborne diseases.[7] The WHO Global Information Management System on Health and Environment (GIMS) project is using maps of weather and disease to identify "hot spots" to serve as an "early warning" for cholera in several countries where they are testing this idea.[7] Weather, environmental, and epidemiological data are also being used for mapping, planning, and creating new predictive models for dengue fever in new geographic areas.[7]

In sub-Saharan Africa, in areas of the "Meningitis Belt," vaccination campaigns are being waged against recurrent epidemics of meningitis, using a vaccine against *N. meningitidis* serogroup-A. A promising strategy uses climate, environmental, and epidemiologic data to develop models to predict the likelihood of future outbreaks in specific areas. This research project, called MERIT (Meningitis Environmental Risk Information Technologies) uses data from these different sources to see if this information can be reliably used as part of the public health response to annual epidemics in affected countries.[7]

Policy Development

The Lancet Commission emphasizes the priority need for primary policy interventions to: decelerate global warming, prevent diseases related to climate change, and strengthen public health systems and infrastructure.[11] The Trust for America's Health found, in 2009, that only five states: California, Maryland, New Hampshire, Virginia, and Washington, included public health in their climate change strategies, suggesting health officials were not included in state-level policymaking, at a time when public health threats related to climate change were well recognized.[38]

Many authors recognize the importance of policy development at a global, national, state, and local level to prevent the public health impact of climate change-related infectious diseases. The WHO has recommended the "Top 10 Actions for National and Local Policy-Makers"[39] to protect public health from climate change. These include recommendations to engage a variety of constituencies and incorporate health impact assessments (HIAs) into policy development related to climate change and public health.[39] HIAs use qualitative, quantitative, and participatory methods to evaluate the health impacts of proposed policies.[40] Other recommended actions include reminders to protect vulnerable populations, such as people living in poverty, older adults, and infants and young children.[39] The WHO stresses the need to use proven public health strategies such as disease surveillance, preparedness, food safety measures, and public education in policies related to health and climate change. In addition, they recommend developing effective education and communication strategies.[39] Additional recommendations for policymakers at all levels include strengthening capacity for research that includes the range of disciplines needed to impact health and climate change.[39] The WHO made analogous recommendations for health professionals, also emphasizing that health professionals should use their scientific knowledge for leadership and advocacy.[41]

CDC recommends strategies such as public health surveillance, improving research, developing public and private partnerships, utilizing public health preparedness plans, identifying vulnerable populations, communicating scientific information about health and climate change, and developing new approaches to predict climate-related health effects.[10]

Research Gaps

A 2010 report from the Interagency Working Group on Climate Change and Health from the National Institute of Environmental Health Sciences provides the following perspective about climate change and health-related policies: "The need for sound science on which to base such policies becomes more critical than ever."[42] In areas of foodborne diseases and nutrition the working group recommends research to identify "sentinel species" that may be especially sensitive to the effects of changing climate and can serve as an early warning.[42] Current surveillance systems used for human and animal health should be connected and research conducted to improve the predictive ability of mathematical models.[42] In addition to research needs related to climate change and risk for chronic diseases, infectious diseases, and injuries, the working group also highlights the importance of strengthening fundamental public health skills and capacity. These recommendations include improving risk communication and public education, determining high-risk populations, strengthening the healthcare and public health systems, and developing better predictive models, all to minimize adverse health outcomes related to a changing climate.[42]

DISCUSSION QUESTIONS: TEMPLATE FOR DISCUSSION

1. Significance of this public health issue:
   a. Why is this health issue important?
   b. How many people does it impact?
   c. How serious is it?
   d. Is it preventable?
2. What is the evidence base for prevention?
3. What specific strategies should be used to achieve progress on this health issue?
   a. What evidence-based approach would you use?
   b. Where would you start if you are an individual citizen; public health professional; healthcare professional; community, state, or federal policymaker?

4. Specific questions for this topic:
   a. What is the evidence for the link between climate change and increases in infectious diseases?
   b. What geographic areas and populations are at greatest risk?
   c. What are additional examples of climate-sensitive diseases?
   d. What diseases are the highest public health concern and why?
   e. What evidence-based policies, if systematically applied, could result in reductions in the public health impacts of climate change and infectious disease?
   f. What barriers prevent better policies to protect public health from being implemented?
5. What is the controversy?
   a. Define the controversy.
   b. Is controversy a good or bad thing? (Does it help or hinder progress?)
6. *Why* is this health issue controversial?
   a. What specific factors are involved?
   b. Do economics, government, scientific uncertainty, or politics play a role?
   c. What is the role of the media?
7. How would you respond to the controversy?

PERSPECTIVES TO CONSIDER

In her article, "We Are All Climate Change Deniers," Mary Pipher argues that we are much more comfortable with "problems that are concrete, close-at-hand, familiar, and require skills and tools that we already possess."[43] Potential health effects of a changing climate are just the opposite—big, distant, and complicated. The wide ranging health effects from extreme heat, hurricanes, droughts and floods, and changing air pollutants may include infectious diseases and also chronic conditions, injuries, access to food and water, and housing.[10]

The complexity of different factors and mechanisms that impact infectious diseases in humans makes precise predictions challenging. For climate-sensitive diseases, ecological factors, temperature, migration, humidity, along with human behaviors and presence of vulnerable populations may all combine to produce different outcomes in different geographic settings.[11,13,16] Despite the complexity and the controversy even in the scientific community about the strength and impact of different contributing and causative factors, there is consensus that public health strategies can help.[10,39] Public health surveillance may signal impending disease outbreaks and has served as a cornerstone of public health investigations. Such systems must be strengthened globally to protect the public and contribute to global awareness of climate sensitive conditions, whether waterborne, vector-borne, or foodborne. The importance of linking different surveillance systems, for example in areas of animal and human health, relates to the global impact of zoonotic diseases, estimated at about three-quarters of emerging and reemerging infections.[36] New partners in meteorology and mapping projects that combine weather-related and infectious disease data have already shown practical applications for meningitis, cholera, and dengue.[7]

In addition, ongoing research and better predictive modeling in interdisciplinary settings is needed to better define the mechanisms and roles of potential mitigating and preventive factors.[11,16,42] From the current discussion of One Health and its benefits,[31,32] entomologists, epidemiologists, climate scientists, microbiologists, meteorologists, veterinarians, healthcare professionals, public health experts, and communication specialists are just some of the experts needed to get a better grasp of biological mechanisms. In addition, public health needs to be at the table in development of policies for the short and long term.[38] Public health leadership is critical not only in research and mitigating the effects of climate change on human health, but more importantly, in preventing them.

FOR ADDITIONAL STUDY

Costello A, Abbas M, Allen A, et al. Managing the health effects of climate change: Lancet and University College London Institute for Global Health Commission. *Lancet.* 2009;373(9676):1693–1733.
Altizer S, Ostfeld RS, Johnson PT, Kutz S, Harvell CD. Climate change and infectious diseases: from evidence to a predictive framework. *Science.* 2013;341(6145):514–519.

REFERENCES

1. Evans M. Brain-eating ameoba case linked to warm water. *AccuWeather.com.* 2013. http://www.accuweather.com/en/weather-news/brain-eatingamoebacaselinkedto/ 15985705. Accessed December 1, 2013.
2. CDC. *Naegleria fowleri*—primary amebic meningoencephalitis (PAM). 2014. http://www.cdc.gov/parasites/naegleria/general.html. Accessed October 5, 2014.
3. MacMath J. CDC looks toward climate change in brain-eating amoeba cases. *AccuWeather.com.* 2013. http://www.accuweather.com/en/weather-news/amoeba-climate-change-cdc/18191791. Accessed December 1, 2013

4. Walsh B. Infectious disease could become more common in a warmer world—especially for plants and animals. *Science.Time.com.* 2013. http://science.time.com/2013/08/02/infectious-disease-could-be-more-common-in-a-warmer-world-especially-for-plants-and-animals/. Accessed December 1, 2013.

5. Climate change and infectious disease 2012. http://chge.med.harvard.edu/topic/climate-change-and-infectious-disease. Accessed December 1, 2013.

6. Karliner J. Protecting public health from climate change. [blog]. *Huffington Post.* 2013. http://www.huffingtonpost.com/health-care-without-harm/protecting-public-health_b_4034160.html. Accessed December 1, 2013.

7. WHO. Atlas of health and climate. 2012. http://www.who.int/globalchange/publications/atlas/en/. Accessed December 1, 2013.

8. NOAA. NOAA: National Climatic Data Center: National Oceanic and Atmospheric Administration. 2014. http://www.ncdc.noaa.gov/. Accessed October 5, 2014.

9. NOAA. Climate change and variability. 2014. http://www.ncdc.noaa.gov/climate-information/climate-change-and-variability. Accessed October 5, 2014.

10. CDC. CDC: Climate change and public health—policy. 2011. http://www.cdc.gov/climateandhealth/policy.htm. Accessed December 1, 2013.

11. Costello A, Abbas M, Allen A, et al. Managing the health effects of climate change: Lancet and University College London Institute for Global Health Commission. *Lancet.* 2009;373(9676):1693–1733.

12. Patz JA, Campbell-Lendrum D, Holloway T, Foley JA. Impact of regional climate change on human health. *Nature.* 2005;438(7066):310–317.

13. CDC. Climate and health program: Health effects 2009. http://www.cdc.gov/climateandhealth/effects/default.htm. Accessed December 1, 2013.

14. Patz JA, Epstein PR, Burke TA, Balbus JM. Global climate change and emerging infectious diseases. *JAMA.* 1996;275(3):217–223.

15. Patz JA, Githeko AK, McCarty, JP, Hussein, S, Confalonieri U, deWet N. Climate change and infectious diseases. *Climate Change and Human Health—Risks and Responses.* Geneva, Switzerland: World Health Organization;2003:103–132.

16. Altizer S, Ostfeld RS, Johnson PT, Kutz S, Harvell CD. Climate change and infectious diseases: From evidence to a predictive framework. *Science.* 2013;341(6145): 514–519.

17. Lafferty KD. The ecology of climate change and infectious diseases. *Ecology.* 2009;90(4):888–900.

18. Gavrilles B. As climate, disease links become clearer, study highlights need to forecast future shifts. *UGA Today.* 2013. http://news.uga.edu/releases/article/climate-disease-links-study-highlights-need-forecast-future-shifts/. Accessed December 1, 2013.

19. CDC. Malaria: *Anopheles* mosquitos. 2012. http://www.cdc.gov/malaria/about/biology/mosquitoes/. Accessed December 1, 2013.

20. CDC. Dengue. 2014. http://www.cdc.gov/Dengue/. Accessed October 5, 2014.

21. NRDC. Infectious diseases: Dengue fever, West Nile virus, and Lyme disease. 2013. http://www.nrdc.org/health/climate/disease.asp. Accessed December 1, 2013.

22. CDC. Meningitis. 2014. http://www.cdc.gov/meningitis/index.html. Accessed October 4, 2014.

23. CDC. Eastern equine encephalitis. 2010. http://www.cdc.gov/easternequineencephalitis/. Accessed December 4, 2013.

24. Climate change may spread North America's deadliest mosquito-borne pathogen. *AccuWeather.com.* 2013. http://m.accuweather.com/en/outdoor-articles/outdoor-living/climate-change-may-spread-nort/18326717. Accessed December 1, 2013.

25. Armstrong PM, Andreadis TG. Eastern equine encephalitis virus—old enemy, new threat. *N Engl J Med.* 2013;368(18):1670–1673.

26. CDC. Lyme disease 2014. http://www.cdc.gov/lyme/. Accessed October 5, 2014.

27. Climate wire and Umair Irfan. Lyme disease pushes Northward. *Scientific American.* 2012. http://www.scientificamerican.com/article.cfm?id=lyme-disease-pushes-northwards. Accessed December 1, 2013.

28. The season of ticks: Could climate change worsen Lyme disease? *Science Daily.* 2009. http://www.sciencedaily.com/releases/2009/04/090426182944.htm. Accessed December 1, 2013.

29. Gatewood AG, Liebman KA, Vourc'h G, et al. Climate and tick seasonality are predictors of *Borrelia burgdorferi* genotype distribution. *Appl Environ Microbiol.* 2009;75(8):2476–2483.

30. Brownstein JS, Holford TR, Fish D. Effect of climate change on Lyme disease risk in North America. *Ecohealth.* 2005;2(1):38–46.

31. CDC. One Health. 2013. http://www.cdc.gov/onehealth/. Accessed December 1, 2013.

32. King LJ, Anderson LR, Blackmore CG, et al. Executive summary of the AVMA One Health Initiative Task Force report. *J Am Vet Med Assoc.* 2008;233(2):259–261.

33. Rosenthal J. Climate change and the geographic distribution of infectious diseases. *Ecohealth.* 2009;6(4):489–495.

34. Rosenthal JP, Jessup CM. Global climate change and health: Developing a research agenda for the NIH. *Trans Am Clin Climatol Assoc.* 2009;120:129–141.

35. Mills JN, Gage KL, Khan AS. Potential influence of climate change on vector-borne and zoonotic diseases: A review and proposed research plan. *Environ Health Perspect.* 2010;118(11):1507–1514.

36. Coker R, Rushton J, Mounier-Jack S, et al. Towards a conceptual framework to support one-health research for policy on emerging zoonoses. *Lancet Infect Dis.* 2011;11(4):326–331.

37. Patz JA, Hahn MB. Climate change and human health: A one health approach. *Curr Top Microbiol Immunol.* 2013;366:141–171.

38. Health problems heat up: Climate change and the public's health. *Trust for America's Health.* 2009. http://healthyamericans.org/reports/environment/. Accessed December 1, 2013.

39. WHO. Protecting health from climate change: Top 10 actions for national and local policy-makers. 2013. http://www.who.int/globalchange/publications/10_actions_Policy_Makers_en.pdf. Accessed December 1, 2013.

40. WHO. Health impact assessment (HIA). 2013. http://www.who.int/hia/en/. Accessed December 1, 2013.

41. WHO. Protecting health from climate change: Top 10 actions for health professionals. 2013. http://www.who.int/phe/10_actions_FINAL.pdf. Accessed December 1, 2013.

42. NIEHS. A human health perspective on climate change. 2010. http://www.niehs.nih.gov/health/materials/a_human_health_perspective_on_climate_change_full_report_508.pdf. Accessed December 1, 2013.

43. Pipher M. We are all climate change deniers *Time.com.* 2013. http://ideas.time.com/2013/07/15/we-are-all-climate-change-deniers/. Accessed December 1, 2013.

CHAPTER 15

Infectious Diseases: Antibiotic Resistance and Public Health

LEARNING OBJECTIVES

- Discuss the public health effects of antibiotic resistance.
- Describe the factors contributing to antibiotic resistance.
- Identify evidence-based policies and practices that can reduce the public health impact of antibiotic resistance.
- Summarize barriers to use of evidence-based strategies to reduce the public health impact of antimicrobial resistance, in the United States and internationally.

THE CONTROVERSY

In January 2014, CBS News in Chicago reported on the largest outbreak to date of a serious antibiotic-resistant infection in northeastern Illinois.[1] Forty-four cases of carbapenem-resistant Enterobacteriaceae (CRE), a bacteria resistant to many antibiotics, were reported to the U.S. Centers for Disease Control and Prevention (CDC).[1,2] In the fall of 2013, CDC reported for the first time actual estimates of numbers of people who are sickened and die each year as a direct result of antibiotic-resistant bacterial infections in the United States.[3,4] Their annual estimates of more than 2 million illnesses and 23,000 deaths represented a starting point to measure prevention progress in the future.[3]

CRE was classified as an "urgent threat" because it is often fatal, it is resistant to nearly all available antibiotic treatments, and it is already found in healthcare settings in 44 states.[3,5] CDC noted a "nightmare scenario" was possible if infections from this bacteria increased,[5] and one CDC official remarked that, "we are getting closer and closer to the cliff."[3] The CDC director urgently called for increased surveillance, preventing unnecessary antibiotic use, and developing new antibiotics or "the medicine cabinet may be empty for patients with life-threatening infections in the coming months and years."[5] CDC estimates that nearly one-half of all antibiotic use in humans is not needed and says that antibiotic use in animals is also a major contributing factor.[3,5] Each day in the United States, 51 tons of antibiotics are used,[6] and between 70 and 80% of all antibiotics are used in animals.[3,6] However, not all agree with this view and a veterinarian writing a blog for *Beef Magazine* argues that "singling out agricultural use of antibiotics is truly a red herring, because everyone who uses antibiotics must be judicious in their use."[7]

BACKGROUND AND SCOPE OF THE PUBLIC HEALTH AND HEALTH POLICY ISSUE

Health Effects and Trends

The threat of some human infections becoming untreatable because pathogens have developed resistance to many categories of antibiotics has become an urgent global public health problem.[4,8] Bacteria, through their ability to adapt, have the capacity to develop resistance to antibiotics used as treatments, which is an escalating problem when antibiotics are used when they are not needed.[9] Experts note that unnecessary use of antibiotics in either humans or animals may allow the selection of pathogens that are resistant to these antibiotics.[10] Over time, this results in infections becoming increasingly difficult if not impossible to treat and even common infections potentially become more serious.[8] In order to quantify, raise awareness, focus public health attention, and to prioritize these threats, CDC published a landmark report in 2013 that contained numerical estimates of antibiotic-resistant infections and categorized them as "urgent," "serious," or "concerning" depending on their extent, severity, and public health impact.[4]

The Lancet Infectious Diseases Commission studied and made recommendations about antibiotic resistance from a global perspective.[11] Antibiotic resistance is now a global public health issue and these authors note the complexity of causes and contributing factors. Low-income and middle-income countries (LMICs) have particular challenges, as antibiotic use is increasing in healthcare settings.[11] However, access to antibiotics to treat common infections (as well as access to newer antibiotics) remains inadequate in many areas of the world, creating an especially precarious balancing act.[11,12]

In the United States, using data from the National Healthcare Safety Network (NHSN) CDC reported that 4.6% of acute-care hospitals had at least one hospital-related infection due to CRE in 2012, which represented a substantial increase since 2001.[13] Globally, healthcare-related infections are increasing in LMICs, with intensive care unit (ICU)-related infections occurring three times as often in developing countries as in the United States and infections related to neonatal ICUs occurring at even higher rates.[11] Examples of antibiotic-resistant infections are reported internationally, for example in Pakistan, India, South Africa, and many other locations and include such bacteria as *Escherichia coli* and hospital-acquired Methicillin-resistant *Staphlococcus aureus* (MRSA).[11]

Allegranzi and colleagues conducted a systematic review and meta-analysis of 220 articles describing healthcare-related infections in developing countries.[12] Infection rates in adult ICUs in developing countries were three times higher than rates in the United States; similarly, surgery-related infections were also much higher.[12] Consequences of these infections globally include higher death rates and longer illnesses, higher treatment costs for resistant infections, and antibiotic-resistant infections hindering the ability to provide other medical treatment (such as chemotherapy) or surgical procedures (such as organ transplantation) that use antibiotics to prevent infections.[11]

CDC estimates 23,000 annual deaths in the United States each year from antibiotic-resistant infections;[4] for Europe this estimate is 25,000 deaths each year.[12] Although accurate data are not available for LMICs, experts suggest these figures may be much higher, and poor health outcomes and deaths are especially likely to be seen in newborn infants.[11] The World Health Organization (WHO) emphasizes that antibiotic-resistant infections cause more severe and prolonged infections, resulting in increased healthcare costs because patients may require longer and more expensive treatment.[14] In 2012, according to the WHO, there were about 450,000 cases of multidrug-resistant tuberculosis (MDR-TB) globally, and antibiotic-resistant infections such as MRSA and Gram-negative bacteria resistant to multiple antibiotics in a wide range of geographic locations.[14] In the 2012 "Options for Action" report, the WHO says "a crisis has been building up over decades" and calls urgently for a coordinated global campaign to reduce antimicrobial resistance.[8]

What Are Antibiotics?

Antibiotics are medications used to treat bacterial infections.[15] Generally, they do this by slowing the bacteria's ability to replicate, so the immune system can fight the infection, or alternatively, they kill the bacteria altogether.[15] Antibiotics are not effective in the treatment of viral infections (the cause of the common cold) or other infections not caused by bacteria.[15] Patients are instructed to finish all prescribed antibiotics to ensure a bacterial infection is successfully treated.[15] A detailed explanation and table of antibiotic categories can be found in CDC's "Antibiotic Resistance Threats in the United States, 2013."[4] The 2013 Lancet Commission report on antibiotic resistance notes the pivotal role antibiotics have played in improvements in medicine, including preventing or treating infections related to surgery, organ transplantation, cancer treatment, and in preterm babies.[11] However, widespread use and misuse also contribute to the development of resistant bacteria. Globally, antibiotic use is increasing and antibiotics are used not only in healthcare settings but also in agriculture, aquaculture, and horticulture. Furthermore, outside of North America and Northern Europe, anywhere from 19% to 100% of all antibiotic use occurs without prescriptions, which is something especially common in LMICs.[11]

Mechanisms of Resistance

According to CDC, use of antibiotics not only stops pathogens that cause illness, but also kills usual bacteria found in the human body allowing the relatively small numbers of pathogens that have developed resistance to antibiotics to multiply[4] (see **Figure 15–1**).

Transfer of antibiotic resistance may occur between bacteria. For example, humans treated with antibiotics may develop small numbers of resistant bacteria in their gastrointestinal tract. Bacteria may be spread to others in the community, and when infection-prevention measures (as simple as hand washing) are not followed, infection may spread in healthcare settings to other patients.[4] Similarly, when animals are treated with antibiotics for any reason, they develop resistant bacteria in their gastrointestinal tracts. These antibiotic-resistant bacteria may spread to humans through animal feces, through fertilizer on crops, contaminated water used for irrigation, or through lapses in safe food handling or cooking[4] (see **Figure 15–2**).

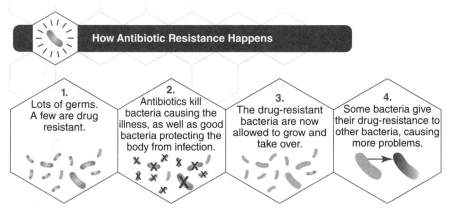

Figure 15–1 How antibiotic resistance happens.

Reproduced from Centers for Disease Control and Prevention. Antibiotic Resistance Threats in the United States, 2013. Available at http://www.cdc.gov/drugresistance/threat-report-2013/pdf/ar-threats-2013-508.pdf

Resistance is related to mutations in bacteria in combination with the selection pressure that occurs when antibiotics are used.[11] Bacteria strains that have mutated to become resistant and are able to survive the effects of the antibiotic used have what is called a "competitive advantage" in the microbial environment.[11] Such resistance genes are carried on chromosomes, and may be also found on structures outside the chromosomes that can also be transferred to other organisms. This process may ultimately result in resistant "clones" that can be widely spread, even globally, in keeping with human activities in our global society, and also influenced by local environmental conditions such as sanitation.[11] Bacteria may become resistant to antibiotics in several ways; all involve transfer of genetic material.[16] They may become resistant by way of mutation in their genes (chromosomal mutation), transfer of genetic material from one bacteria to another by plasmids (called conjugation or transformation), through transposons (other types of DNA—called conjugation), integrons and bacteriophages (called transduction).[16] For example, they may change how well they fit with the antibiotic, make an enzyme that makes the antibiotic ineffective, or reduce the amount of antibiotic that reaches them.[17]

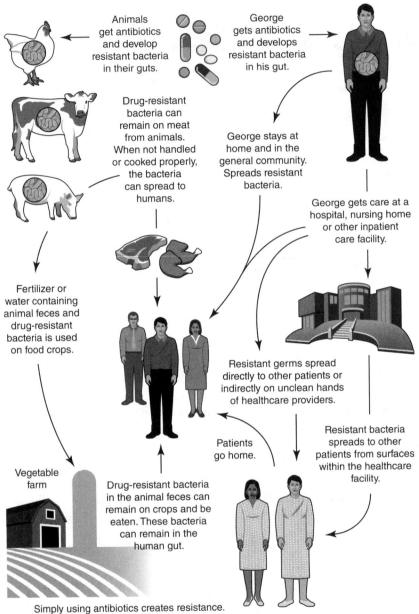

Figure 15–2 Examples of how antibiotic resistance spreads.

Reproduced from Centers for Disease Control and Prevention. Antibiotic Resistance Threats in the United States, 2013. Available at http://www.cdc.gov/drugresistance/ threat-report-2013/pdf/ar-threats-2013-508.pdf

Animal and Human Health Concerns

How does bacterial resistance in animals impact humans? Although complicated and controversial, experts believe that food is the most common source.[11] Resistant bacteria found in animal intestines can contaminate food during slaughter, during other steps in food production, and in home kitchens,[11] utilizing both direct spread (though contact with contaminated food) and indirect spread through water, manure, and contaminated soil.[18] In addition, food is less often produced and consumed locally, and as a result the potential for domestic or global spread of resistant bacteria is very real.[11]

Examples include spread of MRSA from animals to people and also from people to animals.[11] Documented spread of non-typhoid *Salmonella*, *Campylobacter*, and *E. coli* from animals to humans through food products provide additional evidence for connections between animal and human health in resistant infections.[11]

One study in a defined geographic area in Pennsylvania measured the association between human exposure to industrial agriculture (both swine and dairy/veal) and risk of MRSA infections.[19] The investigators studied 446,480 patients in one healthcare system from 2005 to 2010, comparing new MRSA infections documented through electronic health records (case patients). Case patients were compared to control patients to determine the impact of exposure to livestock animals and manure application as potential sources of infection.[19] Important findings included that the highest exposures to swine manure were statistically related to increased risks for community-associated MRSA infections and healthcare-associated MRSA.[19]

Smith and colleagues have used mathematical models to explore the impact of antibiotic use in agricultural settings on antibiotic-resistant infections in humans.[20] Their model suggested that use of antibiotics in agricultural settings speeds up the occurrence of antibiotic-resistant bacteria. Interestingly, they also noticed that this influence was most pronounced when resistant bacteria were increasing in number, implying that limiting antibiotic use might be most effective when resistant bacteria are still few.[20] Other authors highlight evidence that antibiotic-resistant bacteria are associated with food products from animals given antibiotics for "non-therapeutic" purposes and cite substantial evidence of animal-to-human spread of resistant bacteria.[18] The Lancet Commission concluded, "strong circumstantial evidence suggests that resistance genes circulate between people, animals, and the environment."[11]

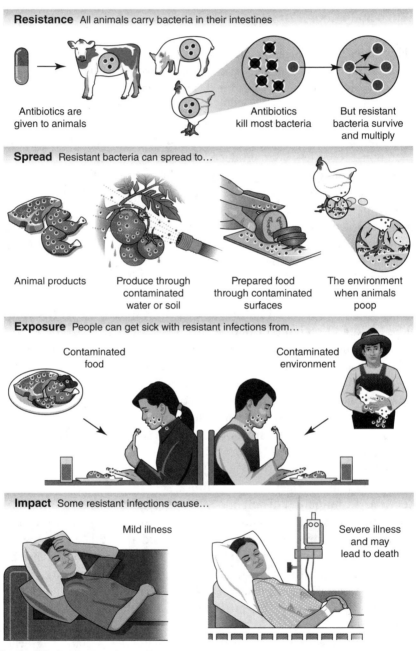

Figure 15–3 Antibiotic resistance in food-producing animals.

Reproduced from Centers for Disease Control and Prevention. National Antimicrobial Monitoring Systems: Antibiotic Use in Food-Producing Animals. Available at http://www.cdc.gov/narms/animals.html

In 1996 in the United States, the National Antimicrobial Resistance Monitoring System for Enteric Bacteria (NARMS) was developed to track how effective antibiotics are for certain intestinal bacteria in humans, meats sold in stores, and animals used for food.[21] The system involved three federal agencies with oversight over these areas: CDC, the U.S. Food and Drug Administration (FDA), and the United States Department of Agriculture (USDA), and the information gives early warnings about antibiotic resistance in these settings.[1] CDC supports reducing inappropriate antibiotic use in both human and animals because of the potential harm to public health[21] (see **Figure 15–3**).

The Infections—Urgent Concerns

CDC has identified three pathogens as "urgent" threats: *Clostridium difficile*, CRE, and drug-resistant *Neisseria gonorrhoeae*.[4] *C. difficile* causes an estimated 250,000 infections, 14,000 deaths (with 90% in people age 65 and older), and excess medical costs in greater than $1 billion each year[4] (see **Figure 15–4**). It causes a serious inflammation of the colon, called colitis, resulting in severe diarrhea. In contrast to some other healthcare-related infections, infections with *C. difficile* have increased by 400% in the period between 2000 and 2007.[22,23] Spread of this infection is often

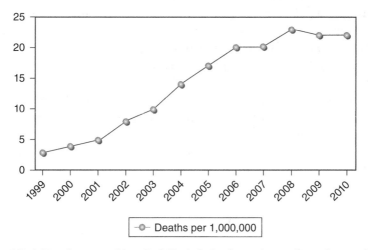

Figure 15–4 Deaths caused by *C. difficile* infections: Age-adjusted rate of *C. difficile* as the primary (underlying) cause of death.

Reproduced from Centers for Disease Control and Prevention. Making Health Care Safer, Stopping *C. difficile* infections. *CDC Vital Signs*. 2012. http://www.cdc.gov/vitalsigns/pdf/2012-03-vitalsigns.pdf

related to health care, especially in older patients who have recently taken antibiotics (making them vulnerable) and contracting the infection from healthcare settings.[22] The infection is then further spread when patients have severe diarrhea and bacteria are spread to others through direct or indirect contact with infectious feces.[22,23] Prevention priorities include tracking infections (surveillance), testing some patients with diarrhea, using antibiotics appropriately, following cleaning and infection control recommendations (including hand washing) to limit spread to others, and being alert to situations where infected patients may be transferred to long-term care facilities.[22]

About 9,000 infections and 600 deaths are attributed each year to CRE infections, such as those from *Klebsiella* and *E. coli* species.[4] Although not as common as some other types of healthcare-related infections, they have increased in the United States in the last 10 years.[24] To date, CRE bacteria have been reported in 42 states and as many as 50% of the bloodstream infections with these pathogens are fatal.[24] The reason that preventing these infections is urgent is they have become resistant to nearly all available antibiotics making them, in essence, untreatable.[24] CRE may spread among patients and is also serious because its resistance to nearly all known antibiotics may be spread to other bacteria.[4,24]

Antibiotic-resistant gonorrhea due to *N. gonorrhoeae* is an urgent threat in a common infection.[4] It has already become resistant to multiple antibiotics and if this continues, it will make it difficult to treat the large number of infections that occur each year in the United States.[4,25] *N. gonorrhoeae* is a sexually transmitted disease and if additional resistance occurs, CDC estimates this infection could result in additional HIV infections (*N. gonorrhoeae* infection makes the spread of HIV more likely), pelvic inflammatory disease (a leading cause of infertility), and increased healthcare costs, estimated at $235 million each year.[4] Prompt and appropriate treatment, careful tracking, ensuring capacity for healthcare and public health laboratory testing, and public education are all needed to prevent and control this infection.[4,25]

The Infections—Serious Concerns

CDC includes a dozen infections in the category of a "serious" threat to public health, including multidrug-resistant *Acinetobacter*, a bacteria resistant to multiple categories of antibiotics that causes pneumonia or infections in the blood of patients who are very ill and is often fatal.[4]

Other examples in this category are drug-resistant tuberculosis, drug-resistant *Salmonella typhi*, drug-resistant *Shigella,* and fluconazole-resistant *Candida,* a fungus.[4]

Drug-resistant *Campylobacter* causes more than 300,000 infections per year and *Campylobacter* of all types cause about 1.3 million infections per year, 13,000 hospitalizations, and more than 100 deaths.[4] Infection with *Campylobacter* causes such symptoms as abdominal pain and cramping, bloody diarrhea, nausea and vomiting, and fever. Complications of infection, although uncommon, can include arthritis and paralysis (called Guillain-Barre syndrome).[4,21] The cause for concern, especially in populations vulnerable to more serious infections (children, people with diseases or treatments causing a reduced ability to fight infections, and older individuals), is the increasing rate of antibiotic resistance, rising from 13% in 1997 to 25% in 2011.[4] Humans can become infected by eating contaminated food (raw or undercooked chicken), drinking raw milk, contact with animals with the bacteria, or from unclean water.[4,21] Public health officials are especially concerned, in the case of this infection, that antibiotic use in animals used for food contributes to the development of antibiotic resistance and subsequent human infection.[4,21]

For MRSA, CDC estimates there are more than 80,000 serious MRSA infections and 11,285 deaths each year from MRSA in the United States; this figure does not include less serious infections that are seen in community and healthcare settings.[4] Often causing a type of skin infection, MRSA can also cause pneumonia and bloodstream infections, and MRSA represents an important cause of serious infections in healthcare settings.[26] The good news related to MRSA is that as a result of specific interventions in healthcare settings, serious (invasive) MRSA infections are decreasing. Interventions designed to prevent blood infections from large intravenous catheters (called central lines) resulted in infection rates cut in half in just 10 years.[4] From the period 2005 to 2011, hospital-related invasive MRSA infections declined by more than 50%, and in total there were about 30,800 fewer MRSA infections in the United States.[27] However, infections in community settings (unrelated to health care) have been increasing over the past decade.[27] In 2011, much smaller declines were seen for MRSA infections in the community, and from a public health perspective additional reduction of MRSA infections must also focus on preventing the infections that are unrelated to health care by using effective public health strategies.[27]

Drug-resistant *Streptococcus pneumoniae,* sometimes called pneumococcus, causes many types of infections such as ear and sinus infections, pneumonia, meningitis, and blood infections.[28] Serious

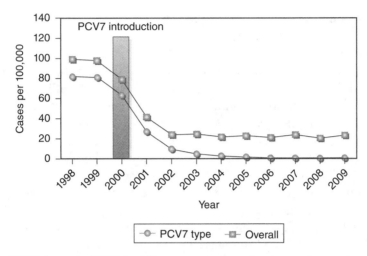

Figure 15–5 Impact of 7-Valent Pneumococcal conjugate vaccine on invasive pneumococcal disease among children <5 years old, 1998–2009.

Reproduced from Centers for Disease Control and Prevention. Pneumococcal Disease: Surveillance and Reporting. http://www.cdc.gov/pneumococcal/surveillance.html

infections (invasive disease) occur when bacteria enter the bloodstream or the fluid around the brain and spinal cord, causing much more serious and sometimes fatal infections.[28] *S. pneumoniae* may now be resistant to commonly used antibiotics, including penicillin and erythromycin; CDC estimates 1.2 million drug-resistant pneumococcal infections, 19,000 hospitalizations, 7,000 deaths, and $96 million in additional medical costs can be attributed to drug-resistant *S. pneumoniae* infections each year in the United States.[4] One of the most important public health strategies involves vaccination with pneumococcal conjugate vaccine (PCV) to prevent infections. This vaccine has prevented invasive disease and has also prevented the spread of some antibiotic-resistant strains.[4] Continued efforts to improve vaccination rates, as well as promoting the appropriate use of antibiotics are essential to combat resistance in *S. pneumoniae*[4,28] (see **Figure 15–5**).

The Infections—Current and Future Concerns

CDC classifies infection with vancomycin-resistant *S. aureus* (VRSA), clindamycin-resistant Group B *Streptococcus*, and erythromycin-resistant Group A *Streptococcus* as "concerning" infections.[4] Group A *Streptococcus* may cause common infections such as sore throat (strep throat), skin infections (impetigo), scarlet fever, rheumatic fever, and more serious infections (invasive GAS disease) when bacteria invade muscle, blood, or lungs.[29] Especially severe GAS infections include a muscle infection called necrotizing fasciitis ("flesh-eating" bacteria), which is fatal in one-quarter to one-third of patients, and a blood infection called Streptococcal toxic shock syndrome (STSS).[4,29] CDC estimates there are currently 1,300 antibiotic-resistant Group A *Streptococcus* infections and 160 deaths from these infections each year in the United States.[4] Although these are small numbers compared to the estimate of 1.0 to 2.6 million annual infections causing strep sore throat each year, GAS has become resistant to important categories of antibiotics needed for effective treatment. Given how common Group A strep infections are, antibiotic resistance will make it more challenging to treat patients who are allergic to penicillin, and some patients with serious GAS infections.[4]

EVIDENCE BASE FOR PREVENTION AND PRACTICE

CDC recommends familiar public health strategies called "Core Actions" to prevent antibiotic resistance: preventing infections (immunizations, hand washing, infection control, food safety), disease surveillance (tracking), "antibiotic stewardship" (appropriate antibiotic use in health care and animals), and calls for development of new antibiotics and laboratory tests.[4] In 2012, the WHO recommended a global strategy with similar elements.[8] The WHO recommends worldwide surveillance of antimicrobial use and resistant bacteria, appropriate use of antibiotics, reducing antibiotic use in animals, preventing and controlling infections in healthcare settings, incentives for the development of new antibiotics, and political commitment to ensure these strategies are systematically implemented.[8] The Lancet Commission recommends similar approaches, including recommendations about global governance and the need for innovation in development of new laboratory tests, vaccines, antibiotics, and other treatments.[11]

Health Care—Improving Antibiotic Prescribing

The public health benefits of appropriate antibiotic prescribing are compelling: reducing antibiotic use by about a third can reduce serious and fatal cases of diarrhea (*C. difficile* infection) by more than 25%.[30] Patients receiving broad-spectrum antibiotics in hospital settings have an increased risk (as much as three times higher) of getting another more serious antibiotic-resistant infection.[30] Furthermore, antibiotic prescribing practices in hospitals varies widely, up to a three-fold difference, across the United States.[30] In 2011 to 2012, the lowest antibiotic prescribing rates were seen in Alaska, California, Colorado, Hawaii, Idaho, Maryland, Minnesota, Montana, Nevada, New Hampshire, New Mexico, Oregon, Vermont, and Washington; the highest prescribing rates were seen in Alabama, Kentucky, Louisiana, Mississippi, Tennessee, and West Virginia.[31] A study conducted in 13 European countries in patients complaining of a cough showed great variation in antibiotic prescribing (from 20% to 90%) that could not be attributed to differences in either patient symptoms or patient populations.[32]

One interesting study looked at the relationship between community antibiotic use and seasons.[33] Using data on United States antibiotic usage and infection surveillance data, investigators conducted a time-series analysis to explore relationships between prescribing certain antibiotics and antibiotic resistance of *E. coli* and MRSA bacteria.[33] They noted that numbers of resistant infections followed antibiotic prescriptions by about a month, implying that on a population level, antibiotic prescribing and sales can result in seasonal changes in antibiotic resistance.[33] Their findings further suggested that hospital-based efforts to ensure appropriate antibiotic use must also be linked with similar efforts in communities to successfully prevent antibiotic-resistant infections.[33]

Previously, antibiotic prescribing for sore throats declined from 80% to 70% in 1993 and then to about 60% in 2000.[34] Despite long-term efforts to reduce unnecessary antibiotic prescribing, in one 2014 study it was estimated that about 60% of adults with sore throats were prescribed antibiotics, a percentage unchanged since 2000.[34] Only about 10% of adults are predicted to have Group A *Streptococcus* (GAS) infection requiring antibiotic treatment and despite the fact that most of these infections are caused by viruses many adult patients were prescribed antibiotics, and sometimes broader-spectrum antibiotics were chosen.[34]

Another study of U.S. adults in outpatient settings, using data from the National Ambulatory and National Hospital Ambulatory Medical Care Surveys, showed that antibiotics were prescribed for 10% of all outpatient visits each year.[35] More than 40% of all antibiotics were prescribed for respiratory conditions, and often broad-spectrum antibiotics were used. The authors concluded from their study that more than one-quarter of prescriptions were for infections where antibiotics were not usually needed.[35] In another study conducted in 12 countries, use of amoxicillin for lower-respiratory tract infections in adult patients (including older patients) who did not have pneumonia resulted in some side effects and no substantial overall clinical impact.[36]

Lawes and colleagues studied the effectiveness of hospital infection control in Scotland, including screening of patients for MRSA when they were admitted to the hospital on subsequent rates of MRSA infections including serious blood infections and death.[37] In the period from 2006 to 2010, they reported significant declines in all *S. aureus* blood infections (41% reduction), deaths (12% reduction), and MRSA blood infections from their combined efforts.[37]

Antibiotic Stewardship

Large medical organizations such as the American College of Physicians (ACP) provide information for health professionals (called ACP Smart Medicine) about antibiotic resistance, causes, and preventive strategies, for example in antibiotic-related *C. difficile* infections.[38] The American Academy of Pediatrics (AAP) published guidelines in 2013 about prescribing antibiotics in children with upper respiratory tract infections.[39] Because of the volume of antibiotic prescriptions written, approaching 50 million annually (or nearly 20% of visits), and the fact that the vast majority of upper respiratory tract infections are due to viral, not bacterial infections, AAP produced guidelines for common infections in children.[39] The "principles" recommended include considering whether or not an infection is bacterial, considering both potential benefits and harms from antibiotic use, and if an antibiotic is chosen, using the most appropriate one.[39]

CDC promotes a national educational campaign, "Get Smart: Know When Antibiotics Work," to educate the public and health professionals about antibiotic prescribing.[40] It includes an extensive and current website with information about what types of infections do and do not require antibiotic treatment, information about antibiotic resistance and how to prevent it, and specific information for health care and also farm settings.[40] Antibiotic stewardship (programs designed to ensure antibiotics are used appropriately and only if needed) can potentially decrease resistance to antibiotics, decrease *C. difficile* infections in healthcare settings, decrease healthcare costs from preventable infections, and improve patient outcomes.[40]

A detailed Cochrane study of 95 hospital inpatient antibiotic stewardship programs assessed their effectiveness in promoting appropriate antibiotic use, reducing antibiotic-resistant infections, and improving patient outcomes.[41] Some programs restricted which antibiotics could be prescribed, others used education and reminders, and some used a combination of these approaches. The programs that used restrictive measures were effective early on, but programs that emphasized an educational approach and restrictive programs both had a similar impact after 6 months.[41] The authors concluded from their extensive review that such antibiotic stewardship programs were associated with a decrease in hospital-related infections, a decline in antibiotic resistance, and better clinical results in patients.[41]

Policy Approaches—Animal and Human Health

In addition to health care, CDC focuses on preventing infections and antibiotic resistance in the community and in food, working with the FDA and USDA to track infections through the National Antimicrobial Resistance Monitoring System (NARMS).[21] This collaborative disease tracking system follows changes in effectiveness of antibiotics in humans, food, and animals to provide information about changes in antibiotic resistance, and links between infections in humans and animals.[21]

In 2005, the FDA banned use of fluoroquinolone antibiotics in poultry and recommended generally against using antibiotics for growth promotion in 2012.[6] In December 2013, the FDA announced a new strategic plan and guidance for companies manufacturing antibiotics used in animals to reduce unnecessary use of antibiotics to promote animal growth.[42] The plan would be phased in and require licensed-veterinarian oversight of antibiotics rather than allowing the over-the-counter (OTC) purchase of antibiotics by animal producers. It also asks companies manufacturing antibiotics for animals to change their labels reflecting the change in use.[42] Some public health experts considered this "the first significant step in dealing with this important public health concern in 20 years."[43] Critics, however, claimed, "The FDA is using a garden hose on a forest fire," and were skeptical that the new guidance would change anything, because the FDA is asking pharmaceutical companies to voluntarily follow their guidance, and in essence, letting the industry regulate itself.[44] The National Chicken Council, although supportive of the FDA's guidance and the process for development and implementation, said, "For those antibiotics that are FDA-approved for use in raising chickens, the majority of them are not used in human medicine and therefore do not represent any threat of creating resistance in humans."[45]

Regulation of antibiotic use in animals is not new; Sweden banned the use in animal food production in 1986 and by 2009 saw a decline from 45 tons to 15 tons of antibiotics sold for this purpose.[10] Denmark, the United Kingdom, and the Netherlands later followed with similar policies. From 1992 to 2008, Denmark experienced more than a 50% decrease in antibiotic use, while swine production increased by nearly 50%. Poultry antibiotic use declined by 90% with a modest increase in production.[10]

Other authors suggest price as a way to limit unnecessary use instead of a ban with a "user fee" for antibiotics use in livestock, pets, crops, and aquaculture.[6] They argue that a ban would increase food prices, especially for lower-income citizens, and would be costly and challenging to enforce (despite the evidence from Europe), whereas a "user fee" would be simpler and create a new source of funds, potentially for new antibiotic development or other related programs.[6] To see whether restrictive antibiotic policies (such as requiring veterinarian prescription or banning use for growth promotion in animals) has an adverse effect on food production, Maron and colleagues conducted a study of policies for antimicrobial use in 17 non-U.S. locations.[46] They concluded that in the long term, food production may not be adversely impacted by these policies, but rather U.S. food production could experience potential trade barriers due to its *less* stringent requirements.[46]

Novel Treatments for Serious Infections

While the long-term goal is to reduce the incidence of antibiotic resistance and prevent these urgent, serious, and concerning infections,[4] the challenges of treating these infections in healthcare settings should not be underestimated. *C. difficile* infections, one of three "urgent" threats, kills 14,000 U.S. patients every year and causes 50,000 infections.[4] Patients who have taken antibiotics (especially for longer periods), killing the normal colon bacteria, are at increased risk.[47] Treatments may mean even more antibiotics, and sometimes the *C. difficile* infection recurs requiring prolonged treatment,[47,48] which is why the infection is so serious to patients, and costly to the healthcare system ($1 million each year).[4]

Many studies have shown the efficacy of using "fecal transplants," giving patients who are seriously ill with *C. difficile* infections, feces from healthy donors using enemas, nasogastric tubes, or colonoscopies to restore normal colon bacteria.[48] Studies have shown the effectiveness of this approach, often called fecal microbiota transplantation (FMT), as superior to antibiotic treatment[49] and both individual studies[50,51] and systematic reviews[52] show a treatment success rate of 90% or higher. The difficulty, until recently, has been in the way the transplants were done, some requiring colonoscopy or other means not well accepted by patients. But in 2014, the National Institutes of Health (NIH) director asks in his blog, "What about poop pills?"[47] Researchers found a way to make purified and concentrated frozen fecal capsules and tested them on 20 patients ranging from 11 to 89 years old. Symptoms were eliminated in 90% of patients, most after the first taking one FMT capsule.[53] Further research is needed in larger groups of patients, and it is likely that researchers will also try to develop these bacteria in laboratory settings.[47]

Development of New Antibiotics

Recognizing the need for multiple initiatives, CDC, WHO, and the Lancet Commission have all included the urgent need for development of new antibiotics as part of an overall global strategy to combat antibiotic resistance.[4,8,11] Cooper and Shlaes write that in the past four decades, only four new antibiotic classes have been developed; they offer concrete policy options for the United States and European Union to collaboratively promote more rapid development of new antibiotics.[54] In the United States, trials to test new drugs, called clinical trials, are conducted in four separate phases in order to study different aspects of a new medication's safety and effectiveness, and compare it to other treatments.[55] Phase III clinical trials use large groups of patients to collect information on side effects, effectiveness, and comparison to other treatments for the same condition.[55] It costs $70 million to conduct the trials for an antibiotic used to treat one disease. This creates a disincentive for pharmaceutical companies, especially smaller ones, from developing such new drugs.[54] In 2009, the London School of Economics suggested a "push-pull" incentive: the "push" component would include government funding for Phase III trials and the "pull" would include government purchase of a defined quantity and expedited review by the FDA, along with 5 additional years of patent protection.[54] Cooper and Shlaes argue that both U.S. and European governments would ultimately experience financial benefits from these investments, given the estimated $20 billion of costs each year to U.S.

hospitals from antibiotic-resistant infections and prevalence of these infections (about 2 million each year) in the European Union.[54] As part of a longer list of recommendations to reduce antimicrobial-resistant infections, the Infectious Diseases Society of America similarly calls for incentives for development of new antibiotics, including grants and tax credits for their research and development.[56]

Future Needs

Many gaps remain in our knowledge about antibiotic-resistant infections and in our basic public health tools to better prevent them. For example, international systems to track antibiotic-resistant infections do not currently exist, and even in the United States, antibiotic use in healthcare, agriculture, or aquaculture is not monitored.[4] Evidence-based programs to reduce unnecessary antibiotic use in healthcare settings are not universal and available technology to better identify antibiotic-resistant pathogens is underutilized.[4] The contribution of the environment is often overlooked: wastewater containing pharmaceuticals, wastewater treatment plants, or runoff of animal manure into surface water may also according to some authors contribute to the spread of bacterial resistance.[11] On a global level, many experts call for a global system of tracking (public health surveillance) of both antibiotic use and resistant organisms.[11]

In addition, lack of widespread immunizations represents an opportunity and a challenge in preventing resistant infections. For example, use of PCV has helped prevent infections and antibiotic resistance in the United States but is far less frequently used in LMICs.[57] Another priority area is development of both new methods and better use of existing laboratory tests for infectious diseases, especially in LMICs. Some experts make the point that availability and better use of existing diagnostic tests for common infectious diseases in every patient could help prioritize needs for antibiotics and be effective on a population level.[11] One interesting approach to educate the public and health professionals about antibiotic use and bacterial resistance has been the development of a "Resistance Map" by the Center for Disease Dynamics, Economics & Policy to allow comparison of between states in the United States and trends over time.[58] This approach is an intriguing way to focus attention of the broad group of stakeholders required to impact antibiotic resistance, and would require consistent surveillance data to be practical for use on a global scale.

DISCUSSION QUESTIONS: TEMPLATE FOR DISCUSSION

1. Significance of this public health issue:
   a. Why is this health issue important?
   b. How many people does it impact?
   c. How serious is it?
   d. Is it preventable?
2. What is the evidence base for prevention?
3. What specific strategies should be used to achieve progress on this health issue?
   a. What evidence-based approach would you use?
   b. Where would you start if you are an individual citizen; public health professional; healthcare professional; community, state, or federal policymaker?
4. Specific questions for this topic:
   a. What is the evidence for the link between inappropriate antibiotic use in humans and animals and increases in antibiotic-resistance in infectious diseases?
   b. What geographic areas and populations are at greatest risk?
   c. What diseases are the highest public health concern and why?
   d. What evidence-based policies, if systematically applied, could result in reductions in the public health impacts of antimicrobial resistance?
   e. What barriers prevent better policies to protect public health from being implemented? In the United States? Globally?
5. What is the controversy?
   a. Define the controversy.
   b. Is controversy a good or bad thing? (Does it help or hinder progress?)
6. *Why* is this health issue controversial?
   a. What specific factors are involved?
   b. Do economics, government, scientific uncertainty, or politics play a role?
   c. What is the role of the media?
7. How would you respond to the controversy?

PERSPECTIVES TO CONSIDER

As with many public health issues, the challenges include gathering all of the stakeholders in a sustained initiative that focuses on prevention. Studies cited remind us that we live in a global society and antibiotic-resistant infections must be prevented on a community, state, national, and global level and not solely in healthcare settings. Some studies suggest that antibiotic use reductions have plateaued at a way-too-high level,[34] suggesting both public and professional education must be sustained. In developing countries, this issues strikes a delicate balancing act between overuse and lack of access in many countries and especially in rural locations.[11] CDC's efforts in the United States to quantify the magnitude and severity of this public health issue,[4] will serve as a foundation to measure progress moving forward. Despite the size and complexity of this issue, there is striking consensus on a global level,[4,8,11,56] regarding the strategies, systems, and actions needed to improve public health.

FOR ADDITIONAL STUDY

Laxminarayan R, Duse A, Wattal C, et al. Antibiotic resistance—the need for global solutions. *Lancet Infect Dis.* 2013;13(12):1057–1098.

WHO. The evolving threat of antimicrobial resistance: Options for action. 2012. http://whqlibdoc.who.int/publications/2012/9789241503181_eng.pdf.

REFERENCES

1. CBS Chicago. Outbreak of drug-resistant bacteria linked to Lutheran General Hospital 2014. http://chicago.cbslocal.com/2014/01/06/outbreak-of-drug-resistant-bacteria-linked-to-lutheran-general-hospital/. Accessed Janaury 17, 2014.
2. CDC. Notes from the field: New Delhi Metallo-β-Lactamase–Producing *Escherichia coli* associated with endoscopic retrograde cholangiopancreatography—Illinois, 2013. *MMWR.* 2014. http://www.cdc.gov/mmwr/preview/mmwrhtml/mm6251a4.htm. Accessed January 17, 2014.
3. Tavernise S. Antibiotic-resistant infections lead to 23,000 deaths a year, CDC finds. *The New York Times.* 2013. http://www.nytimes.com/2013/09/17/health/cdc-report-finds-23000-deaths-a-year-from-antibiotic-resistant-infections.html. Accessed December 8, 2013.
4. CDC. Antibiotic resistance threats in the United States, 2013. 2013. http://www.cdc.gov/drugresistance/threat-report-2013/pdf/ar-threats-2013-508.pdf. Accessed December 5, 2013.
5. Editorial. The antibiotic resistance crisis. *The New York Times.* 2013. http://www.nytimes.com/2013/09/18/opinion/the-antibiotic-resistance-crisis.html. Accessed January 3, 2014.
6. Hollis A, Ahmed Z. Preserving antibiotics, rationally. *N Engl J Med.* 2013;369(26): 2474–2476.
7. Sjeklocha D. Antimicrobial resistance needs a team solution. *Beef Magazine.com.* 2013. http://beefmagazine.com/blog/antimicrobial-resistance-needs-team-solution. Accessed January 17, 2014.

8. WHO. The evolving threat of antimicrobial resistance: Options for action. 2012. http://whqlibdoc.who.int/publications/2012/9789241503181_eng.pdf. Accessed January 18, 2014.

9. WHO. 10 Facts on antimicrobial resistance. 2012. http://www.who.int/features/factfiles/antimicrobial_resistance/en/. Accessed December 8, 2013.

10. Mackie B. Lessons from Europe on reducing antibiotic use in livestock. *BCMJ.* 2011. http://www.bcmj.org/council-health-promotion/lessons-europe-reducing-antibiotic-use-livestock. Accessed January 17, 2014.

11. Laxminarayan R, Duse A, Wattal C, et al. Antibiotic resistance—the need for global solutions. *Lancet Infect Dis.* 2013;13(12):1057–1098.

12. Allegranzi B, Bagheri Nejad S, Combescure C, et al. Burden of endemic health-care-associated infection in developing countries: systematic review and meta-analysis. *Lancet.* 2011;377(9761):228–241.

13. Jacob JT, et al. Vital signs: Carbapenem-resistant *Enterobacteriaceae. MMWR.* 2013; 62(09):165–170. http://www.cdc.gov/mmwr/preview/mmwrhtml/mm6209a3.htm. Accessed January 18, 2014.

14. WHO. Antimicrobial resistance fact sheet. 2014. http://who.int/mediacentre/factsheets/fs194/en/. Accessed October 20, 2014.

15. MedlinePlus: Antibiotics. 2013. http://www.nlm.nih.gov/medlineplus/antibiotics.html. Accessed January 17, 2014.

16. Giedraitiene A, Vitkauskiene A, Naginiene R, Pavilonis A. Antibiotic resistance mechanisms of clinically important bacteria. *Medicina.* 2011;47(3):137–146.

17. Jacoby GA, Archer GL. New mechanisms of bacterial resistance to antimicrobial agents. *N Engl J Med.* 1991;324(9):601–612.

18. Marshall BM, Levy SB. Food animals and antimicrobials: Impacts on human health. *Clin Micro Rev.* 2011;24(4):718–733.

19. Casey JA, Curriero FC, Cosgrove SE, Nachman KE, Schwartz BS. High-density livestock operations, crop field application of manure, and risk of community-associated methicillin-resistant *Staphylococcus aureus* infection in Pennsylvania. *JAMA Int Med.* 2013;173(21):1980–1990.

20. Smith DL, Harris AD, Johnson JA, Silbergeld EK, Morris JG, Jr. Animal antibiotic use has an early but important impact on the emergence of antibiotic resistance in human commensal bacteria. *Proc Natl Acad Sci U S A.* 2002;99(9):6434–6439.

21. CDC. National Antimicrobial Resistance Monitoring System (NARMS). 2013. http://www.cdc.gov/narms Accessed January 17, 2014.

22. CDC. Making health care safer: Stopping *C. difficile* infections. *CDC Vital Signs.* 2012. http://www.cdc.gov/VitalSigns/Hai/StoppingCdifficile/. Accessed January 17, 2014.

23. CDC. Healthcare-associated infections (HAIs): *Clostridium difficile* infection. 2013. http://www.cdc.gov/HAI/organisms/cdiff/Cdiff_infect.html. Accessed January 17, 2014.

24. CDC. Making health care safer: Stop infections from lethal CRE germs now. *CDC Vital Signs.* 2013. http://www.cdc.gov/vitalsigns/pdf/2013-03-vitalsigns.pdf. Accessed December 8, 2013.

25. CDC. Sexually transmitted diseases (STDs): Antibiotic-resistant gonnorrhea. 2013. http://www.cdc.gov/std/Gonorrhea/arg/default.htm. Accessed January 17, 2014.

26. CDC. Methicillin-resistant *Staphylococcus aureus* (MRSA) infections. 2013. http://www.cdc.gov/mrsa/. Accessed October 20, 2014.

27. Dantes R, Mu Y, Belflower R, et al. National burden of invasive methicillin-resistant *Staphylococcus aureus* infections, United States, 2011. *JAMA Int Med.* 2013;173(21): 1970–1978.

28. CDC. Pneumoccal disease. 2014. http://www.cdc.gov/pneumococcal/index.html. Accessed October 20, 2014.

29. CDC. Group A Streptococcal (GAS) disease. 2014. http://www.cdc.gov/groupastrep/index.html. Accessed October 20, 2014.

30. CDC. Making health care safer: Antibiotic Rx in hospitals: Proceed with caution *CDC Vital Signs.* 2014. http://www.cdc.gov/vitalsigns/antibiotic-prescribing-practices/index.html. Accessed October 20, 2014.

31. CDC. Antibiotic prescribing rates by state across the U.S. (2011/2012). 2012. http://www.cdc.gov/media/releases/2012/images/dpk-antibiotics-week-prescribing-rate.html. Accessed January 18, 2014.

32. Butler CC, Hood K, Verheij T, et al. Variation in antibiotic prescribing and its impact on recovery in patients with acute cough in primary care: Prospective study in 13 countries. *BMJ.* 2009;338:b2242.

33. Sun L, Klein EY, Laxminarayan R. Seasonality and temporal correlation between community antibiotic use and resistance in the United States. *Clin Inf Dis.* 2012;55(5): 687–694.

34. Barnett ML, Linder JA. Antibiotic prescribing to adults with sore throat in the United States, 1997–2010. *JAMA Int Med.* 2014;174(1):138–140.

35. Shapiro DJ, Hicks LA, Pavia AT, Hersh AL. Antibiotic prescribing for adults in ambulatory care in the USA, 2007–09. *J Antimicrob Chemother.* 2014;69(1):234–240.

36. Little P, Stuart B, Moore M, et al. Amoxicillin for acute lower-respiratory-tract infection in primary care when pneumonia is not suspected: A 12-country, randomised, placebo-controlled trial. *Lancet Inf Dis.* 2013;13(2):123–129.

37. Lawes T, Edwards B, Lopez-Lozano JM, Gould I. Trends in *Staphylococcus aureus* bacteraemia and impacts of infection control practices including universal MRSA admission screening in a hospital in Scotland, 2006–2010: Retrospective cohort study and time-series intervention analysis. *BMJ Open.* 2012;e000797;1–17.

38. ACP. ACP smart medicine: *Clostridium difficile*-associated diarrhea. 2014. http://smartmedicine.acponline.org/content.aspx?gbosId=216. Accessed October 20, 2014.

39. Hersh AL, Jackson MA, Hicks LA. American Academy of Pediatrics Committee on Infectious Diseases. Principles of judicious antibiotic prescribing for upper respiratory tract infections in pediatrics. *Pediatrics.* 2013;132(6):1146–1154.

40. CDC. Get smart: Know when antibiotics work. 2014. http://www.cdc.gov/getsmart/. Accessed October 20, 2014.

41. Davey P, Brown E, Charani E, et al. Interventions to improve antibiotic prescribing practices for hospital inpatients. *Cochrane Database Syst Rev.* 2013;4:1–208.

42. US FDA. FDA News Release: FDA takes significant steps to address antimicrobial resistance. 2013. http://www.fda.gov/NewsEvents/Newsroom/PressAnnouncements/ucm378193.htm. Accessed January 17, 2014.

43. Tavernise S. FDA restricts antibiotics use for livestock. *The New York Times.* 2013. http://www.nytimes.com/2013/12/12/health/fda-to-phase-out-use-of-some-antibiotics-in-animals-raised-for-meat.html?_r=0. Accessed December 8, 2013.

44. Rosenberg M. Dream on! Is the FDA really phasing antibiotics out of meat? *Counterpunch.* 2013. http://www.counterpunch.org/2013/12/24/is-the-fda-really-phasing-antibiotics-out-of-meat/. Accessed January 17, 2014.

45. NCC Statement on FDA Final Guidance #213 and Veterinary Feed Directive Proposal. *National Chicken Council: Press Release and Statement.* 2013. http://www.nationalchickencouncil.org/ncc-statement-fda-final-guidance-213-veterinary-feed-directive-proposal/. Accessed January 17, 2013.

46. Maron DF, Smith TJ, Nachman KE. Restrictions on antimicrobial use in food animal production: An international regulatory and economic survey. *Glob Health.* 2013;9:48.

47. Collins F. You won't believe what's in these pills. *NIH Director's Blog.* 2014. http://directorsblog.nih.gov/2014/10/21/you-wont-believe-whats-in-these-pills/. Accessed October 22, 2014.

48. Malani P. Fecal transplant pill effective against recurrent *Clostridium difficile* infection. *news@JAMA.* 2013. http://newsatjama.jama.com/2013/10/04/fecal-transplant-pill-effective-against-recurrent-clostridium-difficile-infection/. Accessed December 8, 2013.

49. van Nood E, Vrieze A, Nieuwdorp M, et al. Duodenal infusion of donor feces for recurrent *Clostridium difficile. N Engl J Med.* 2013;368(5):407–415.

50. Rohlke F, Stollman N. Fecal microbiota transplantation in relapsing *Clostridium difficile* infection. *Thera Ad Gas.* 2012;5(6):403–420.

51. Youngster I, Sauk J, Pindar C, et al. Fecal microbiota transplant for relapsing *Clostridium difficile* infection using a frozen inoculum from unrelated donors: A randomized, open-label, controlled pilot study. *Clin Inf Dis.* 2014;58(11):1515–1522.

52. Gough E, Shaikh H, Manges AR. Systematic review of intestinal microbiota transplantation (fecal bacteriotherapy) for recurrent *Clostridium difficile* infection. *Clin Inf Dis.* 2011;53(10):994–1002.

53. Youngster I, Russell GH, Pindar C, Ziv-Baran T, Sauk J, Hohmann EL. Oral, capsulized, frozen fecal microbiota transplantation for relapsing *Clostridium difficile* infection. *JAMA.* 2014; 312(17):1772–1778.

54. Cooper MA, Shlaes D. Fix the antibiotics pipeline. *Nature.* 2011;472(7341):32.

55. NIH. Clinical Trials.gov—Clinical trial phases. 2008. http://www.nlm.nih.gov/services/ctphases.html. Accessed January 20, 2014.

56. Spellberg B, Guidos R, Gilbert D, et al. The epidemic of antibiotic-resistant infections: A call to action for the medical community from the Infectious Diseases Society of America. *Clin Inf Dis.* 2008;46(2):155–164.

57. Laxminarayan R, Heymann DL. Challenges of drug resistance in the developing world. *BMJ.* 2012;344:e1567.

58. CDDEP. Center for disease dynamics, economics & policy: Resistance map. 2013. http://www.cddep.org/map. Accessed January 18, 2014.

CHAPTER 16

Preventing Firearm Injuries— A Public Health Issue

LEARNING OBJECTIVES

- Discuss the public health impact of firearm injuries in the United States.
- Identify statistics for types of injuries, prevalence, epidemiology, and geographic variation.
- Identify populations at increased risk for firearms injuries, both homicides and suicides.
- Describe the role of advocacy organizations in the development and implementation of evidence-based policies to prevent firearm injury.
- Critically evaluate the evidence for programs and policies to reduce firearm injuries and death in the United States.
- Propose priority research areas to address current gaps.
- Propose evidence-based strategies to reduce the public health impact of firearm injuries.

THE CONTROVERSY

On December 14, 2012, a young man, after first killing his mother, forcibly entered the Sandy Hook Elementary School in Newtown, CT and killed 20 young children and 6 adults, then killed himself using semiautomatic pistols and a semiautomatic rifle.[1] In recent years, only the 2007 Virginia Tech shootings, when a single gunman killed 32 people before killing himself, claimed more lives.[1] Pictures of terrified children, grieving parents, and the all-too-many questions of a peaceful community flooded the national news, as the nation collectively searched for answers, again. At a memorial service, President Obama said, "We can't tolerate this anymore. We are not doing enough and we have to change."[2] Observers noted the occasion marked the fourth time the President had addressed grieving communities and saw a change in the tone of his remarks, as he seemed to take an "enough is enough" approach, promising "I'll use whatever power this office holds . . ." and emphasizing the need for stronger efforts to prevent such events in the future.[2]

A week later, as public discussion of potential solutions, including new laws, grew louder, the National Rifle Association (NRA) announced a plan to have armed security officers (including retired law enforcement officers and volunteers) in every school in the United States.[3] The proposed program was called the National School Shield program and would be financed in part by the NRA. In the media announcement, the NRA vice president stated, "The only thing that stops a bad guy with a gun is a good guy with a gun," and further argued that lack of enforcement, the media, and violent video games played a critical role.[3] Although armed security officers in schools were already being used in some large U.S. cities, the proposal was met with mixed reactions. Some called the proposal "delusional," and the parent of a child in the Newtown, CT school system said simply, "I think people are smarter than that."[3]

In January, 2013 the White House released a plan entitled: "Now is the Time: The president's plan to protect our children and our communities by reducing gun violence."[4] The plan included closing loopholes in background checks, bans on military-style assault weapons and high-capacity magazines, improving school safety, and improving access to mental health services.[4] However, on the 1-year anniversary of the Newtown shootings, there was little evidence of a "tipping point" having been reached. Although there were many new laws passed at the state level, they included both more and fewer restrictions on firearms.[5] Federal policy activity remained at a standstill and despite an impassioned plea by Gabrielle Giffords,[6] representative from Arizona from 2007 to 2012 and herself a shooting victim, U.S. Senate proposals were making no headway. As of June 2013, the U.S. House had not taken up these measures.[7,8]

What did the American public think? A poll conducted by the Washington Post/Pew Research Center found that after the Newtown shootings, 90% of respondents supported some type of universal background checks, though far fewer, about half, were distressed when the Senate did not pass these measures.[8] During this time, new advocacy organizations were formed, such as Moms Demand Action, the Sandy Hook Promise, the Campaign to Unload, and Americans for Responsible Solutions, formed by Gabrielle Giffords and Mark Kelly.[7] Lobbying in Congress was also intense: gun control groups spent $1.6 million in 2013 (a 500% increase over their spending in 2012), while opponents of gun control measures spent $6.2 million; both figures were reported by the Sunlight Foundation.[7]

However, state laws saw much activity in just a year's time, with 1,500 state firearm bills introduced across the country since December 14, 2012.[5] Of these, *The New York Times* reported that 109 became state laws, with 39 "tightening" gun restrictions and 70 laws "loosening" gun restrictions.[5] A State University of New York (SUNY Cortland) professor remarked, "I think both Republicans and Democrats, by and large, would rather the gun issue would go away. . . Neither party really wants to latch on to this issue."[7]

Mass shootings are not new in the United States, and the history of these shootings, whether in schools, worksites, or public places, can be found in a variety of Web-based sources,[9–11] including *Mother Jones*[10] and *The Washington Post* Wonk blog.[11] Sources of information include data from media sources, sociologists, economists, but only an occasional public health researcher.[11] In a *JAMA* editorial[12] describing the strengths and limitations of a research study to determine whether states with more firearm laws had fewer firearm-related deaths,[13] the author observed "it is as if the scientists have both hands tied behind their backs," referring to the collective efforts of the scientific community to determine "what works?" to prevent firearm injuries.[12] Sparse research has been published by very few investigators since the 1990s, following what was described as a "clash between public health scientists and the NRA."[14] At this time, the Center for Disease Control and Prevention's (CDC) program funding was cut and redirected. The impact on CDC's research program was characterized by one firearm injury researcher as a "near-death experience."[12,14]

BACKGROUND AND SCOPE OF THE PUBLIC HEALTH AND HEALTH POLICY ISSUE

Data and Statistics—The Epidemiology of Firearm Injuries

In 2013, CDC reported on fatal firearm homicides and suicides in some large U.S. cities in the time periods from 2006–2007 and 2009–2010.[15] Using data from WISQARS (Web-based Injury Statistics Query and Reporting System),[16] the National Vital Statistics System

(NVSS), and population data from the U.S. Census Bureau, CDC analyzed fatal injuries (homicides and suicides) for cities such as Atlanta, Baltimore, Boston, Chicago, New York, Los Angeles, and Washington, DC, including the 50 largest (most populous) U.S. metropolitan statistical areas (MSAs) in their analysis. From 2009 to 2010, there were 38,126 firearm-related suicides and 22,571 firearm-related homicides in U.S. residents.[15]

From 2009 to 2010, homicide was the 15th leading cause of death for people of all ages and the second leading cause of death in adolescents and young adults (ages 10 to 19).[15] Overall, 68% of homicides were due to firearm injuries; for adolescents and young adults, the figure was 83%.[15] Suicide is the 10th leading cause of death in the U.S. and the third leading cause of death for 10 to 19 year olds; 51% of all suicides and 40% of suicides in adolescents and young adults were attributed to firearm injuries.[15]

Since 2006–2007, data shows that more than 75% of MSAs had a decreased homicide rate, and more than 75% had an increased suicide rate.[15] In addition, rates of firearm-related homicides and suicides showed variation across the U.S. in 2009–2010. For example, firearm-related homicides ranged from a low of 1.1 per 100,000 residents per year (San Diego–Carlsbad, CA) to a high of 19.0 per 100,000 residents per year (New Orleans–Metairie, LA).[15] Firearm-related suicides ranged from a low of 1.6 per 100,000 residents per year (New York–Newark–Jersey City, NY-NJ-PA) to a high of 11.4 per 100,000 residents per year (Las Vegas–Henderson–Paradise, NV).[15] The authors note the importance of using data to monitor trends in firearm injuries, and to assess the impact and effectiveness of prevention and policy approaches.[15]

Studies of injuries and death from firearms, using national public health surveys such as the Behavioral Risk Factor Surveillance System (BRFSS), have reported higher rates of homicides in men, women, and children occurring in states with higher rates of firearm ownership.[17] Although these associations are statistically significant, the authors note that findings from these types of studies do not determine cause and effect, but rather generate hypotheses for additional detailed study.[17]

A comprehensive summary of firearm injuries that reviews available data and its limitations is published by the Firearm and Injury Center at Penn (FICAP).[18] A 2011 summary notes that 13 U.S. data systems are housed in different federal agencies. Data from the National Violent Death Registry System (NVDRS), from CDC, is available for 16 states.[19] There are limitations of available data for use in research and to determine effectiveness of prevention strategies. Most of the national data systems are not connected, there is sparse community-level data, and a paucity of data about less-serious injuries.[18] Currently available data sources include CDC's National Center for Health Statistics data in the National Vital Statistics System (NVSS), WISQARS, National Electronic Injury Surveillance System (NEISS) data about nonfatal injuries (from 91 U.S. hospitals), the NVDRS, the Federal Bureau of Investigation (FBI) Uniform Crime Reporting (UCR), Bureau of Justice Statistics (BJS), U.S. Bureau of Alcohol, Tobacco, Firearms, and Explosives (firearm manufacturing and sales), World Health Organization (WHO), and others.[18]

Based on the FICAP report, each year between 1980 and 2007, there were about 32,300 firearm-related deaths in the United States, making these injuries the second leading cause of death from injury in the United States, exceeded only by motor vehicle injuries.[18] In young people, aged 15 to 24 years, firearm-related homicide is the second leading cause of death and firearm-related suicide is the third leading cause of death.[18] In addition, firearm deaths (including both homicides and suicides) vary across the United States: Louisiana, Alaska, Mississippi, and Alabama have the highest death rates and Hawaii, Massachusetts, Rhode Island, and New York have the lowest.[18] Deaths from firearms are seen in both urban and rural areas in the United States with firearm-related homicides higher in cities and firearm-related suicides and injuries higher in rural settings.[18] Data from WISQARS highlights geographic variation in the United States for both firearm-related suicide and homicide deaths[16] (see **Figures 16–1** and **16–2**).

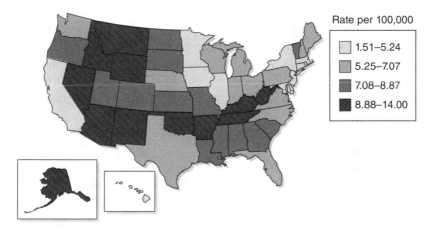

Figure 16–1 Age-adjusted death rates for firearm suicide, US, 2004–2010.

Reproduced from CDC Injury Prevention and Control: Data and Statistics (WISQARS). Available at http://www.cdc.gov/injury/wisqars/index.html

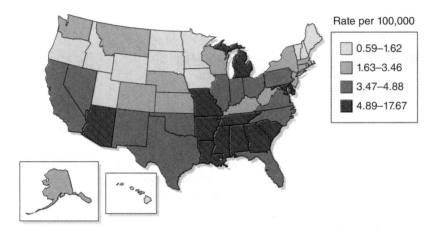

Figure 16–2 Age-adjusted death rates for firearm homicide, US, 2004–2010.

Reproduced from CDC Injury Prevention and Control: Data and Statistics (WISQARS). Available at http://www.cdc.gov/injury/wisqars/index.html

International Comparisons

A comparison of homicide rates from the 1990s of 26 high-income countries, using a simple comparison between firearm homicide rates and firearm availability, showed a statistically significant association between the availability of firearms and firearm-related homicides.[20] The United Nations Office on Drugs and Crime (UNODC) homicide statistics, covering 207 countries and territories and using both public health and criminal justice data, facilitates comparison of intentional firearm-related homicide rates between the United States and other countries.[21] An analysis of this data in *The Washington Post* notes the U.S. firearm homicide rate is 4 times higher than that of Turkey and Switzerland, and about 20 times higher than rates in many other developed countries.[22] The highest rates of firearm homicides are found in Honduras, with 68.4 firearm homicides per 100,000 people, about 20 times higher than the U.S. rate.[22,23]

In a provocative interactive map using available data on firearm homicides from a variety of sources (only some from government organizations), an author from *The Atlantic CityLab* provides visual comparisons between major U.S. cities and other countries.[23] For example, Washington, DC's firearm homicide rate is higher than that of Brazil, and Baltimore's rate is similar to that of Guatemala.[23] Detroit's rate is similar to El Salvador, and New Orleans (62.1 firearm homicides per 100,000 people) would

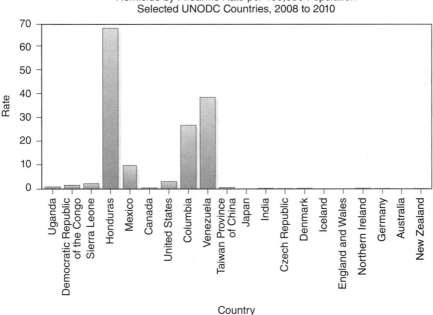

Figure 16–3 United Nations Office on Drugs and Crime (UNODC): Homicide by firearm rates.

Data from UNODC Homicide Statistics 2014. Available at http://www.unodc.org/unodc/en/data-and-analysis/homicide.html

rank number two in the world, if it were a country.[23] Available data from the UNODC demonstrates differences in firearm homicide rates among countries[21] (see **Figure 16–3**).

Suicide and Firearms

Data from 2002 show firearm suicide rates as higher than homicide rates and higher in men.[24] Although firearm suicide rates are highest in older people, people under age 55 have the highest absolute numbers of firearm-related suicides (two-thirds).[24] Data from the second Injury Control and Risk Survey, a U.S. household telephone survey conducted in 2001–2003, suggested that when people who have firearms in their home are suicidal, their plan more often included a firearm.[25] In another 2004 study conducted in the Northeast United States, having household firearms was associated with higher suicide rates.[26] Other authors emphasize that suicide attempts with firearms are more often fatal (91%) than attempts using other means.[27]

In addition, studies show that most people who survive a suicide attempt do not ultimately die from suicide.[27] The time between thinking and planning a suicide attempt is often very short—less than 5 minutes in 40% of attempts in one published study and 10 minutes or less in 50% attempts in another study.[27] Another author reports that 70% of people took under 1 hour to try to kill themselves after making their decision.[28] The public health implications of these studies are readily apparent, because of the short interval between a suicide decision and the attempt itself and the often time-limited nature of many suicide attempts.[28] Many studies provide evidence for a connection between household firearms and risk of suicide,[28] and support for recommendations that promote the safe household storage of firearms.[29] Reviews of the published literature about suicide prevention conclude that physician education and limiting or delaying access to lethal means are effective strategies to prevent suicide.[27,30]

Firearm Injuries in Children

In U.S. children, firearm injuries are the second leading cause of death.[31] However, less published data is available for the public health impact of nonlethal firearm injuries in children. Researchers from the Yale School of Medicine published a study of children's hospitalizations due to firearm injuries, which concluded that each day in the United States in 2009, 20 children and adolescents were hospitalized from a firearm injury.[31,32] Using 2009 data from the Kids' Inpatient Database, Leventhal and colleagues quantified the number of firearm injuries in young people (less than 20 years of age) and found 7,391 hospitalizations. The most common reason for hospitalization was from an assault.[31] Adolescents aged 15 to 19 had the highest rate of hospitalization, nearly 90% of hospitalizations were in males, and black males were hospitalized 10 times more often. Although suicide attempts were the least frequent reason for hospitalization from a firearm injury, 35% of these individuals died in the hospital.[31]

Some journalists suggest the numbers of fatal injuries are underestimated.[33] Using available data and specifically including medical examiner reports, *The New York Times* published a review of 259 child firearm deaths in children younger than 15, in eight states, such as California, Georgia, North Carolina, and Ohio.[33] They concluded that the number of accidental shootings in children, either by their own hand or that of another child, was about double what was actually reported because of how these data are collected and categorized.[33]

How Many People in the United States Own Firearms?

Data from a 2004 national firearms survey of 2,770 adults in the United States suggests that 38% of households (42 million) and 26% of individuals (57 million adults) report owning a firearm.[34] Rifles and shotguns (long guns) comprised about 60% of the guns owned, and 77% of long gun owners reporting "sport shooting" as the primary reason for owning a gun.[34] When compared to a decade prior, a small increase was noted in the proportion of firearms that were handguns, representing about 40% of the firearms owned, often for self-defense (46%).[34] In this survey, firearms owners were more likely to be male, white, middle-aged, from rural areas, and more commonly in the southern and midwestern parts of the United States.[34] Gun ownership in the United States is not evenly distributed: nearly half (48%) of individual gun owners own four or more firearms, and 65% of the total firearms in the United States are owned by 20% of gun owners.[34] In a review of literature from 1992 to 2002 about firearm storage in homes, it was estimated that 25% of firearms in U.S. households were kept loaded, and only about half of these were stored locked.[35] Hemenway, in a review of published scientific studies, concluded "the health risk of a gun in the home is greater than the benefit," especially for women, children, and those at risk for suicide.[36]

Mental Illness and the Media

In September 2013, two days after the shooting at the Washington Navy Yard, in Washington, DC, a Gallup poll showed Americans believed the largest contributors to mass shootings were "failure of the mental health system" (48%), "easy access to guns" (40%), "drug use" (37%), and "violence in movies, video games, music lyrics" (29%).[37] When compared to a similar poll conducted in December 2012 after the Newtown, CT shootings that reported 58% believed "laws governing the sale of firearms should be made stricter," only 49% believed this in the fall of 2013.[37]

McGinty and colleagues published the results of a randomized online study of news stories with differing information about a mass shooting, mental illness, and firearm restrictions and compared them to a control group.[38] Their findings from a national sample of 1,797 individuals, suggested media coverage of mass shootings, while increasing support for firearm restrictions, also resulted in more negative views about people with mental illness.[38]

In December 2013, during a time of intense public discussion about the role of mental illness in firearm violence, a consortium of leading researchers, practitioners, and advocates in firearm injury prevention and mental health, called the Consortium for Risk-Based Firearm Policy, released a report called "Guns, Public Health and Mental Illness: An Evidence-Based Approach for State Policy."[39] In this report, the authors conclude that most people diagnosed with mental illness do not commit violent acts, although at certain specific times "small subgroups of individuals with serious mental illness are at elevated risk of violence."[39] In addition, they highlight the greatly increased risk of suicide (50% of U.S. firearm-related deaths) in individuals with depression.[39]

The consortium recommended that policy changes emphasize preventing temporary firearm access in people at increased risk for dangerous behavior using evidence-based criteria.[39] Examples of elevated risks would include individuals convicted of a violent misdemeanor, those with restraining orders for domestic violence, individuals with multiple DUIs or controlled substance misdemeanors in a 5-year period.[39] They also recommended strengthening state laws to prohibit firearm access after "short-term involuntary hospitalization" for mental illness, and ensure that the process to restore firearms is clear.[39] The consortium's third recommendation involves law enforcement mechanisms to protect individuals who are an "immediate threat" to themselves or to protect others in such situations.[39]

The Director of the Institute of Law, Psychiatry, and Public Policy at the University of Virginia, and a Consortium member, added, "Most people with serious mental illness are not violent, and they account for only 4 percent of violent crimes . . . mental illness is only part of the problem, and so it is only part of the solution."[40]

EVIDENCE BASE FOR PREVENTION AND PRACTICE

Gun Buy-Back Programs—Do They Work?

One popular but controversial policy strategy used in some U.S. cities involves gun "buy-back" programs, in which public or private organizations offer to pay cash or provide other monetary incentives such as gift cards to persuade individuals (whose identities are not revealed) to turn in guns, which are later destroyed.[41] One published study from 2002 evaluated whether firearms gathered in a 1994–1996 buy-back program in Milwaukee County, WS were similar to those used to commit homicides and suicides in the same geographic location.[42] The authors reported that of the 941 handguns gathered from the buy-back program the types were unlike those related to homicides and suicides in the same geographic location during the same time period.[42] For example, more than three-quarters of the handguns from the buy-back program were small caliber, in sharp contrast to the same caliber handguns' use in homicides (24%) and suicides (32%), a statistically significant difference.[42] In addition, while semiautomatic pistols were involved in two-thirds of homicides, they represented only one-third of guns in the buy-back program, a statistically significant difference.[42] The authors concluded "limited resources for firearm injury prevention programs may be better spent in other ways."[42]

A more recent (2013) publication described the assessment of a buy-back program in Hartford, CT where 464 firearms were collected over a 4-year period.[43] The authors noted the small percentage of firearms collected, compared to the numbers sold—more than 91,000 each year. They further reported that firearm-related deaths did not change over the study period and concluded "a gun buy-back program alone is not likely to produce a measurable decrease in firearm injuries and deaths."[43]

This point is similarly emphasized by other authors.[41,44] Gun buy-back programs in the United States may result in return of an estimated 1,000 guns; this number is miniscule in comparison to numbers of guns sold and owned.[41] In contrast, a 1997 gun buy-back program in Australia, part of the National Firearms Agreement (NFA), reduced the total firearms in Australia by about 20%, a reduction of more than 650,000 firearms.[44] In addition, in a long-term and comprehensive evaluation of Australia's program published in 2010, firearm-related suicides dropped by nearly 80%.[44] The data on firearm-related homicides also showed a decline, but because overall numbers were small, the authors could not be certain it was solely due to the program.[44]

Braga and Wintemute evaluated the two programs in Boston, one starting in 1993–1994 and another beginning in 2006. The 1993–1994 buy-back program began at a time of high firearm-related violence in Boston, offered $50 per gun recovered, gathered 2,158 total firearms, and was conducted by city police, the County District Attorney, and a nonprofit agency.[41] After another period of increased firearm violence, another buy-back program was implemented, but this time Boston's mayor, Police Department, and faith-based and other community organizations initiated a new buy-back program named "Aim for Peace."[41] It was different from the earlier programs and included $200 gift cards for returning a handgun, included "drop-off" locations in places such as churches, instead of relying just on police department locations, and included a communications strategy aimed at Boston young people, blanketing the city's public transportation system.[41]

This time the program gathered 1,019 firearms (more than half were hand guns) and recovered (based on Bureau of Alcohol, Tobacco, and Firearms tracing) more firearms purchased in the prior 3 years or along Interstate 95, suggestive of illegal sales.[41] Furthermore, gun violence decreased 30% (from 2006 to 2010) in Boston after this program was implemented.[41] However, study investigators could not separate out the specific effect of the 2006 gun buy-back program because other effective community prevention programs were implemented during the same time period.[41] The authors concluded that buy-back programs "can be an important element in a broader community-based effort to prevent violence."[41]

Can We Make "Safer" Guns?

In the prevention of motor vehicle injuries and fatalities, improved road design, guard rails, seat belts, air bags, and rear brake lights in cars, along with laws to prevent alcohol-impaired drivers, have all been used to prevent injuries and deaths. "Why, if we have childproof aspirin bottles, don't we have childproof guns?" asked one study author.[33] Some wonder whether the design of firearms, called "smart guns," could reduce firearm injuries.[33] First proposed in 2010, with examples found in companies such as Safe Gun Technology (SGTi),[45] many substantive barriers remain to commercial viability of this technology, and it is not yet known whether people would buy "smart guns."[33] According to *The New York Times*, an Australian company partnering with Taurus International Manufacturing, Colt's Manufacturing Company, and Smith & Wesson all dropped their efforts to develop this technology after controversy and financial challenges.[33]

Physicians' Role?

Another area of controversy includes physician conversations with patients about firearms their home. The 2013 President of the American Academy of Pediatrics (AAP) said, "We ask patients about all kinds of things. Doctors ask about the setting on the water heater and whether family cyclists wear bike helmets."[46] Physicians who care for older patients may elect to discuss firearms in light of the high rates of suicide in older men.[46] The American College of Physicians (ACP) recommends the following: "physicians are encouraged to discuss with their patients the risks that may be associated with having a firearm in the home. . ."[47] However, lawmakers in Florida passed a law in 2011 restricting such conversations between doctors and patients,[46] and similar measures have been proposed in legislatures in seven other states.[48] Despite legal challenges, in 2014, the U.S. Court of Appeals for the 11th Circuit upheld the Florida Privacy of Firearms Owners Act, with one judge writing (in a 2-1 majority opinion) that, "good medical care does not require inquiry or record-keeping regarding firearms when unnecessary to a patient's care."[49,50]

Physician organizations, such as the AAP, the American Medical Association (AMA), and the ACP have published comprehensive policy statements about firearm injuries and death.[47,51,52]

Policy Studies

There is evidence that social factors and policies may play a role in urban firearm violence. A study published in 2010 evaluated the impact of specific policy and program changes on homicide rates in New York City in the 1990s.[53] Prevention and social service policies that reduced cocaine and alcohol use, increased availability of public assistance, and added more policing for misdemeanor crimes (called "broken windows" policing), resulted in declines in homicide rates in a variety of age groups.[53] A 2013 cross-sectional study evaluated whether states with more firearm laws had fewer firearm-related deaths.[13] Using the WISQARS data and a score to grade firearm-related laws, investigators noted that the states with the most laws had statistically fewer firearm suicide and homicide rates and lower firearm-related fatalities overall.[13]

Arguments for a Public Health Approach

In a 2014 policy position paper, the ACP articulates nine strategies to reduce deaths and injuries from firearms, advocating a public health approach to prevent firearm injuries and deaths.[47] Investigators at FICAP emphasize that firearm injuries are preventable, especially impact young people, and must be approached from a community perspective.[18]

CDC's four-step sequence for a public health approach includes using data to define the problem, finding risk and protective factors, designing and trying different prevention approaches, and promoting widespread use of strategies that work (evidence-based approaches).[54,55] Hemenway and Miller argue that a public health approach to reduce firearm violence has five components: is population-based, emphasizes prevention, uses a systems approach, is comprehensive, and emphasizes collective responsibility.[55]

Characteristics of a public health approach include making changes in the surrounding environment rather than emphasizing changing individual behavior.[55] One example is the dramatic progress in reducing motor vehicle fatalities that included changes in road and motor vehicle design, speed limits, and laws designed to reduce driving under the influence of alcohol.[55] Such an approach applied to the public health issue of firearm injuries would include creating high-quality data systems to measure progress in different geographic areas of the United States over time, provide insight into new prevention strategies, and evaluate policies and programs.[55]

For example, the NVDRS[19] that is available in 18 states could be expanded across the United States.[56] Many authors describe well-documented gaps in data and research funding[12,48] and the limitations of published ecological studies. They call for research that is comprehensive, sustained, and includes program and policy evaluation.[12] Using the example of the National Transportation Safety Board, some authors cite the need for new transdisciplinary research models, use of multidisciplinary teams, new methods, and specific research strategies to prevent "rampage violence."[57]

Many experts contrast progress in reducing firearm-related injuries and deaths with progress seen in other areas of public health that have utilized a public health approach, such as motor vehicle injuries, tobacco prevention and control, and unintentional childhood poisoning.[48,58] CDC emphasizes that it is essential to use a public health approach in violence prevention to evaluate prevention strategies and widely promote "what works."[54]

Should We Think About Firearm Injuries as Epidemics?

Malcolm Gladwell, author of *The Tipping Point*, a book he characterizes as "an intellectual adventure story," describes numerous example of "epidemics" related to the positive spread of ideas as well as for behaviors such as suicide that spread in much the same way that infectious diseases are characterized as contagious.[59] He describes the epidemic of teenage suicide in the 1970s and 1980s in the South Pacific islands of Micronesia, where suicide rates were 10 times higher than elsewhere. He suggests that mass shootings following Columbine followed a similar copycat pattern, implying that these episodes of firearm-related injury may be different from firearm-related injuries in other settings.[59]

Another author suggests media dramatization glamourizes such events and potentially contributes to additional events, citing (as did Gladwell) post-Columbine examples.[60] Other authors in the peer-reviewed literature use the epidemic analogy as well, arguing that firearm injuries in the United States were *epidemic* (higher than baseline levels and/or increasing) in the mid-1980s to 1990s and are currently *endemic* (ongoing at some ongoing level).[61]

Examples might include infectious diseases of many types and noninfectious conditions, such as motor vehicle injuries and obesity. Christoffel describes three potential cumulative risks of *endemic* conditions: public health issues may arise in new locations, a condition may increase and become *epidemic* again, and over time, ongoing injury or illness caused by *endemic* public health issues creates a cumulative disease burden.[61]

Other authors editorialize that we need to "unlearn gun violence," changing behavioral norms in local communities as a way to prevent future epidemics of gun violence.[62] He cites a program called Save our Streets (SOS) in which employed outreach workers (familiar with gun violence) are responsible for finding the "disease carriers," individuals at high-risk for violent gun behavior.[62] The outreach workers engage with them to try to prevent episodes of gun violence. "Violence interrupters" try to calm community disruptions that might precipitate violence, and staff members try to interrupt violent revenge when a shooting does happen.[62] In 2010, just a year after the Chicago program began, shootings declined in the small program area from 28 to 13, and evaluation showed a significant impact from the program.[62]

Future Directions—Research Needs

In January 2014, ABC News queried firearm researchers about what questions they would like to answer if funding existed.[63] Some examples of questions provided by research experts included:

"Does gun safety education work to reduce firearm injuries among children?"

"Does gun violence in the mass media make kids more likely to want to shoot a gun? Do our youth want to imitate media characters that use guns?"

"How do we communicate the risks of guns in a credible, honest way and inspire families to think about gun safety, regardless of their political views."[63]

DISCUSSION QUESTIONS: TEMPLATE FOR DISCUSSION

1. Significance of this public health issue:
   a. Why is this health issue important?
   b. How many people does it impact?
   c. How serious is it?
   d. Is it preventable?
2. What is the evidence base for prevention?
3. What specific strategies should be used to achieve progress on this health issue?
   a. What evidence-based approach would you use?
   b. Where would you start if you are an individual citizen; public health professional; healthcare professional; community, state, or federal policymaker?
4. Specific questions for this topic:
   a. How does the study of mental health relate to this discussion?
   b. What is the role of the NRA? What are the roles of public health advocacy organizations?
   c. What does research tell us about effective public health approaches to prevent firearm-related injuries and deaths?
   d. Are there gaps in research? What types of additional research are needed?
5. What is the controversy?
   a. Define the controversy.
   b. Is controversy a good or bad thing? (Does it help or hinder progress?)
6. *Why* is this health issue controversial?
   a. What specific factors are involved?
   b. Do economics, government, scientific uncertainty, or politics play a role?
   c. What is the role of the media?
7. How would you respond to the controversy?

PERSPECTIVES TO CONSIDER

The most noticeable aspect of this public health issue is the paucity of data and research about the risks and protective factors for firearm injuries, in different geographic locations and settings, as well as what policies and programs will likely work best and could be systematically applied. Compared to many other areas of public health, when searching for data and statistics on the public health impact of firearm injury, it is easy to find in-depth investigative research efforts by *The Washington Post*[11] and *The New York Times*,[5] making the lack of peer-reviewed research even more apparent. Funding plummeted for this research at CDC in the 1990s,[12,14] and the number of researchers actively working in this field remains small.

Why is adequate funding and conducting peer-reviewed research so important? Because despite what we currently know, there are still many questions, and finding specific community-based programs, educational efforts, and policy initiatives—all part of a public health approach—must be guided by evidence-based practice. The use of ecological studies and comparisons with other states and countries is helpful but limited[12] and may not reveal the nuances and differences in approaches needed in different settings and locations. Researchers have noted many questions that need answers and would help in collective efforts to prevent more injuries and deaths.[63] Are firearm homicide deaths from mass shootings and inner city violence amenable to the same approaches? Will approaches that work in Boston or San Diego be successful in New Orleans or Las Vegas? When we are publically focused on horrific mass shootings, does the media help or make it worse? These are just some of the questions, as political and advocacy issues remain so polarized. Moving ahead with successful approaches or changes in policy is even challenging to discuss.

However, no discussion of research gaps suggests standing by, watching, and waiting. In 2009–2010, there were 38,126 firearm-related suicides and 22,571 firearm-related homicides in U.S. residents, and CDC reported more than 75% of the U.S. major metropolitan areas they studied showed an increased suicide rate.[15] Many studies remind us of the near-immediate but often transient nature of suicide attempts,[27,28] which provides a potentially life-saving opportunity to intervene, especially important when firearms are used.

Efforts to prioritize a research focus, targeting specific aspects of firearm violence, may ultimately help prevent injuries and deaths. It seems apparent, even in the presence of intense and ongoing controversy, areas such as suicide and unintentional injury prevention (accidents) may benefit by systematically raising awareness on an individual and population level. While policy debates continue, public health and healthcare professionals must use existing data, support the call for more research and evidence-based initiatives, and move forward with the same basic approaches used to improve public health in many other areas.

FOR ADDITIONAL STUDY

> Firearm and Injury Center at Penn (FICAP). Firearm injury in the U.S. 2011. http://www.uphs.upenn.edu/ficap/resourcebook/pdf/monograph.pdf.

REFERENCES

1. Barron J. Nation reels after gunman massacres 20 children at school in Connecticut. *The New York Times.* 2012. http://www.nytimes.com/2012/12/15/nyregion/shooting-reported-at-connecticut-elementary-school.html?_r=2&. Accessed April 5, 2014.
2. Cillizza C. President Obama's enough-is-enough Newtown speech. *The Washington Post* 2012. http://www.washingtonpost.com/blogs/the-fix/wp/2012/12/16/president-obamas-enough-is-enough-newtown-speech/. Accessed April 4, 2014.
3. Lichtblau E, Rich M. N.R.A. envisions 'a good guy with a gun' in every school. *The New York Times.* 2012. http://www.nytimes.com/2012/12/22/us/nra-calls-for-armed-guards-at-schools.html. Accessed April 6, 2014.
4. Now is the Time: The President's plan to protect our children and our communities by reducing gun violence. 2013. http://www.whitehouse.gov/sites/default/files/docs/wh_now_is_the_time_full.pdf. Accessed April 4, 2014.
5. State gun laws enacted in the year since Newtown. *The New York Times.* 2013. http://www.nytimes.com/interactive/2013/12/10/us/state-gun-laws-enacted-in-the-year-since-newtown.html. Accessed April 4, 2014.
6. Giffords G. A Senate in the Gun Lobby's Grip. *The New York Times.* 2013. http://www.nytimes.com/2013/04/18/opinion/a-senate-in-the-gun-lobbys-grip.html?_r=0. Accessed March 12, 2014.
7. James F. Newtown anniversary marked by gun control stalemate. *NPR.org.* 2013. http://www.npr.org/blogs/itsallpolitics/2013/12/13/250808035/newtown-anniversary-marked-by-gun-control-stalemate. Accessed April 4, 2014.
8. Abdullah H. Has the moment passed? Why gun control push fizzled. *CNN.com.* 2013. http://www.cnn.com/2013/06/12/politics/guns-revisited/. Accessed April 4, 2014.
9. Shen A. A timeline of mass shootings in the US since Columbine. *Thinkprogress.* 2012. http://thinkprogress.org/justice/2012/12/14/1337221/a-timeline-of-mass-shootings-in-the-us-since-columbine/. Accessed April 4, 2014.
10. Follman M, Aronsen G, Pan D. A guide to mass shootings in America. *Mother Jones.* 2014. http://www.motherjones.com/politics/2012/07/mass-shootings-map. Accessed April 4, 2014.

11. Klein E. Twelve facts about guns and mass shootings in the United States. *Wonkblog.* Vol 2014: *The Washington Post.* 2013. http://www.washingtonpost.com/blogs/wonkblog/wp/2012/12/14/nine-facts-about-guns-and-mass-shootings-in-the-united-states/. Accessed April 4, 2014.

12. Wintemute GJ. Responding to the crisis of firearm violence in the United States: Comment on "firearm legislation and firearm-related fatalities in the United States". *JAMA Int Med.* 2013;173(9):740.

13. Fleegler EW, Lee LK, Monuteaux MC, Hemenway D, Mannix R. Firearm legislation and firearm-related fatalities in the United States. *JAMA Int Med.* 2013;173(9): 732–740.

14. Luo M. N.R.A. stymies firearms research, scientists say. *The New York Times.* 2011. http://www.nytimes.com/2011/01/26/us/26guns.html. Accessed April 4, 2014.

15. CDC. Firearm homicides and suicides in major metropolitan areas — United States, 2006–2007 and 2009–2010. *MMWR.* 2013. http://www.cdc.gov/mmwr/preview/mmwrhtml/mm6230a1.htm. Accessed April 4, 2014.

16. CDC. Injury Prevention and Control: Data and Statistics (WISQARS). 2014. http://www.cdc.gov/injury/wisqars/index.html. Accessed October 22, 2014.

17. Miller M, Hemenway D, Azrael D. State-level homicide victimization rates in the US in relation to survey measures of household firearm ownership, 2001–2003. *Soc Sci Med.* 2007;64(3):656–664.

18. FICAP. Firearm injury in the U.S. *FICAP: Firearm & Injury Center at Penn.* 2011. http://www.uphs.upenn.edu/ficap/resourcebook/pdf/monograph.pdf. Accessed April 4, 2014.

19. CDC. Injury Prevention and Control: National Violent Death Reporting System. 2014. http://www.cdc.gov/violencePrevention/NVDRS/index.html. Accessed October 22, 2014.

20. Hemenway D, Miller M. Firearm availability and homicide rates across 26 high-income countries. *J Trauma.* 2000;49(6):985–988.

21. UNODC Homicide Statistics 2014. http://www.unodc.org/unodc/en/data-and-analysis/homicide.html. Accessed October 22, 2014.

22. Fisher M. Chart: The U.S. has far more gun-related killings than any other developed country. *The Washington Post.* 2012. http://www.washingtonpost.com/blogs/worldviews/wp/2012/12/14/chart-the-u-s-has-far-more-gun-related-killings-than-any-other-developed-country/. Accessed April 4, 2014.

23. Florida R. Gun violence in U.S. cities compared to the deadliest nations in the world. *The Atlantic CityLab.* 2013. http://www.citylab.com/politics/2013/01/gun-violence-us-cities-compared-deadliest-nations-world/4412/. Accessed October 22, 2014.

24. Romero MP, Wintemute GJ. The epidemiology of firearm suicide in the United States. *J Urban Health.* 2002;79(1):39–48.

25. Betz ME, Barber C, Miller M. Suicidal behavior and firearm access: Results from the second injury control and risk survey. *Suicide Life Threat Behav.* 2011;41(4):384–391.

26. Miller M, Hemenway D, Azrael D. Firearms and suicide in the northeast. *J Trauma.* 2004;57(3):626–632.

27. Lewiecki EM, Miller SA. Suicide, guns, and public policy. *Am J Public Health.* 2013;103(1):27–31.

28. Miller M, Hemenway D. Guns and suicide in the United States. *N Engl J Med.* 2008;359(10):989–991.

29. Miller M, Azrael D, Hemenway D, Vriniotis M. Firearm storage practices and rates of unintentional firearm deaths in the United States. *Accident Anal Prev.* 2005;37(4):661–667.

30. Mann JJ, Apter A, Bertolote J, et al. Suicide prevention strategies: A systematic review. *JAMA.* 2005;294(16):2064–2074.

31. Leventhal JM, Gaither JR, Sege R. Hospitalizations due to firearm injuries in children and adolescents. *Pediatrics.* 2014;133(2):219–225.

32. Kim C. Nearly 10,000 American children are injured or killed by guns every year *MSNBC.* 2014. http://www.msnbc.com/the-last-word/the-toll-gun-violence-children. Accessed April 4, 2014.

33. Luo M, McIntire M. Children and guns: The hidden toll. *The New York Times.* 2013. http://www.nytimes.com/2013/09/29/us/children-and-guns-the-hidden-toll.html?emc=edit_th_20130929&nl=todaysheadlines&nlid=67811076. Accessed March 12, 2014.

34. Hepburn L, Miller M, Azrael D, Hemenway D. The US gun stock: Results from the 2004 national firearms survey. *Inj Prev.* 2007;13(1):15–19.

35. Miller M. One third of households in the USA own firearms which are often stored unsafely. *Evid-Based Healthcare Pub Health.* 2005;9(1):23–25.

36. Hemenway D. Risks and benefits of a gun in the home. *Am J Lifestyle Med.* 2011:1–11.

37. Saad L. Americans fault mental health system most for gun violence: Half say gun laws should be stricter, down from 58% after Newtown. *GALLUP Politics.* 2013. http://www.gallup.com/poll/164507/americans-fault-mental-health-system-gun-violence.aspx. Accessed April 4, 2014.

38. McGinty EE, Webster DW, Barry CL. Effects of news media messages about mass shootings on attitudes toward persons with serious mental illness and public support for gun control policies. *Am J Psych.* 2013;170(5):494–501.

39. Consortium for Risk-Based Firearm Policy. Guns, public health and mental illness: An evidence-based approach for state policy. 2013. http://www.jhsph.edu/research/centers-and-institutes/johns-hopkins-center-for-gun-policy-and-research/publications/GPHMI-State.pdf. Accessed April 4, 2014.

40. Levin A. Violence risk, not mental illness, should guide gun access. *Psychiatric NEWS.* 2013. http://psychnews.psychiatryonline.org/newsArticle.aspx?articleid=1812238. Accessed April 4, 2014.

41. Braga AA, Wintemute GJ. Improving the potential effectiveness of gun buyback programs. *Am J Prev Med.* 2013;45(5):668–671.

42. Kuhn EM, Nie CL, O'Brien ME, Withers RL, Wintemute GJ, Hargarten SW. Missing the target: A comparison of buyback and fatality related guns. *Injury Prev.* 2002;8(2):143–146.

43. Marinelli LW, Thaker S, Borrup K, et al. Hartford's gun buy-back program: Are we on target? *Conn Med.* 2013;77(8):453–459.

44. Leigh A, Neill C. Do gun buybacks save lives? Evidence from panel data. *Am Law Econ Rev.* 2010;12(2):509–557.

45. Safe Gun Technology 2013. http://sgti9154.wpengine.com/. Accessed April 4, 2014.

46. Hensley S. Doctors' questions about guns spark a constitutional fight. *SHOTS: Health News from NPR.* 2013. http://www.npr.org/blogs/health/2013/07/17/203031144/doctors-questions-about-guns-spark-a-constitutional-fight. Accessed April 4, 2014.

47. Butkus R, Doherty R, Daniel H. Reducing firearm-related injuries and deaths in the United States: Executive summary of a policy position paper from the American College of Physicians. *Ann Intern Med.* 17 2014;160(12):858–860.

48. Kellermann AL, Rivara FP. Silencing the science on gun research. *JAMA.* 2013; 309(6):549–550.

49. Hamblin J. The questions doctors can't ask. *The Atlantic.* 2014. http://www.theatlantic .com/health/archive/2014/08/doctors-cant-ask-about-guns/375566/. Accessed October 22, 2014.

50. Sherman P, McNamara R. Censorship in your doctor's office. *The New York Times.* 2014. http://www.nytimes.com/2014/08/02/opinion/censorship-in-your-doctors-office.html. Accessed October 22, 2014.

51. AAP. American Academy of Pediatrics gun violence policy recommendations. 2012. http://www.aap.org/en-us/advocacy-and-policy/federal-advocacy/Documents/ AAPGunViolencePreventionPolicyRecommendations_Jan2013.pdf. Accessed April 4, 2014.

52. AMA. Violence prevention. 2014. http://www.ama-assn.org/ama/pub/advocacy/topics/ violence-prevention.page. Accessed October 22, 2014.

53. Cerda M, Messner SF, Tracy M, et al. Investigating the effect of social changes on age-specific gun-related homicide rates in New York City during the 1990s. *Am J Public Health.* 2010;100(6):1107–1115.

54. CDC. The public health approach to violence orevention. 2013. http://www.cdc.gov/ violenceprevention/overview/publichealthapproach.html. Accessed April 4, 2014.

55. Hemenway D, Miller M. Public health approach to the prevention of gun violence. *N Engl J Med.* 2013;368(21):2033–2035.

56. Barber C, Azrael D, Hemenway D. A truly national National Violent Death Reporting System. *Injury Prev.* 2013;19(4):225–226.

57. Harris JM, Jr., Harris RB. Rampage violence requires a new type of research. *Am J Public Health.* 2012;102(6):1054–1057.

58. Mozaffarian D, Hemenway D, Ludwig DS. Curbing gun violence: Lessons from public health successes. *JAMA.* 2013;309(6):551–552.

59. Gladwell M. The tipping point: Q and A with Malcolm. 2014. http://gladwell.com/ the-tipping-point/the-tipping-point-q-and-a/. Accessed April 5, 2014.

60. Hundal S. Copycat killers. *The Guardian.* 2006. http://www.theguardian.com/ commentisfree/2006/oct/04/copycatkillers. Accessed April 5, 2014.

61. Christoffel KK. Firearm injuries: Epidemic then, endemic now. *Am J Public Health.* 2007;97(4):626–629.

62. Nocera J. Unlearning gun violence. *The New York Times.* 2013. http://www.nytimes. com/2013/11/12/opinion/nocera-unlearning-gun-violence.html. Accessed April 4, 2014.

63. Pearle L. Unanswered questions gun violence researchers would tackle if they had the money. *ABC News.* 2014. http://abcnews.go.com/US/unanswered-questions-gun-violence-researchers-tackle-money/story?id=22322439. Accessed April 4, 2014.

CHAPTER 17

Preventing Injuries: Concussions in Sports

LEARNING OBJECTIVES

- Discuss the public health impact of concussions in the United States.
- Describe the epidemiology of concussions.
- Identify populations at increased risk for concussions.
- Critically evaluate evidence-based guidelines and their potential applications.
- Propose priority research areas to address current gaps.
- Propose evidence-based prevention strategies to reduce the public health impact of concussions.

THE CONTROVERSY

In the July 2005 issue of the medical journal *Neurosurgery*, Dr. Bennett Omalu and colleagues described the autopsy results of a retired professional football player who had had difficulties with his memory, changes in mood, and symptoms similar to those of patients diagnosed with Parkinson's disease.[1] In 2002, "Iron" Mike Webster, Pittsburg Steelers' and National Football League Hall of Fame football star, died of cardiovascular disease at age 50, 12 years after retiring from 17 years playing on the line of scrimmage, often called "the pit."[2] The Allegheny County Medical Examiner, Dr. Omalu, a neuropathologist, performed the autopsy and focused special attention on the brain.[2] Dr. Omalu and colleagues concluded the autopsy "highlights potential long-term neuro-degenerative outcomes in retired professional National Football League players subjected to repeated mild traumatic brain injury," and recommended additional study of this "emergent professional sport hazard."[1]

301

A subsequent letter to the same journal by Casson and colleagues disagreed with the report, calling for retraction of the article."[3] And that was just the beginning.

On May 14, 2009, with support from a broad coalition of stakeholders, including the Centers for Disease Control and Prevention, the Seattle Seahawks, and many others, Washington State's Governor Christine Gregoire signed House Bill 1824, the Zackery Lystedt Law, billed as the "nation's toughest youth athlete return-to-play law."[4] The bill was named after Zack Lystedt who, in 2006, at age 13 had a life-threatening brain injury during a football game. After hitting his head, he returned to play after a brief respite and then experienced a second hit to his helmet.[5] Years later, in 2011, he walked slowly with a cane at his high school graduation ceremony.[6] Washington House Bill 1824, inspired by his story, directed that youth with suspected concussions be removed from play, emphasizing "when in doubt, sit them out."[4] It required educational information and policies for coaches, athletes, and parents and required parents to sign an information sheet about concussion each season. The bill required medical clearance (in writing) from a "licensed healthcare provider trained in the evaluation and management of concussion, " before they could return to play.[4] Since then, 47 states and the District of Columbia have passed laws, called "return-to-play laws," to prevent concussions in youth or high school sports.[7]

In October 2009, the NFL Commissioner was summoned to testify before the House Judiciary Committee about the role of playing professional football and later mental impairment.[8] His refusal to acknowledge the connection brought a strong rebuke from Representative Linda T. Sanchez of California, saying ". . . and it sort of reminds me of the tobacco companies pre-'90s when they kept saying, 'Oh, there's no link between smoking and damage to your health.'"[8] Despite the controversial hearing, there was agreement that how the NFL manages brain injuries in professional football players would resonate with youth and high school sports. Representative Mike Quigley of Illinois agreed "the norms of the NFL, for better or worse, become the norms of high school football players."[8]

Despite laws passed and intense media scrutiny of head injuries from youth to professional athletes, not all agree on the severity of the problem. A survey of 300 fathers (all former football players) about their children's participation in tackle football revealed some surprising findings. Nearly half believed "there is too much hype over concussions in sports."[9]

BACKGROUND AND SCOPE OF THE PUBLIC HEALTH AND HEALTH POLICY ISSUE

What Is a Concussion?

According to the Centers for Disease Control and Prevention (CDC), a concussion is part of a larger category of traumatic brain injuries (TBI).[10] A concussion may be caused by any direct impact to the head, or impact to other parts of the body that causes the head to move rapidly back and forth.[10] Concussions may occur in a wide range of competitive sports and also in recreational activities.[11] As early as 1928, boxers were described as "punch drunk," referring to what we now know as signs and symptoms of dementia pugilistica.[12,13] More recently, some experts estimate that in the United States more than 1.5 million people have mild TBIs each year.[13] In addition, knowledge has expanded about potential risks of concussion from participation in athletics and recreational activities, short-term and long-term health implications, and underlying pathophysiology, although many scientific questions remain.[13] Widespread public awareness has resulted from the work of federal agencies, such as CDC, health and sports-related organizations, as well as policymakers.[7] Experts note that most concussions heal on their own within short time periods, with 80–90% resolving in 7–10 days, sometimes taking longer in children and adolescents.[14] However, brain vulnerability during this time creates risks from a second recurrent injury, and potential for long-term effects of repeated concussions is a serious concern. In addition, the ability to rapidly diagnose concussions during actual athletic or recreational events remains a practical challenge.[15]

Signs, Symptoms, and Diagnosis

CDC recommends two critical considerations in recognizing concussions: a bump or direct impact to the head or other part of the body that results in quick head movement and changes in physical or cognitive behavior.[11] Examples of athletes' symptoms might include headache, difficulty with balance, having trouble concentrating, and a wide range of other symptoms that might include not "feeling right."[11] Signs of concussion that may be noticed by parents or coaches include brief loss of consciousness, trouble thinking or forgetting things, changes in mood or behavior, or confusion.[11] Some signs and symptoms may not appear immediately, but instead occur hours or days after experiencing an injury. For this reason, education for health professionals, athletes, parents, coaches and school officials stresses the importance of having a high index of suspicion after head or body impact that may lead to concussion.[11] Recommendations after a possible or suspected concussion in athletes (or participants in recreational activities) include removing the athlete from play right away, requiring evaluation by a health professional with training and experience in diagnosing concussions, waiting until they have no symptoms and are cleared by a health professional to return.[11]

Several key facts highlight the importance of preventing concussions.[7] First, concussions are most common in children and adolescents, who may also take more time than adults to heal from their injury.[7] Second, anyone who has experienced a concussion is at higher risk of having another concussion in the future. Finally, early recognition, response, and appropriate management of concussions can help prevent long-term injury or death.[7]

What Is Second Impact Syndrome?

Second impact syndrome (SIS) was described in 1973 in two young athletes with concussions who later died after a second, but very mild, head injury, and again in 1984 following the death of a college football player.[16,17] SIS is characterized by a second head injury, rapidly-occurring brain swelling, and a conspicuous lack of brain bruising.[16] Accurate statistics and epidemiological data are lacking, and the phenomenon itself remains controversial.[17] However, the severity of this condition has focused research and attracted public health attention, in particular, influencing decisions about returning athletes to play after a concussion.[16,17]

After a head injury causing a concussion, symptoms such as headache, confusion, and memory loss may occur, as well as swelling of the brain. However, there are usually protective features in the brain, called "auto-regulatory" mechanisms (such as changes in blood flow to the brain) that prevent rapid, severe, and potentially fatal brain swelling.[17] Research suggests that as a result of injury, brain metabolism may be impacted for as long as 10 days, and these changes in blood flow and brain metabolism may contribute to conditions in which the brain is more "vulnerable" to a second injury.[17] Research into the rare SIS suggests failure of the usually protective auto-regulatory mechanisms in the brain; after a "second impact," rapid brain swelling may sometimes cause death in as fast as 2 to 5 minutes.[17]

One notable observation, although debated, is that a minor injury may be sufficient to trigger this cascade of events, especially in children.[17] Differences in SIS, compared to brain swelling seen in most severe head injuries, feature a failure of the brain's auto-regulation from a seemingly minor second injury, especially an injury to the head. This second injury causes the production of stress hormones, a rise in blood pressure, and rapid and severe brain swelling.[16] Authors call for additional research to more accurately determine the subsequent risk of SIS in individuals with concussions, paying particular attention to return-to-play guidelines for athletes, especially children and adolescents.[17]

Data and Statistics—Epidemiology

Concussions are more likely in children and teens. Children and teens may also need more time to heal completely.[18] There are an estimated 173,285 traumatic brain injuries (TBIs) each year requiring emergency care in children, adolescents, and young adults up to age 19, including both recreational and athletics-related injuries.[18] In addition, over a 10-year period, emergency department (ED) visits in this same age group increased by 60%. Football, bicycling, basketball, soccer, and playground activities are the sports and recreational activities resulting in the most ED visits for TBIs; specific contributing sports or activities varies by age and gender.[11,18] CDC has published extensive resources for athletes, parents, coaches, school officials, and health professionals, such as "Heads Up: Concussion in High School Sports" tool kit.[10,19]

CDC estimates there were more than 200,000 ED visits for sports and recreation-related concussions and other TBIs each year (from 2001 to 2005). Of these, nearly two-thirds (65%) were seen in children and adolescents under age 18.[20] A sample from the Canadian National Population Health Survey, showed similar demographic findings, reporting more than 54% of concussions were sports-related, and more likely to occur in males and younger people.[21]

Using data from the National Electronic Injury Surveillance System—All Injury Program (NEISS-AIP), a program of the U.S. Consumer Product Safety Commission, CDC described trends and patterns of nonfatal TBIs from sports and recreational activities from 2001 to 2009.[20] During this time period, there was a 62% (statistically significant) increase in ED visits from 153,375 to 248,418 each year. Numbers of ED visits that resulted in hospitalizations, reflecting more serious TBIs, did not increase significantly over this same time period.[20] Of the estimated 173,285 annual ED visits during this time period for sports and recreation-related nonfatal TBIs, about 71% were in males and 70.5% in children and adolescents aged 10 to 19 years.[20] However, CDC concluded that increased awareness of concussions may be responsible for increased ED visits because a parallel increase in more serious injuries requiring hospitalization was not seen.[20]

What Specific Sports and Activities Are Associated with Concussions?

In one study, the most common sports and recreational activities resulting in the highest *number* of ED visits for TBIs included bicycling, football, playground activities, basketball and soccer, all common sports, and recreational activities.[20] (see **Figure 17–1**). However, when looking at the data a different way, activities in which TBIs were responsible for more than 10% of the usual injuries seen, horseback riding, ice skating,

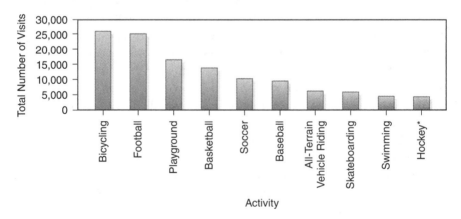

*includes ice hockey, field hockey, roller hockey, and street hockey

Figure 17–1 Numbers of emergency department visits for nonfatal traumatic brain injuries, United States, 2001–2009.

Data from Centers for Disease Control and Prevention. Nonfatal Traumatic Brain Injuries Related to Sports and Recreation Activities Among Persons Aged ≤19 Years—United States, 2001–2009. *MMWR*. 2011. Available at http://www.cdc.gov/MMWR/preview/mmwrhtml/mm6039a1.htm?s_cid=mm6039a1_w.

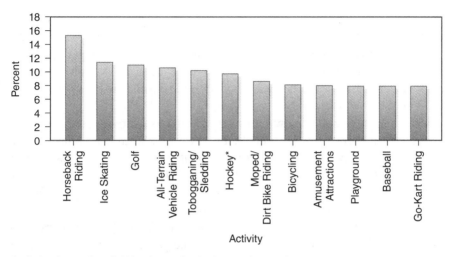

*includes ice hockey, field hockey, roller hockey, and street hockey

Figure 17–2 Percentage of emergency department injury visits that were traumatic brain injuries, United States, 2001–2009.

Data from Centers for Disease Control and Prevention. Nonfatal Traumatic Brain Injuries Related to Sports and Recreation Activities Among Persons Aged ≤19 Years—United States, 2001–2009. *MMWR.* 2011. Available at http://www.cdc.gov/MMWR/preview/ mmwrhtml/mm6039a1.htm?s_cid=mm6039a1_w.

golf (includes golf cart-related injuries), all-terrain vehicles, and sledding had higher *rates* of TBIs[20] (see **Figure 17–2**).

In addition, TBI ED visits were related to age and gender: for younger children, playground injuries were causes of TBIs, whereas for older children and adolescents, football and bicycling were the source of TBIs for boys, and soccer, basketball, and bicycling for girls.[20]

A study of 25 schools in a large public school system in the United States by Lincoln and colleagues described concussion risk in a dozen different high-school sports in both boys and girls, including such sports as football, basketball, lacrosse, soccer, softball and baseball, field hockey, and cheerleading.[22] When the authors compared academic years 1997–1998 and 2007–2008, they found an overall incidence rate of concussion of 24 per 100,000 athletes. Concussion rates increased over this time period in all of the sports studied, but the study authors were not able to distinguish whether this was due to an actual increase or related to widespread increases in education and awareness.[22] Half of all concussions in this study could be attributed to football, which also had the highest incidence rate (60 per 100,000). Soccer had the second highest incidence rate of concussion (35 per 100,000) and resulted in the most concussions among girls sports. However, what was surprising in this study was when the authors compared sports that were similar in both boys and girls, such as basketball and soccer, they found the risk of concussion in girls was twice as high as in boys.[22]

Another published review by Laker looked at different sports, position played in that sport, gender, and other factors.[23] This study emphasized the need to look at both how common or popular a sport is (e.g., basketball or soccer) leading to a high overall number of concussions, and rates of concussions in specific sports where participation may not be as high. By such comparisons, football may have a greater *number* of concussions, but women's ice hockey has a higher *rate* of concussion.[23] This review also reported details of how, when, and where concussions occurred. More than 75% of concussions were from player-to-player contact, whereas 15.5% were from contact with the ground, turf, gym, or other playing surface.[23] Nearly 80% of concussions were in games and competitions. In addition, some positions in athletics may carry higher risks for concussions, such as quarterbacks, linebackers, and running backs in football, batters in baseball and softball, and goalkeepers in soccer.[23]

Another large study of concussions used data from the National High School Sports-Related Injury Surveillance System, High School RIO (Reporting Information Online), an Internet-based system, to study 1,936 concussions among high school athletes in 20 sports, from 2008–2010.[24] These authors again noted higher rates of concussion in competition than in practice, the highest numbers of concussions from football, girls' soccer, boys' wrestling, and girls' basketball, and the highest rates of concussions from football, boys' ice hockey, and boys' lacrosse. Again, when sports were similar in boys and girls, concussion rates in girls were higher.[24]

Soccer Heading—A Common Question

One question arising frequently relates to the risk from repeated soccer "heading." Soccer balls may travel as fast as or faster than 50 miles per hour, and during soccer practice players may head the ball more than 30 times, and 6 to 12 times in games.[25] A 2003 study summarized the results of neurocognitive testing in 60 male soccer players (a mix of high school to professional) and 12 controls who did not play soccer. Greater lifetime amount of heading (rather than level of current play) was associated with poorer scores related to general brain functioning, attention, concentration, and "cognitive flexibility."[26] A decade later, Lipton and colleagues published a study of 37 amateur soccer players in New York City (average age about 31 and 78% male), and found these amateur players had headed soccer balls from 32 to 5,400 times (median 432 times) over the past year.[27] Using magnetic resonance imaging and computerized cognitive testing, investigators found that more heading (not a history of concussion) was associated with white matter brain abnormalities as well as poorer results on cognitive tests.[27] Soccer players heading between 885 and 1,550 times per year, in this study, showed abnormal white matter patterns, and poorer memory scores were associated with soccer players heading more than 1,800 times per year.[25] The study's lead author said, "Our study provides compelling evidence that brain changes resembling mild traumatic brain injury are associated with frequently heading a soccer ball over many years."[25]

Other types of body contact may also increase risks for concussion. In a study designed to determine whether body checking increased concussion risk in youth ice hockey, investigators looked prospectively at concussion risks in Canadian Pee Wee hockey leagues.[28] Emery and colleagues studied ice hockey players (ages 11 to 12) in leagues that did (Alberta, Canada) or did *not* (Quebec, Canada) allow body checking. In a study of 2,154 hockey players during the 2007–2008 season, investigators found that playing in a league that allowed checking was associated with an increased injury risk three times higher than in leagues that did not allow checking.[28] Risk for concussion was nearly four times higher (incidence rate ratio 3.88) and more than three and one-half times higher for severe concussion (incidence rate ratio 3.61) in leagues that allowed body checking.[28]

EVIDENCE BASE FOR PREVENTION AND PRACTICE

Some particular areas of controversy in youth, high school, and collegiate athletics include defining when an athlete can return to play, use of many published guidelines (more than 20 exist) for concussion management, risk of second impact syndrome (SIS), and potential risk of long-term and permanent cognitive impairments from concussion.[29] Experts maintain that the best preparation includes "knowing your athletes," keeping health-related data, using effective communication, anticipating the possibility of concussions, and keeping up-to-date with evidence-based recommendations for prevention, early identification, and management of concussions.[29]

Are Helmets Effective in Preventing Concussions?

Helmets are widely perceived to protect the heads of athletes both young and adult, and are intended to reduce skull fractures and more serious brain injuries; however, a 2014 study questioned their effectiveness against concussions.[30] A preliminary report from the *Los Angeles Times* about a study presented at the American Academy of Neurology's annual meeting compared 10 commonly used football helmets by simulating forces similar to those that cause concussions.[30] To test the helmets, the investigators put motion sensors on the heads of crash dummies wearing football helmets and exposed them to 12-mile-per-hour impacts. Comparing the crash dummies with and without football helmets, they estimated that the helmets only produced a 20% reduction in concussion risk, which varied by helmet brand.[31] "All of them were terrible," one study author noted and emphasized the need for proper tackling technique, strict officiating, and muscle strengthening in football, instead of solely relying on helmets.[30] Sensors on the crash dummy helmets were designed to measure both linear forces (contributing to skull fractures) and rotational forces (contributing to concussions). Skull fracture risk was reduced by 60–70% and brain bruising was reduced by 70–80% from wearing football helmets in this study.[31,32]

With increasing awareness about concussions, many argue against helmets as a panacea in some sports, particularly women's lacrosse. Rules in women's lacrosse emphasize safety and no body contact, and are thus dramatically different from the men's version of the same sport.[33,34] The president of US Lacrosse, the national governing body of both men's and women's lacrosse said, "Everybody looks at equipment intervention as the end-all, be-all—but it's not, and the football discussion bears this out . . . the picture of a helmet on a kid makes them feel better, but it's more complicated than that." US Lacrosse supports education of players, parents, and coaches, and strictly enforcing game rules designed for player safety.[33,34] The 2013 Consensus Statement on Concussion in Sport found "no good clinical evidence that currently available protective equipment will prevent concussion, although mouth guards have a definite role in preventing dental and orofacial injury."[14] Similar findings were reported by the Institute of Medicine committee in 2013.[35]

What Can We Learn from Canadian Pee Wee Hockey?

Based on a *JAMA* study[28] that evaluated rates of concussion in Canadian youth hockey Pee Wee players (aged 11 to 12 years) who played in leagues that either did and did not allow body checking, USA Hockey enacted a new rule to raise the age group in which body checking is allowed, from Pee Wee (age 12 and under) to Bantam (age 14 and under); the rule change became effective in the 2011–2012 ice hockey season.[36] Through not without controversy, with some "wondering if their beloved game was turning into hockey lite," other coaches at the youth level observed, "It puts parents at ease, that's for sure."[37] In a follow-up study to the Canadian Pee Wee hockey study, Emery and colleagues investigated the commonly asked question of whether or not injuries in players at the older Bantam level were different in players who did or did not have 2 years of prior body checking experience at the younger Pee Wee level.[38]

Emery and colleagues conducted a similar comparison in nearly 2,000 Bantam youth players (aged 13 to 14 years) in the Alberta and Quebec leagues.[38] They found no differences between total injuries and concussions in players with and without previous body checking experience.[38] In addition, there were no differences in rates of severe concussion injury (more than 10 days' time loss). However the authors did find a reduction in injuries lasting more than 7 days in the Bantam players with checking experience (incidence rate ratio 0.67 with 95% CI = 0.46 to 0.99).[38] The authors suggested that current findings be balanced against results of their previous study, when injury and concussion risks were three times higher in 11 and 12 year olds when body checking was allowed.[28] USA Hockey, in its "points of emphasis" for ice hockey rules from 2013–2014 through 2016–2107 seasons highlights their standard of play for body checking, aims to promote player skill development, and emphasizes enforcement of the standard.[39]

Policy Approaches and Consensus Guidelines

In late 2012, consensus guidelines were published following the 4th International Conference in Sport, in Zurich, Switzerland, and in 2013, updated guidelines were published by the American Academy of Neurology (AAN).[14,15,40] The "Consensus Statement on Concussion in Sport" is a comprehensive summary of expert recommendations, covering diagnosis, neuropsychological (NP) testing, management, special populations such as children and adolescents, and injury prevention.[14] The AAN updated their 1997 guidelines in 2013, using evidence-based criteria to develop recommendations in such areas as risk factors, diagnostic tools, factors predicting long-term consequences, and effectiveness of current treatment strategies.[40] They studied the evidence for factors such as age, level of competition, sex, weight, type of sport, equipment, and position played and whether they increased or decreased concussion risk.[40] They also studied assessment tools and checklists of concussion symptoms, determining sensitivity and specificity of identifying concussion with available tests. They suggest that neuropsychological tests to identify concussions (whether paper or computer-based), to evaluate memory, cognitive processing speed, and reaction time are "likely useful."[40] They also concluded that there was "insufficient data" to determine whether or not currently used treatments speed healing or prevent adverse outcomes in the future.[40] An online Sports Concussion Toolkit contains resources for patients, coaches and athletic trainers, and health professionals.[41]

An editorial discussing both strengths and limitations of these updated guidelines, emphasizes areas of agreement between the two: immediate removal from play when concussion is suspected, evaluation by an appropriately trained health professional, and return to play only after complete resolution, using a gradual approach.[14,15,40] Always erring on the side of protecting players is consistently recommended. Preventive measures including rule changes, use of appropriate protective equipment, and ongoing education for health professionals, coaches, parents, players, and school officials are all emphasized as part of comprehensive efforts to best manage and prevent concussions.[15]

The Institute of Medicine and National Research Council published a report in October 2013, called "Sports-Related Concussions in Youth: Improving the Science, Changing the Culture," after convening a committee of experts to review scientific evidence about concussion in children, adolescents, and young adults.[35] The committee recommended a national surveillance system managed by CDC to provide better data for research on the numbers, types, cause, and severity of concussions.[35] Research was recommended to identify specific changes in the brain following concussion, develop objective measures to diagnose concussion, and determine evidence-based treatment and management strategies.[35] Additionally, research was recommended on short-term and long-term effects of multiple concussions from long-term population studies.[35] The committee recommended additional study of effective ways to improve safety in youth sports, including "changing the culture" of athletics to support concussion reporting.[35] A *Lancet* editorial agreed that "a multidisciplinary effort on a grand scale is needed."[42]

CDC recommends primary prevention strategies, emphasizing skills and safe practices in athletics, following rules, strict officiating, and emphasis on sportsmanship.[20] Recommendations for secondary prevention and detecting concussions as early as possible include raising awareness of signs and symptoms such as through their HEADS UP concussion campaign.[19] Similar to other consensus guidelines, CDC recommends that athletes with a suspected concussion be immediately removed from play, evaluated by an experienced health professional, and cleared by a trained professional before they resume the sport or activity, with special emphasis on children and adolescents.[20]

CDC has also published a guide called "Get a Heads Up on Concussion in Sports Policies" designed for parents, coaches, and schools.[7] As awareness of the importance of preventing, identifying, and managing concussions has grown, so has the number of laws and policies enacted by states in the United States. For example, between 2009 and 2013, 47 states and the District of Columbia passed laws (sometimes called "return-to-play" laws) related to preventing concussions in youth or high school sports.[7] The National Conference of State Legislatures has created a map of states that have enacted such laws, and maintains an updated list of these laws, by state, with descriptions of the legislation.[7,43] The majority of these laws contain three action steps based on the 2008 International Concussion Consensus Statement, including: educating coaches, parent, and athletes; immediately removing injured athletes from play; and requiring permission from a healthcare professional to return to play, never on the same day.[7] How well are prevention and education efforts working? CDC reported a 60% increase in ED visits for concussion over an 8-year period, attributed in large part to increased awareness.[44]

DISCUSSION QUESTIONS: TEMPLATE FOR DISCUSSION

1. Significance of this public health issue:
   a. Why is this health issue important?
   b. How many people does it impact?
   c. How serious is it?
   d. Is it preventable?

2. What is the evidence base for prevention?
3. What specific strategies should be used to achieve progress on this health issue?
   a. What evidence-based approach would you use?
   b. Where would you start if you are an individual citizen; public health professional; healthcare professional; community, state, or federal policymaker?
4. Specific questions for this topic:
   a. How does the story of chronic head injury in the NFL help with developing prevention strategies in athletics for children and adolescents?
   b. What are the most pressing research questions?
   c. What is the role of a "culture of competition" in athletics today? Can safety and competition coexist?
5. What is the controversy?
   a. Define the controversy.
   b. Is controversy a good or bad thing? (Does it help or hinder progress?)
6. *Why* is this health issue controversial?
   a. What specific factors are involved?
   b. Do economics, government, scientific uncertainty, or politics play a role?
   c. What is the role of the media?
7. How would you respond to the controversy?

PERSPECTIVES TO CONSIDER

The NFL story is a sad one that has generated tremendous national controversy in a sport watched and played by thousands of children and young adults.[2] However, like a study of adverse outcomes in occupational settings, the NFL's experience provided a glimpse of potential long-term and devastating outcomes from repeated exposures to head and body contact and accelerated a national discussion of prevention strategies. Zackery Lystedt's tragic injury and recovery provided inspiration for many strong state laws to prevent traumatic brain injury in young athletes.[6] CDC's data suggest increased awareness about concussions,[20] and if this continues, we might expect to see more concussions reported, but without corresponding increases in the numbers of serious head injuries.

Some of the more recent consensus guidelines, especially those that are evidence-based, point to huge gaps in our knowledge in such areas as diagnostic testing, treatment, and management. They also highlight misperceptions about the effectiveness of protective equipment (such as helmets) in some specific sports.[14,40] Much more research is needed in many areas, including pathophysiology and molecular changes, SIS, gender and age differences, and short- and long-term effects of multiple concussions.[13]

From a public health perspective, it is essential to focus prevention efforts both on sports with large numbers of injuries and on sports that have higher *rates* of concussion.[20] Training, proper technique, rules development and enforcement, and coaching education all become urgent priorities in an environment where more young people are participating and competition increases. Experts are calling for more short- and long-term research in all of these areas as well as changes to athletic culture, especially in youth sports.[35]

There are also gaps in our knowledge about policy approaches. Some authors stress the need for more practical guidelines, based on current knowledge.[13,15] Many controversial questions arise from current literature, especially as it relates to potential risks in children and adolescents. For example, from the literature about soccer heading,[26,27] should youth soccer consider policy changes for young players, analogous to steps taken in youth hockey?

At the current time, most experts recommend a cautious approach that protects the child, adolescent, or young adult.[7,14,20,40] Removing athletes from sports immediately after a possible concussion, ensuring expert health evaluation, and return to play gradually and only with health professional clearance, all make sense, given what we currently know. For now, the best rule remains, "when in doubt, sit them out."[7]

FOR ADDITIONAL STUDY

League of denial: The NFL's concussion crisis. [video]. PBS Frontline. 2013. http://www.pbs.org/wgbh/pages/frontline/league-of-denial/

REFERENCES

1. Omalu BI, DeKosky ST, Minster RL, Kamboh MI, Hamilton RL, Wecht CH. Chronic traumatic encephalopathy in a National Football League player. *Neurosurgery.* 2005;57(1):128–134; discussion 128–134.
2. League of denial: The NFL's concussion crisis. [video]. PBS Frontline. 2013. http://www.pbs.org/wgbh/pages/frontline/league-of-denial/. Accessed April 28, 2014.

3. Casson IR, Pellman EJ, Viano DC. Chronic traumatic encephalopathy in a National Football League player. *Neurosurgery.* 2006;58(5):E1003; author reply E1003; discussion E1003.

4. Zackery Lystedt Law-House Bill 1824. 2013. http://www.tbiwashington.org/tbi_wa/bill1824.shtml. Accessed May 5, 2014.

5. Marvex A. Lystedt lays down law on concussions. *Fox Sports.* 2012. http://msn.foxsports.com/nfl/story/zack-lystedt-bring-awareness-nfl-concussion-issue-lystedt-law-052012. Accessed May 5, 2014.

6. Mickool S.The story behind the Zackery Lystedt law: The Washington teenager who inspired groundbreaking health and safety legislation. *Seattle Magazine.* 2012. http://www.seattlemag.com/article/story-behind-zackery-lystedt-law. Accessed May 5, 2014.

7. CDC. Get a heads up on concussion in sports policies. 2013. http://www.cdc.gov/concussion/pdf/HeadsUpOnConcussionInSportsPolicies-a.pdf. Accessed May 5, 2014.

8. Schwarz A. N.F.L. scolded over injuries to its players. *The New York Times.* 2009. http://www.nytimes.com/2009/10/29/sports/football/29hearing.html?_r=0. Accessed May 5, 2014.

9. Nearly half of dads believe there is too much hype around concussions. *Concussion Policy & the Law.* 2012. http://concussionpolicyandthelaw.com/2012/10/12/nearly-half-of-dads-believe-there-is-too-much-hype-around-concussions/. Accessed October 2, 2014.

10. CDC. Injury prevention & control: Traumatic brain injury. 2013. http://www.cdc.gov/concussion/. Accessed May 5, 2014.

11. CDC. Concussion in sports 2013. http://www.cdc.gov/concussion/sports/. Accessed May 5, 2014.

12. Corsellis JA. Boxing and the brain. *BMJ.* 1989;298(6666):105–109.

13. DeKosky ST, Ikonomovic MD, Gandy S. Traumatic brain injury: Football, warfare, and long-term effects. *Minn Med.* 2010;93(12):46–47.

14. McCrory P, Meeuwisse W, Aubry M, et al. Consensus statement on concussion in sport—the 4th International Conference on Concussion in Sport held in Zurich, November 2012. *Clin J Sport Med.* 2013;23(2):89–117.

15. *The Lancet Neurology.* Time for a gamechanger in the management of concussion. *Lancet Neurol.* 2013;12(5):415.

16. Wetjen NM, Pichelmann MA, Atkinson JL. Second impact syndrome: Concussion and second injury brain complications. *J Am Coll Surg.* 2010;211(4):553–557.

17. Bey T, Ostick B. Second impact syndrome. *Western J Emerg Med.* 2009;10(1):6–10.

18. CDC. Concussion in sports and play: Get the facts 2011. http://www.cdc.gov/concussion/sports/facts.html. Accessed November 4, 2014.

19. CDC. HEADS UP. 2014. http://www.cdc.gov/headsup/index.html Accessed November 4, 2014.

20. CDC. Nonfatal traumatic brain injuries related to sports and recreation activities among persons aged ≤19 Years—United States, 2001–2009. *MMWR.* 2011. http://www.cdc.gov/MMWR/preview/mmwrhtml/mm6039a1.htm?s_cid=mm6039a1_w. Accessed May 5, 2014.

21. Gordon KE, Dooley JM, Wood EP. Descriptive epidemiology of concussion. *Pediatric Neurol.* 2006;34(5):376–378.

22. Lincoln AE, Caswell SV, Almquist JL, Dunn RE, Norris JB, Hinton RY. Trends in concussion incidence in high school sports: A prospective 11-year study. *Am J Sports Med.* 2011;39(5):958–963.

23. Laker SR. Epidemiology of concussion and mild traumatic brain injury. *PMR.* 2011;3(10 Suppl 2):S354–358.

24. Marar M, McIlvain NM, Fields SK, Comstock RD. Epidemiology of concussions among United States high school athletes in 20 sports. *Am J Sports Med.* 2012;40(4):747–755.

25. Albert Einstein College of Medicine Yeshiva University. Frequent soccer ball "heading" may lead to brain injury. *Science Daily.* 2013. http://www.sciencedaily .com/releases/2013/06/130611082233.htm. Accessed May 5, 2014.

26. Witol AD, Webbe FM. Soccer heading frequency predicts neuropsychological deficits. *Arch Clin Neuropsych.* 2003;18(4):397-417.

27. Lipton ML, Kim N, Zimmerman ME, et al. Soccer heading is associated with white matter microstructural and cognitive abnormalities. *Radiology.* 2013;268(3):850–857.

28. Emery CA, Kang J, Shrier I, et al. Risk of injury associated with body checking among youth ice hockey players. *JAMA.* 2010;303(22):2265–2272.

29. Standaert CJ, Herring SA, Cantu RC. Expert opinion and controversies in sports and musculoskeletal medicine: Concussion in the young athlete. *Arch Phys Med Rehabil.* 2007;88(8):1077–1079.

30. Healy M. Football helmets and concussion: A new study opens new questions. *Los Angeles Times.* 2014. http://articles.latimes.com/2014/feb/17/science/la-sci-sn-football-helmets-concussion-20140217. Accessed April 28, 2014.

31. Football helmets do little to prevent concussions, study finds. *Fox News.* 2014. http://www.foxnews.com/health/2014/02/18/football-helmets-do-little-to-prevent-concussions-study-finds/. Accessed April 28, 2014.

32. How well do football helmets protect players from concussions? *ScienceDaily.* 2014. http://www.sciencedaily.com/releases/2014/02/140217200751.htm. Accessed April 28, 2014.

33. US Lacrosse. Why Women's lacrosse is not played with additional protective equipment. 2012. http://www.uslacrosse.org/Portals/1/documents/pdf/participants/ coaches/safety-issues-in-girls-and-womens-lacrosse.pdf. Accessed May 5, 2014.

34. Schwarz A. A case against helmets in lacrosse. 2011. http://www.nytimes.com/2011/ 02/17/sports/17lacrosse.html?pagewanted=all. Accessed May 5, 2014.

35. Graham R, Rivara FP, Ford MA, Spicer CM, Eds. *Sports-related concussions in youth: Improving the science, changing the culture.* Washington DC: National Academies Press; 2014.

36. Sebastian L. USA Hockey changes age of legal body checking. *Pittsburgh Youth Hockey Network.* 2011. http://penguins.nhl.com/club/page.htm?id=69640. Accessed May 5, 2014.

37. Mahler D. Changing checking: Coaches and players evaluate new youth hockey rules on hitting. *Valley News.* 2013. http://www.vnews.com/home/4221074-95/checking-hockey-players-game. Accessed May 5, 2014.

38. Emery C, Kang J, Shrier I, et al. Risk of injury associated with bodychecking experience among youth hockey players. *CMAJ.* 2011;183(11):1249–1256.

39. USA Hockey. USA Hockey official playing rules, points of emphasis 2013–14 through 2016–17 playing seasons. http://assets.ngin.com/attachments/document/0040/ 8294/2013-17_USA_Hockey_Rule_Change_Summary.pdf. Accessed May 5, 2014.

40. Giza CC, Kutcher JS, Ashwal S, et al. Summary of evidence-based guideline update: Evaluation and management of concussion in sports: Report of the Guideline Development Subcommittee of the American Academy of Neurology. *Neurology.* 2013;80(24):2250–2257.
41. AAN.com. American Academy of Neurology sports concussion toolkit. 2014. https://www.aan.com/go/practice/concussion. Accessed May 5, 2014.
42. Concussion in sport: Fair play for young people. *Lancet.* 2013;382(9904):1536.
43. National Conference of State Legislatures (NCSL). Traumatic brain injury legislation. 2014. http://www.ncsl.org/research/health/traumatic-brain-injury-legislation.aspx. Accessed May 5, 2014.
44. Zinser L. Report indicates an increase in concussion awareness. 2011. http://www.nytimes.com/2011/10/07/sports/report-shows-rise-in-er-visits-for-concussions-among-young.html?_r=0. Accessed May 5, 2014.

CHAPTER 18

HIV and AIDS:
The Fourth Decade

LEARNING OBJECTIVES

- Describe the status of the HIV/AIDS pandemic.
- Discuss the most prominent controversies in HIV prevention and treatment.
- Identify challenges associated with finding a cure for HIV.
- Critically assess the evidence for the effectiveness of treatment as prevention.
- Propose evidence-based prevention strategies to reduce HIV infection in the United States and internationally.

THE CONTROVERSY

Dr. Anthony Fauci, director of the National Institute of Allergy and Infectious Diseases (NIAID) at the National Institutes of Health, delivered a grim media message: a rural Mississippi baby girl believed cured of HIV, now showed evidence of infection.[1,2] The physician who took care of the baby was crushed. "It felt very much like a punch to the gut," she said.[2] In March 2013, the baby was reported "apparently cured," when she was found to be free of HIV infection 2 years after her birth.[3] "In Medical First, a Baby With H.I.V Is Deemed Cured," proclaimed *The New York Times*.[4] When the baby was born, her mother had had no prenatal care during her pregnancy and tested positive for HIV at the hospital near the time of the baby's birth.[3] To reduce risks that babies will be born infected with HIV, known HIV-infected mothers in the United States usually receive anti-HIV medications during their pregnancy.[5] However, because the mother's HIV status was not known until just before the baby's birth, the baby was at very high risk for infection with HIV.[3] Her physician, Dr. Gay, decided to begin full HIV treatment, using three drugs, rather than the customary preventive regimen, because of this risk.[3] There were skeptics. Experts pointed out that it may be difficult to determine if a baby is infected right away, because the HIV antibodies from her mother may be detected in her blood.[3,4] However, in this instance, the amount of HIV found in the baby's blood followed a pattern that was more typical of someone who is HIV infected and responds to treatment.[3]

The baby was lost to medical follow-up after she was 1.5 years old, but when she was tested at nearly 2 years of age, HIV was still not detected in her blood by clinical laboratory tests, the child's status termed a "functional cure."[3] However, after 27 months without treatment for HIV (called antiretroviral therapy), the girl tested positive for HIV.[2] Findings had already been published in the NEJM in 2013.[6] Enthusiasm for the "Mississippi baby's" apparent cure was high;[5] findings were presented at a national medical conference in Atlanta,[7] and the article was subsequently cited frequently in the medical and scientific literature.

A second baby born in Los Angeles, CA called the "LA baby," reported as "possibly cured" in March 2014, at 9 months of age, continues antiretroviral treatment and is followed closely.[8,9] This baby was also treated aggressively with three treatment drugs after birth, but experts hesitated to term her "cured" as she remained on medications.[9]

A cure had only been described in one previous patient, known as the "Berlin Patient," a patient with HIV infection and acute myelogenous leukemia who underwent a stem-cell transplant,[10–12] His new stem cells contained a mutation, uncommon in the general population, called the CCR5-delta32 mutation, which is known to confer genetic resistance to HIV infection.[12]

Challenges in achieving a cure are in part due to "reservoirs" of HIV-1 infection in various cells and locations in the body,[13] such as in intestinal tissue, which remain functionally hidden from treatment.[10] Even though not detected in the blood, HIV virus may be lying in wait in lymph nodes, brain, liver, kidney, gastrointestinal, or heart tissues.[14]

Meanwhile, in 2014, scientists successfully tested the feasibility of editing genes in the CCR5 receptor and then giving the cells back to 12 patients infected with HIV.[15] The potential benefit of making genetic changes in immune cells (called T-cells) from HIV patients is that researchers can then give patients an *acquired* genetic ability to fight HIV infection.[12] One patient who participated in this trial said, "It makes me very excited. Hopeful, and it makes me want to . . . shout out to the world that there could be an end to this."[12]

BACKGROUND AND SCOPE OF THE PUBLIC HEALTH AND HEALTH POLICY ISSUE

History

The history of the HIV and AIDS pandemic began in 1981 when the U.S. Centers for Disease Control and Prevention (CDC) reported five previously healthy young men in Los Angeles, CA were infected with *Pneumocystis carinii* pneumonia, an infection usually seen in individuals with compromised immune systems.[16] After the initial report, there were more case reports from New York City and San Francisco and in the next 18 months, major risk factors for Acquired Immunodeficiency Syndrome (AIDS) were identified and published.[17] AIDS was characterized by loss of CD4+ T cells, critical parts of the immune system needed to defend against many infections.[18] In addition to men who have sex with men (MSM), AIDS was reported in patients with hemophilia, injection-drug users, and infants born to mothers with AIDS.[18] An epidemic of AIDS was also reported in Africa, notably affecting women. Two years later, a retrovirus was found to be the cause of AIDS, and the virus named human immunodeficiency virus (HIV).[18] The history of the AIDS pandemic has been described in many publications,[18–21] and progress since 1981 has also been fraught with controversies in such areas as prevention, treatment, research, and advocacy for funding. In the fourth decade, there is much evidence of progress, but extensive needs in the United States and globally remain in these same major areas.[18]

Epidemiology and Statistics

CDC tracks trends in HIV and AIDS through public health surveillance, defined as "the ongoing, systematic collection, analysis, interpretation, and dissemination of data regarding a health-related event."[22] CDC previously tracked trends in AIDS, as a proxy for HIV infection, before the advent of highly active antiretroviral therapy (HAART) in 1996, which necessitated development of systems to monitor HIV infection.[22] States then began tracking HIV infection, and all states in the United States had confidential name-based systems for HIV reporting to CDC in place by 2008, in order to be able to monitor progress in preventing and treating HIV infections nationally.[22]

Another type of available testing called *serologic testing algorithm for recent HIV seroconversion* (STARHS) helps determine whether or not infections are newly acquired (in the past 5 months). This testing is used in 25 areas of the United States to monitor HIV infection trends.[22,23] There are also tracking systems in place to collect information about HIV risk behaviors, called the MMP (Medical Monitoring Project) and NHBS (National HIV Behavioral Surveillance system).[22] Since 1985, CDC has also funded National HIV Prevention Monitoring and Evaluation (NHM&E) program, working with health-related organizations and health departments to collect data to help evaluate prevention programs.[22] Detailed information about these data systems and trends in HIV infection can be found on the CDC website.[22]

In November 2013, CDC estimated 1,144,500 people over the age of 13 are living with HIV infection in the United States.[24] They also estimate that nearly 16%, (180,900 people) are not aware that they are infected. In addition, there are about 50,000 new infections each year, a figure that has not changed since the mid-1990s.[23] In 2010, 47,500 were infected with HIV and 15,529 people died from AIDS.[23,24] The risk for HIV infection is not spread evenly, with some populations, such as MSM infected more often.[23] Blacks/African Americans had 44% of new HIV infections, and Hispanics/Latinos had 21% of new HIV infections in the United States in 2010, which is out of proportion to their representation in the United States population[23] (see **Figure 18–1**).

In 2010, CDC reported 29,800 new infections among MSM, 63% of all new HIV infections, a significant increase since 2008.[24] Although new infections in white MSM were higher (11,200 in 2010) than in black MSM (10,600) overall, the highest number of new infections (4,800) in MSM was in young black/African American MSM aged 13 to 24.[24] From the National HIV Surveillance System (NHSS) and NHBS, CDC reported in 2013 that across the United States, 50% or more of new HIV infections were in MSM. Further, the percentage of MSM having unprotected sex in the past year increased significantly from 2005 to 2011 (48% to 57%; $p < 0.001$).[25] This same trend has been noted in MSM in Canada, Britain, the Netherlands, France, and Australia.[26]

In the United States, only about two-thirds of MSM report HIV testing in the past year,[25] a relevant finding because being tested for HIV is associated with engaging in less-risky behaviors, no matter what the test results show.[26] Although just theories, experts observe that current young men have not personally witnessed deaths from AIDS, so common in the earlier years of the epidemic, and the availability of antiretroviral drugs

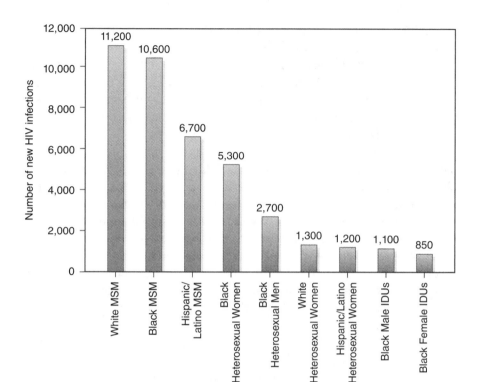

Subpopulations representing 2% or less of the overall US epidemic are not reflected in this chart.

Figure 18–1 Estimated new HIV infectious in the United States, 2010.

Data from Centers for Disease Control and Prevention. HIV in the United States: At A Glance. Available at http://www.cdc.gov/hiv/statistics/basics/ataglance.html

may also alter the perception of severity of risk, even if infected. "Young guys are less worried. HIV has become a chronic disease," observed one HIV researcher.[26]

One-fifth of new HIV infections in 2010 were in women, and Black/ African American and Hispanic/Latino women were especially impacted.[27] New infections in women have decreased significantly from 2008 (12,000 new infections) to 2010 (9,500 new infections), a decline of 21%.[24] New HIV infections also specifically decreased in black women in the period from 2008 to 2010, declining from 7,700 to 6,100 infections, although it is too soon to determine whether this is a longer-term trend.[23] One critical issue affecting women with HIV is access to care: in the period from 2009 to 2010, just over half of women with HIV (53%) were actively involved in health care for HIV and only 42% showed viral suppression, evidence of ongoing and effective treatment.[27]

HIV infection also varies geographically, with higher rates often seen in urban areas.[28] In 2008, the rate of HIV infections (which is the number of HIV infections divided by the population, expressed as number of cases per 100,000 population), showed highest rates in the northeast and south.[28] (see **Figure 18–2**).

HIV infections are also unevenly distributed by age.[29,30] In 2010, 31% of new HIV infections were in people aged 25–34 years (14,500 infections), 26% of new infections were in people aged 13–24 years (12,200); CDC has identified youth (defined as ages 13–24) as a priority group for prevention and treatment.[29] Of infections in youth, 80% are in young men, 60% are in African American individuals, 20% in Hispanic and Latino individuals, and 20% are in white young people.[29] Furthermore, 87% of young men overall became infected through male-to-male sex and 86% of young women became infected through heterosexual sex.[29] An estimated 60% of young people infected with HIV are unaware of their infection, thus not getting treatment.[29]

In 2010, 24% of new HIV infections were in individuals aged 35–44 years (11,300 infections). Further, 15% or 7,100 new infections were in people aged 45–54 years and 5% or 2,500 new infections were in people age 55 and

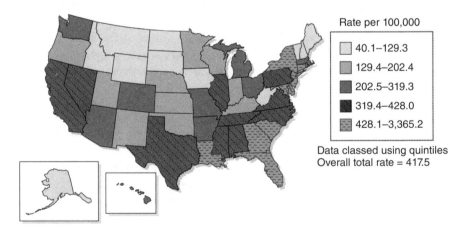

Figure 18–2 Rates of persons aged 18–64 years living with a diagnosis of HIV infection, year-end 2008—United States.

Reproduced from Centers for Disease Control and Prevention. HIV and AIDS in the United States by Geographic Distribution. Available at http://www.cdc.gov/hiv/statistics/basics/geographicdistribution.html

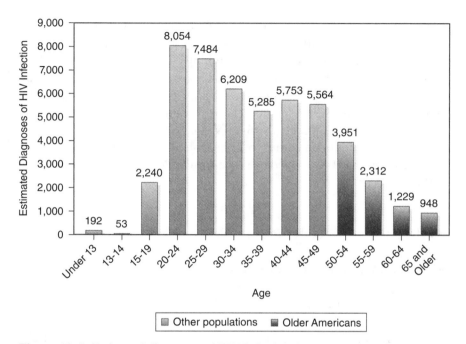

Figure 18–3 Estimated diagnoses of HIV infection, by age 2011, United States.

Reproduced from Centers for Disease Control and Prevention. HIV among Older Americans. Available at http://www.cdc.gov/hiv/pdf/library_factsheet_HIV_%20 AmongOlderAmericans.pdf

older.[23] Because of these statistics, older Americans (age 50 or older) are also a priority for HIV prevention and treatment, and have the same risk factors as other age groups.[30] In 2010, nearly 20% of the 1.1 million people living with HIV infection in the US were aged 55 or older, and in contrast to younger people with HIV infection, older individuals are diagnosed later and have a shorter time period between their diagnosis and progression to AIDS[30] (see **Figure 18–3**).

Recommendations for HIV Testing

CDC recommends HIV testing for adolescents and adults, at least once, as a routine part of health care, as part of the National HIV/AIDS strategy goal to "ensure 90 percent of Americans with HIV are aware of their status and that more people are linked to care within 3 months of their diagnosis."[31] The U.S. Preventive Services Task Force (USPSTF) also recommends HIV screening for adolescents, adults, and pregnant women as a part of clinical preventive care.[32] HIV testing is essential for both prevention and treatment. By linking people with HIV infection to health care, HIV-infected patients benefit from effective treatment. In addition, early treatment can reduce the risk of transmitting HIV by 96%, as virus levels are greatly reduced.[31] According to CDC, about 180,000 people (16% of those infected with HIV) do not know they are infected.[31] Despite these recommendations, over half of all adults in the United States have never had an HIV test and over one-third of MSM have not been tested in the past year.[31]

EVIDENCE BASE FOR PREVENTION AND PRACTICE

Advances in Treatment as Prevention

In the mid-1990s, discovery and widespread use of highly active antiretroviral therapy (HAART) resulted in reductions in HIV/AIDS deaths in developed countries.[18] In addition, huge benefits were also seen in HIV-infected pregnant women, as use of these drugs during their pregnancies resulted in fewer HIV-infected infants.[18,33] Such prevention efforts are estimated to have prevented the deaths of more than 1 million children globally[34] (see **Figure 18–4**).

Part of the international response to the growing HIV/AIDS pandemic included the 2001 Declaration of Commitment on HIV/AIDS from the United Nations General Assembly, updated in 2011, and the President's Emergency Plan for AIDS Relief (PEPFAR) in 2003, intensifying the resources and multidisciplinary efforts focused on the pandemic.[18] In 2001, the Joint United Nations Programme on HIV/AIDS (UNAIDS) estimated 29.1 million people were living with HIV infection, a figure that increased to 34.2 million in 2011.[18] However, during this decade, both the numbers of new infections and deaths decreased. In 2011, 2.5 million people had new HIV infections, down 22% in the past 10 years, and deaths from HIV/AIDS declined by 26% from 2.3 million in 2005 to 1.7 million in 2011.[18] From 1995 to 2012, the widespread use of antiretroviral therapy (ART) in low- and middle-income counties has prevented 5.4 million deaths.[34]

CDC, U.S. Department of Health and Human Services, and National Institutes of Health publish regularly updated guidelines for HIV prevention and treatment.[35,36] Access to ART for HIV-infected individuals is essential for longer lives, fewer new infections, and improved quality of life.[37]

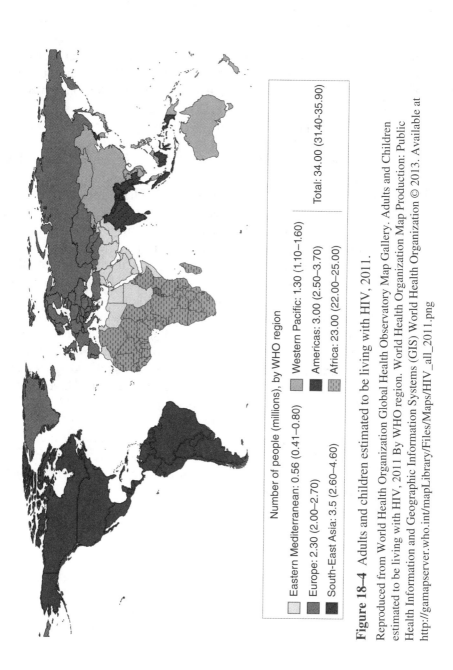

Figure 18–4 Adults and children estimated to be living with HIV, 2011.

Reproduced from World Health Organization Global Health Observatory Map Gallery. Adults and Children estimated to be living with HIV, 2011 By WHO region. World Health Organization Map Production: Public Health Information and Geographic Information Systems (GIS) World Health Organization © 2013. Available at http://gamapserver.who.int/mapLibrary/Files/Maps/HIV_all_2011.png

In addition, as these medications reduce virus levels, they also reduce risk of HIV transmission.[37] At least 26 medications are currently licensed for treatment of HIV[18] and experts remain optimistic about the potential for HIV to be managed as a chronic condition rather than a fatal illness, as was common in the earlier decades of the epidemic.[21] However, this is not without practical challenges such as the need to take multiple daily medications for life, potential chronic side effects, costs, and the knowledge that these drugs manage the infection if taken optimally but are not curative.[21]

In addition, essential to this treatment strategy is having an HIV test and the ability to access medications and health care; currently less than one-third of HIV-infected individuals are receiving optimal care.[37] As of 2011, CDC reports that for every 100 people in the United States living with HIV, 80 know they are infected, 62 receive HIV care, 41 receive ongoing HIV care, 36 receive ART, and 28 have low levels of detectable HIV.[37] These figures demonstrate huge gaps in knowledge, access, and receipt of HIV-related prevention and care in the United States. In 2014, international treatment recommendations emphasized that after a diagnosis of HIV infection, ART is recommended for all adults.[38]

The HIV Prevention Trials Network conducted a randomized, controlled trial, called HPTN 052 in nine countries: Gaborone, Botswana; Kisumu, Kenya; Lilongwe and Blantyre, Malawi; Johannesburg and Soweto, South Africa; Harare, Zimbabwe; Rio de Janeiro and Porto Alegre, Brazil; Pune and Chennai, India; Chiang Mai, Thailand; and Boston.[39] Investigators enrolled 1,763 couples with one HIV-infected partner and tested the ability of ART to reduce HIV infection, comparing the outcomes after giving ART right away or later in the course of their infection. The study found that use of early ART dramatically decreased sexual transmission of HIV, as well as certain HIV-related clinical conditions, implying benefits to both individuals and the entire community.[39]

Pre-Exposure Prophylaxis

In 2012, CDC summarized the pre-exposure prophylaxis (PrEP) as an additional way to prevent HIV in people *not* infected with HIV, to be used along with other established HIV prevention methods.[40] Two different antiretroviral medications (tenofovir disoproxil fumarate [TDF or tenofovir]) and emtricitabine (FTC) are taken each day in a single pill to prevent HIV. The U.S. Food and Drug Association (FDA) approved the single pill containing these two medications in 2004 for HIV treatment, under the brand name Truvada. The FDA approved Truvada for PrEP in July 2012.[40]

Strong supportive research included a multinational study, released in 2010.[40] Investigators found that using this daily pill (containing tenofovir and emtricitabine), combined with established prevention methods such as condoms, HIV testing, and counseling, resulted in greatly increased protection (44%) from HIV infection in MSM.[40] Protection from HIV infection was even better in individuals consistently taking the medication: risk of HIV infection declined by 90% in MSM who had any level of the medication found in their blood (a measure of medication use).[40]

In heterosexually active men and women, two studies released in July 2011 affirmed safety and effectiveness of PrEP.[40] The TDF2 study found 62% reduction in risk of new HIV infection in heterosexual men and women not infected with HIV.[40] The Partners PrEP study looked at circumstances in which one partner was infected with HIV and how effective PrEP was in reducing subsequent risk of HIV infection if taken by the noninfected partner. Using the two combined medications, risk of HIV infection was reduced by 75% and reduced by about two-thirds if tenofovir alone was used, and it worked equally well in men and women.[40] All of these studies confirmed that protection levels against HIV infection were directly related to how well study participants followed the daily medication regimen, with as much as a 90% reduction in risk for HIV infection if medications were taken regularly.[40]

CDC released interim guidelines in 2012,[40] which were updated in 2014.[41] In all of the research trials to date, risk of HIV infection was as much as 92% lower with consistent use of these daily medications.[41] Guidelines recommended that healthcare providers consider the use of PrEP in individuals who are HIV negative and "at substantial risk for HIV infection," including risk factors for sexual transmission and use of injection drugs.[41] Other prevention methods such as consistent use of condoms, regular HIV testing, reducing risk behaviors for sexual activity or injection drug use, were also included in the PrEP recommendations. The 2014 guidance emphasized again, the importance of taking PrEP every day to be maximally effective.[41]

But despite these scientific findings, PrEP remains controversial, with less-than-expected interest.[42] Based on the science, the highly effective daily prevention pill could help with reducing some of the nearly 50,000 annual new HIV infections. However, in a period of 26 months, only 1,774 people filled Truvada prescriptions for HIV prevention, with one-half of the prescriptions filled by women.[42] Boston medical experts wondered if the idea of taking a pill was "flying in the face of community norms," where condom use has been the standard recommendation for many years.[42] Others noted serious, but rare, side effects and an annual cost of nearly $13,000.[42,43] The AIDS Healthcare Foundation of Los Angeles, CA even tried to dissuade the FDA from approving the combination pill for prevention, worrying users might in fact engage in riskier sexual behaviors, a concern not confirmed by research studies.[42] In other cities, such as New York, despite the data on prevention effectiveness, the debate is even louder, with Truvada's use stigmatized in some communities and some activists calling it just "a party drug."[43] Despite the ongoing controversy, one expert remained optimistic, saying, "It's going to take time."[42]

Following the 2014 International AIDS Conference,[44] a series of updated HIV recommendations were published in *JAMA*.[38,45,46] In addition to updated recommendations for prevention and treatment, authors emphasized advances in prevention since the beginning of the AIDS pandemic. At first such recommendations emphasized clean needles and condoms, but later also included guidelines for HIV testing, methods to prevent transmission to infants from HIV-infected mothers through use of ART, male circumcision, and PrEP.[45,46,47] These updated recommendations outlined critical roles of behavioral and medical approaches and emphasized the need to systematically link both to ongoing clinical care.[45,46]

Renewed Interest in a Cure

Some of the questions and controversies surrounding research for an HIV cure stem from the fact that ART treatment does not eliminate HIV infection, due to the presence of "reservoirs" of infection in various body locations that are resistant to or hidden from treatment.[48] Where these reservoirs are located and how they actually work may help in the development of pharmacologic or genetic strategies for the future.[48] Recent, but short-lived reports of potential "functional cures" have sparked a renewed interest in the possibility of an HIV cure.[2–6] Reports of the apparent cure of an HIV-infected patient following stem-cell transplantation for acute myleogenous leukemia continues to be referenced (called the "Berlin patient," as the treatment was in Berlin, Germany).[10,11]

First published in 2009 in the *NEJM*, the 40-year-old HIV-infected patient developed acute leukemia.[10] Seven months after his leukemia diagnosis and treatment failure, he received an allogeneic stem-cell transplantation from a matched donor who had two genetic copies (homozygous) for the CCR5-delta32 allele. In order to be infected with HIV-1, two receptors are needed, one called a CD4 receptor and another called a chemokine receptor, usually CCR5.[10] If a patient is homozygous for the 32-bp deletion in the CCR5 allele, present in about 1–3% of the population, the individual is genetically resistant to HIV infection.[10,14] He relapsed again and received a second transplant from the same donor, which resulted in a complete remission from the leukemia and he is still in remission after 20 months.[10] Genetic testing determined that the patient now had acquired the donor's homozygous genotype for the CCR5-delta32 allele. Further, HIV-1 RNA was not detectable in the patient during the entire follow-up period, despite the fact that HAART had been stopped.[10] A follow-up publication in 2011 further suggested the patient had been "cured."[11]

In a 2014 publication, two HIV-infected patients who underwent allogeneic stem cell transplantation were studied.[49] The authors found that while HIV-1 infection was initially undetectable, it recurred 12 and 32 weeks after ART was stopped, attributed to persistent HIV reservoirs in the body.[49] Many questions about the nature and function of the hidden pockets of HIV infection plague efforts to achieve complete cures and have prompted some to ask, "Are We Making Progress?"[50] At the same time, experts are suggesting new strategies for potential treatment approaches.[50,51]

Another innovative pilot study tried to imitate naturally occurring genetic resistance to HIV infection.[15] This approach involved editing genes for the CCR5 receptor with an enzyme called a zinc-finger nuclease (ZFN) and then reinfusing the CD4 T cells into the same HIV-infected patients.[15] Named "zinc fingers" because a zinc atom holds two protein pieces together, ZFNs are man-made proteins that can turn genes on or off and they are also a tool used to find specific genetic locations.[52] The 2014 trial was conducted in 12 patients to determine whether the procedure was safe, and did not focus on effectiveness of the treatment. Although one severe transfusion reaction occurred, the treatment was judged to be feasible.[15] Whether this new treatment can be effective remains a pressing research question for future studies.[53] Dr. Anthony Fauci, director of NIAID said, "It's a great strategy."[54]

Challenges in HIV Prevention

Challenges remain in identifying what specific combination of approaches (and how they are implemented) will be most effective, in an environment characterized by new scientific advances in HIV prevention.[55,56] According to experts, the most important risk factor for HIV transmission is the level of HIV virus or *viral load*.[18,57] The rationale for treatment as prevention is ART, which can reduce the HIV virus to levels that are not clinically detectable, thus reducing potential for virus transmission.[18,39] Global challenges to more effective prevention and treatment of the HIV pandemic include the fact that only about one-quarter of HIV-infected individuals have access to ART, especially challenging in lower-income countries.[18] In addition, effective prevention strategies are not reaching most individuals; in 2008, these programs reached less than half of injection-drug users and only 40% of MSM.[18]

However experts also note that international progress to date has been achieved without a successful vaccine against HIV.[34] Vaccine development and trials have been challenging. A 2013 published report showed the DNA/rAd5 vaccine was not effective in preventing HIV-1 infection.[58] However, a 2009 trial in Thailand of 16,042 young and healthy men and women of the vaccines ALVAC and AIDSVAX showed a "modest benefit" in reducing HIV risk in a heterosexual population.[59] Vaccine development against HIV has been particularly difficult, as broadly neutralizing antibodies (BNAbs) needed for adequate protection are made in only some HIV-infected individuals after several years, when HIV genetic material is firmly in place and "latent reservoirs" established.[34] One of the challenges to both vaccine development and eliminating the virus entirely through treatment is the presence of these hidden HIV virus reservoirs in the bodies of infected individuals.[34] However, despite these hurdles, current efforts to develop effective vaccines are characterized as "dynamic."[34] The Director of the NIAID in the United States writes that an HIV vaccine is indeed necessary to best combat the AIDS pandemic and editorializes that development and use of an effective vaccine side-by-side with other effective prevention strategies is ultimately needed.[34]

The Future of HIV Prevention

CDC estimates that more than 350,000 HIV infections have been prevented and new HIV infections in the United States have decreased by at least two-thirds since the 1980s.[60] Their focus for using the best evidence-based strategies is called "High-Impact Prevention," and builds on the National HIV/AIDS Strategy published in 2010.[61,62] Goals of the national strategy include measurable targets and action steps for reducing new HIV infections, improving access to care and health outcomes for people with HIV, and reducing health disparities related to HIV infection.[61] CDC's

High-Impact Prevention approach includes setting priorities and focusing efforts where HIV is most common (including geographic areas and specific populations), combining evidence-based prevention methods, and improving public education about HIV.[60]

Geographic focus, increased HIV testing, and ensuring the best use of evidence-based prevention are all part of this strategy.[60] For example, in Houston, TX five neighborhoods with high rates of HIV offered enhanced testing, health services, and education. The city of Los Angeles, TX similarly identified 5 "hot spots" for focused prevention and treatment. New York City is using the Antiretroviral Treatment and Access to Services (ARTAS) approach to improve access to treatment services.[60]

Many factors contribute to challenges in reducing the number of new HIV infections in the United States, currently estimated at about 50,000 per year.[24] For example, individuals infected with HIV now live longer now because of the advances and availability of antiretroviral drugs.[24] In 2014, CDC Director explained it this way: "It's like what the Red Queen said to Alice: 'You have to run faster and faster to stay in the same place.' When you go from one million infected to 1.2 million, you have to do better and better just to stay steady."[26]

DISCUSSION QUESTIONS: TEMPLATE FOR DISCUSSION

1. Significance of this public health issue:
   a. Why is this health issue important?
   b. How many people does it impact?
   c. How serious is it?
   d. Is it preventable?
2. What is the evidence base for prevention?
3. What specific strategies should be used to achieve progress on this health issue?
   a. What evidence-based approach would you use?
   b. Where would you start if you are an individual citizen; public health professional; healthcare professional; community, state, or federal policymaker?
4. Specific questions for this topic:
   a. What are the most important priorities for HIV prevention? What populations experience disproportionate risks and why?
   b. Why do a substantial proportion of new infections occur in both younger and older populations?

    c. What changes can be expected in prevention and treatment of HIV from the Patient Protection and Affordable Care Act?

    d. How should resources be allocated between prevention, treatment, and finding a cure?

5. What is the controversy?

    a. Define the controversy.

    b. Is controversy a good or bad thing? (Does it help or hinder progress?)

6. *Why* is this health issue controversial?

    a. What specific factors are involved?

    b. Do economics, government, scientific uncertainty, or politics play a role?

    c. What is the role of the media?

7. How would you respond to the controversy?

PERSPECTIVES TO CONSIDER

Although CDC reminds us that new HIV infections have declined more than two-thirds since the peak of the epidemic,[23] there are still nearly 50,000 new infections each year, a stubborn figure in the recent past.[23,24] People are living longer with HIV as a result of treatment advances and improvements in HIV-related care.[24] At the same time new advances are forthcoming in prevention and treatment, challenges remain in reaching populations and geographic areas at highest risk, and in engaging individuals and entire communities in HIV prevention.[25,27–30] Controversy over PrEP is ongoing, and how treatment-as-prevention strategies are best used in combination with other prevention approaches remains a priority for current research and practice.[40–42]

What will the fourth decade of HIV and AIDS bring?[18] With the current level of energy, enthusiasm, and optimism toward new prevention methods,[41,60] vaccines,[34] and innovative treatment approaches,[15,63] it is hoped these strategies, combined with ongoing global commitment, will collectively reduce the public health impact of HIV.

FOR ADDITIONAL STUDY

Volberding PA, Deeks SG. Antiretroviral therapy and management of HIV infection. *Lancet.* 2010;376(9734):49–62.

Piot P, Quinn TC. Response to the AIDS pandemic–a global health model. *N Engl J Med.* 2013;368(23):2210–2218.

Mathers BM, Cooper DA. Integrating HIV prevention into practice. *JAMA.* 2014;312(4):349–350.

REFERENCES

1. Le Coz E. HIV again found in Miss. girl who was medical first. *The Clarion-Ledger.* 2014. http://www.clarionledger.com/story/news/2014/07/10/hiv-relapses-in-miss-girl-thought-to-be-cured/12486167/. Accessed November 4, 2014.
2. Cha AE. Child thought cured of HIV tests positive for the virus. *The Washington Post.* 2014. http://www.washingtonpost.com/national/health-science/child-thought-cured-of-hiv-tests-positive-for-the-virus/2014/07/10/686ec2ec-085e-11e4-a0dd-f2b22a257353_story.html. Accessed July 26, 2014.
3. Brown D. Baby born with HIV is apparently cured with aggressive drug treatment. *The Washington Post.* 2013. http://www.washingtonpost.com/national/baby-born-with-hiv-is-apparently-cured-with-aggressive-drug-treatment/2013/03/03/ec6bfb76-8454-11e2-98a3-b3db6b9ac586_story.html. Accessed July 26, 2014.
4. Pollack A, McNeil DG, Jr. In medical first, a baby with H.I.V. is deemed cured. *The New York Times.* 2013. http://www.nytimes.com/2013/03/04/health/for-first-time-baby-cured-of-hiv-doctors-say.html?pagewanted=all&_r=0. Accessed July 26, 2014.
5. Child once thought "cured" of HIV tests positive. *CBS News.* 2014. http://www.cbsnews.com/news/mississippi-child-once-thought-cured-of-hiv-tests-positive/. Accessed July 26, 2014.
6. Persaud D, Gay H, Ziemniak C, et al. Absence of detectable HIV-1 Viremia after treatment cessation in an infant. *N Engl J Med.* 2013;369(19):1828–1835.
7. Young S. Researchers: Toddler cured of HIV. *CNN Health.* 2013. http://www.cnn.com/2013/03/03/health/hiv-toddler-cured/. Accessed July 26, 2014.
8. Second HIV-positive baby may be cured of AIDS. *CBS News.* 2014. http://www.cbsnews.com/news/second-hiv-positive-baby-may-be-cured-of-aids/. Accessed July 26, 2014.
9. McNeil DG, Jr. Early treatment is found to clear H.I.V. in a 2nd baby. *The New York Times.* 2014. http://www.nytimes.com/2014/03/06/health/second-success-raises-hope-for-a-way-to-rid-babies-of-hiv.html. Accessed July 26, 2014.
10. Hütter G, Nowak D, Mossner M, et al. Long-term control of HIV by CCR5-Delta32/Delta32 stem-cell transplantation. *N Engl J Med.* 2009;360(7):692–698.
11. Allers K, Hütter G, Hofmann J, et al. Evidence for the cure of HIV infection by CCR5Δ32/Δ32 stem cell transplantation. *Blood.* 2011;117(10):2791–2799.
12. Jaslow R. New advance: Engineered immune cells seem to block HIV. *CBS News.* 2014. http://www.cbsnews.com/news/gene-therapy-engineer-t-cells-block-hiv/. Accessed July 26, 2014.
13. Delobel P, Sandres-Saune K, Cazabat M, et al. Persistence of distinct HIV-1 populations in blood monocytes and naive and memory CD4 T cells during prolonged suppressive HAART. *Aids.* 2005;19(16):1739–1750.
14. Levy JA. Not an HIV cure, but encouraging new directions. *N Engl J Med.* 2009;360(7):724–725.
15. Tebas P, Stein D, Tang WW, et al. Gene editing of CCR5 in autologous CD4 T cells of persons infected with HIV. *N Engl J Med.* 2014;370(10):901–910.
16. CDC. Pneumocystis pneumonia—Los Angeles. *MMWR.* 1981. http://www.cdc.gov/mmwr/preview/mmwrhtml/june_5.htm. Accessed August 1, 2014.
17. CDC. First report of AIDS *MMWR.* 2001. http://www.cdc.gov/mmwr/preview/mmwrhtml/mm5021a1.htm. Accessed August 1, 2014.

18. Piot P, Quinn TC. Response to the AIDS pandemic–a global health model. *N Engl J Med.* 2013;368(23):2210–2218.
19. Wilson J. Timeline: AIDS moments to remember. *CNN Health.* 2013. http://www.cnn.com/2013/03/04/health/timeline-hiv-aids-moments/. Accessed August 1, 2014.
20. AVERT. Averting HIV and AIDS: History of HIV and AIDS in the US. 2014. http://www.avert.org/history-hiv-aids-us.htm. Accessed August 1, 2014.
21. Volberding PA, Deeks SG. Antiretroviral therapy and management of HIV infection. *Lancet.* 2010;376(9734):49–62.
22. CDC. What CDC is saying about surveillance. 2013. http://www.cdc.gov/hiv/statistics/surveillance/index.html. Accessed July 26, 2014.
23. CDC. New HIV infections in the United States. *CDC Fact Sheet.* 2012. http://www.cdc.gov/nchhstp/newsroom/docs/2012/hiv-infections-2007-2010.pdf. Accessed July 26, 2014.
24. CDC. HIV in the United States: At a glance. 2013. http://www.cdc.gov/hiv/statistics/basics/ataglance.html. Accessed July 26, 2014.
25. CDC. HIV testing and risk behaviors among gay, bisexual, and other men who have sex with men—United States. *MMWR.* 2013. http://www.cdc.gov/mmwr/preview/mmwrhtml/mm6247a4.htm. Accessed July 26, 2014.
26. McNeil DG, Jr. Rise in unprotected sex by gay men spurs H.I.V. fears. *The New York Times.* 2013. http://www.nytimes.com/2013/11/28/health/unprotected-sex-among-gay-men-on-the-rise-health-officials-say.html. Accessed July 26, 2014.
27. CDC. HIV among women. *CDC Fact Sheet.* 2014. http://www.cdc.gov/hiv/pdf/risk_women.pdf. Accessed July 26, 2014.
28. CDC. HIV and AIDS in the United States by geographic distribution. 2012. http://www.cdc.gov/hiv/statistics/basics/geographicdistribution.html. Accessed July 26, 2014.
29. CDC. HIV among youth in the US. *CDC Vital Signs.* 2012. http://www.cdc.gov/vitalsigns/hivamongyouth/. Accessed July 26, 2014.
30. CDC. HIV among older Americans. *CDC Fact Sheet.* 2013. http://www.cdc.gov/hiv/pdf/library_factsheet_HIV_%20AmongOlderAmericans.pdf. Accessed July 26, 2014.
31. CDC. HIV Testing in the United States. *CDC Fact Sheet.* 2014. http://www.cdc.gov/nchhstp/newsroom/docs/HIV-Testing-US-508.pdf. Accessed July 26, 2014.
32. USPSTF. Screening for HIV. 2013. http://www.uspreventiveservicestaskforce.org/uspstf/uspshivi.htm. Accessed July 26, 2014.
33. Sperling RS, Shapiro DE, Coombs RW, et al. Maternal viral load, zidovudine treatment, and the risk of transmission of human immunodeficiency virus type 1 from mother to infant. Pediatric AIDS Clinical Trials Group Protocol 076 Study Group. *N Engl J Med.* 1996;335(22):1621–1629.
34. Fauci AS, Marston HD. Ending AIDS–is an HIV vaccine necessary? *N Engl J Med.* 2014;370(6):495–498.
35. DHHS. Panel on antiretroviral guidelines for adults and adolescents. Guidelines for the use of antiretroviral agents in HIV-1-infected adults and adolescents. 2014. http://aidsinfo.nih.gov/contentfiles/lvguidelines/adultandadolescentgl.pdf. Accessed August 1, 2014.
36. CDC. Guidelines and recommendations. 2014. http://www.cdc.gov/hiv/guidelines/. Accessed August 1, 2014.
37. CDC. New hope for stopping HIV. *CDC Vital Signs.* 2011. http://www.cdc.gov/vitalsigns/hivtesting/. Accessed August 1, 2014.

38. Gunthard HF, Aberg JA, Eron JJ, et al. Antiretroviral treatment of adult HIV infection: 2014 recommendations of the International Antiviral Society-USA Panel. *JAMA.* 2014;312(4):410–425.

39. Cohen MS, Chen YQ, McCauley M, et al. Prevention of HIV-1 infection with early antiretroviral therapy. *N Engl J Med.* 2011;365(6):493–505.

40. CDC. PrEP: A New Tool for HIV prevention: *CDC Fact Sheet.* 2012. http://www.cdc.gov/hiv/pdf/prevention_PrEP_factsheet.pdf. Accessed July 26, 2014.

41. CDC. Pre-exposure prophylaxix (PrEP) for HIV prevention. *CDC Fact Sheet.* 2014. http://www.cdc.gov/hiv/pdf/PrEP_fact_sheet_final.pdf. Accessed August 1, 2014.

42. Tuller D. A resisted pill to prevent H.I.V. *The New York Times.* 2013. http://www.nytimes.com/2013/12/31/health/a-resisted-pill-to-prevent-hiv.html?src=recg&_r=0. Accessed July 26, 2014.

43. Crary D. Truvada, HIV prevention drug, divides gay community. *Huffington Post.* 2014. http://www.huffingtonpost.com/2014/04/07/truvada-gay-men-hiv_n_5102515.html. Accessed July 26, 2014.

44. AIDS 2014: 20th International AIDS Conference; Melbourne, Australia: Stepping up the pace. 2014. http://www.aids2014.org/. Accessed July 26, 2014.

45. Marrazzo JM, del Rio C, Holtgrave DR, et al. HIV prevention in clinical care settings: 2014 recommendations of the International Antiviral Society-USA Panel. *JAMA.* 2014;312(4):390–409.

46. Mathers BM, Cooper DA. Integrating HIV prevention into practice. *JAMA.* 2014;312(4):349–350.

47. Tobian AA, Serwadda D, Quinn TC, et al. Male circumcision for the prevention of HSV-2 and HPV infections and syphilis. *N Engl J Med.* 2009;360(13):1298–1309.

48. Johnston R, Barre-Sinoussi F. Controversies in HIV cure research. *J Internat AIDS Soc.* 2012;15(1):16.

49. Henrich TJ, Hanhauser E, Marty FM, et al. Antiretroviral-free HIV-1 remission and viral rebound after allogeneic stem cell transplantation: Report of 2 cases. *Ann Intern Med.* 2014;161(5):319–327.

50. Lewin SR, Deeks SG, Barre-Sinoussi F. Towards a cure for HIV–are we making progress? *Lancet.* 2014;384(9939):209–211.

51. Lewin SR. Finding a cure for HIV: Much work to do. *Ann Intern Med.* 2014;161(5):368–369.

52. Wade N. In new way to edit DNA, hope for treating disease. *The New York Times.* 2009. http://www.nytimes.com/2009/12/29/health/research/29zinc.html?pagewanted=all. Accessed August 1, 2014.

53. Kay MA, Walker BD. Engineering cellular resistance to HIV. *N Engl J Med.* 2014;370(10):968–969.

54. Grady D. Study gives hope of altering genes to repel H.I.V. *The New York Times.* 2014. http://www.nytimes.com/2014/03/06/health/study-gives-hope-of-altering-genes-to-repel-hiv.html. Accessed August 1, 2014.

55. Padian NS, McCoy SI, Karim SS, et al. HIV prevention transformed: The new prevention research agenda. *Lancet.* 2011;378(9787):269–278.

56. Sullivan PS, Carballo-Dieguez A, Coates T, et al. Successes and challenges of HIV prevention in men who have sex with men. *Lancet.* 2012;380(9839):388–399.

57. Quinn TC, Serwadda D. The future of HIV/AIDS in Africa: A shared responsibility. *Lancet.* 2011;377(9772):1133–1134.

58. Hammer SM, Sobieszczyk ME, Janes H, et al. Efficacy trial of a DNA/rAd5 HIV-1 preventive vaccine. *N Engl J Med.* 2013;369(22):2083–2092.
59. Rerks-Ngarm S, Pitisuttithum P, Nitayaphan S, et al. Vaccination with ALVAC and AIDSVAX to prevent HIV-1 infection in Thailand. *N Engl J Med.* 2009; 361(23):2209–2220.
60. CDC. The Future of HIV prevention *CDC Fact Sheet.* 2013. http://www.cdc.gov/nchhstp/newsroom/docs/HIVFactSheets/Future-508.pdf. Accessed July 26, 2014.
61. National HIV/AIDS strategy 2010. http://aids.gov/federal-resources/national-hiv-aids-strategy/nhas-fact-sheet.pdf. Accessed August 1, 2014.
62. AIDS.gov overview. 2014. http://aids.gov/federal-resources/national-hiv-aids-strategy/overview/. Accessed August 1, 2014.
63. Fauci AS, Marston HD, Folkers GK. An HIV cure: Feasibility, discovery, and implementation. *JAMA.* 2014;312(4):335–336

CHAPTER 19

Radiation—Benefits and Risks of Medical Imaging

LEARNING OBJECTIVES

- Describe trends in population exposure to ionizing radiation from medical sources.
- Discuss contributing factors and public health impact of increased use of medical imaging in the United States.
- Identify populations at risk from increasing radiation exposure from medical sources.
- Describe the role of professional and government organizations in the development and implementation of evidence-based policies to prevent unnecessary exposure to medical sources of ionizing radiation.
- List and discuss research gaps.
- Propose evidence-based strategies that may be effective in reducing risks from medical imaging while preserving clinical benefits.

THE CONTROVERSY

In 2009, the U.S. Food and Drug Administration (FDA) investigated three hospitals in California and one in Alabama. Over 300 patients received huge radiation doses—equal to several thousand chest X-rays—from one type of computed tomography (CT) scan, called a perfusion CT.[1] In one prominent Los Angeles, CA hospital, a patient began to lose clumps of hair following a head CT scan, and it was later discovered that 206 patients received between 8 and 10 times the usual radiation dose for this type of CT scan.[2] Another patient, reported in the *NEJM,* received 100 times the usual head CT dose, and although the excessively high dose was shown on the CT scanner, it was not recognized as being too high by personnel performing the scan.[3] As of 2010, more than 378 U.S. patients had received excessive doses from CT-perfusion scans.[3]

A professor of radiology in the Institute for Healthcare Improvement "Safety First" blog told a story about a young patient who had a CT scan to help determine whether or not she had appendicitis.[4] An incidental finding from her scan, sometimes called "incidentalomas,"[5] included a lung nodule of "unknown malignant potential." The patient then had a CT scan every few months to follow the size of the nodule, despite the fact she lived in a geographic area of the United States where a common cause of lung nodules is a fungal infection called histoplasmosis.[4] CT scans, while providing detailed and quick imaging, also deliver radiation doses between 100 and 500 times higher than customary X-rays.[3] From these combined imaging studies, at a young age, the patient had accumulated a radiation exposure associated with an elevated future cancer risk of 1 in 400.[4]

While advances in medical technology, specifically imaging techniques such as CT scanning, have allowed much earlier diagnosis, there is growing concern their increased use may also contribute to future harm, especially in children.[3,6] "Radiation, like alcohol, is a double-edged sword," says one author, referring to the benefits and risks from medical imaging.[6] Others are more frank. "We Are Giving Ourselves Cancer" says the title of a *New York Times* op-ed by two medical experts in the field of cardiology and radiology.[7] As population exposures to medical radiation have increased by six times or more since the 1980s, these experts said, "We are silently irradiating ourselves to death."[7]

One commonly cited study predicts that 29,000 excess cancer diagnoses and 14,500 more deaths will occur during the lives of patients who received CT scans in 2007.[7,8] The National Cancer Institute describes the "Downside of Diagnostic Imaging" due to increasing per capita radiation exposure from medical imaging, which has doubled worldwide in recent decades.[9] Increases in radiation exposure from medical imaging are highest in the United States, and experts note that no single governmental or professional organization has authority to monitor the way scans are utilized or to report patient-exposure data.[3,9]

BACKGROUND AND SCOPE OF THE PUBLIC HEALTH AND HEALTH POLICY ISSUE

Radiation 101

Ionizing radiation (IR) is one form of radiation. IR produces ions and derives from both natural and man-made sources.[10,11] IR produces ions by breaking bonds or moving electrons in molecules or atoms, as the IR passes through tissue, air, or water.[10] Examples of IR include alpha and beta particles, gamma and X-rays, neutrons and other particles.[10] There are a variety of excellent sources of information about IR,[12–16] including RadTown USA, a virtual community on the the U.S. Environmental Protection Agency (EPA) website,[17] and the Health Physics Society's published information about doses from types of medical imaging.[18]

There are several commonly used units for radiation. The energy deposited per unit mass, or *absorbed dose*, is measured in grays (Gy).[19] The absorbed dose multiplied by a weighting factor to adjust for the biological effects of different types of radiation is used to calculate a *dose equivalent*, which is measured in Sieverts (Sv).[13,19] For medical imaging, 1 Gy is equal to 1 Sv because the weighting factor is 1.[19]

The estimated annual U.S. population exposure to radiation is about 6.2 millisieverts (mSv).[20] (Other authors, using a variety of sources, estimate this annual population exposure as 5.6 mSv.)[15] About 50% of the annual per capita radiation exposure in the United States is from natural sources, such as air (cosmic), ground (terrestrial), water, food, or building materials. The annual average per capita exposure from natural background sources is about 3.1 mSv, with about two-thirds of this attributed to radon and thoron gases, and cosmic, terrestrial, and internal sources comprising the rest.[20] The other 50% (or another 3.1 mSv annual per capita annual exposure) is from man-made sources, which includes medical, occupational, or commercial products, with nearly all of the man-made exposure coming from medical imaging.[20] CT scans contribute about 1.5 mSv each year.[20] Exposure to medical sources of IR has increased dramatically in the U.S. population since the 1980s, with radiation exposure from medical sources increasing by more than seven times as of 2006[21] (see **Figure 19–1**).

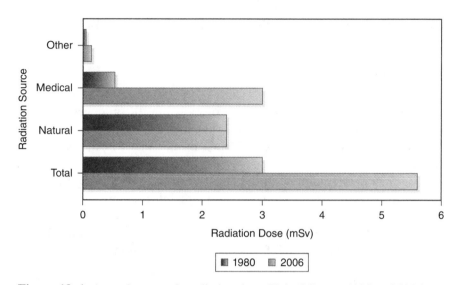

Figure 19-1 Annual per captia radiation dose, United States, 1980 and 2006.
Data from Linet MS, Slovis TL, Miller DL, et al. Cancer risks associated with external radiation from diagnostic imaging procedures. *CA: a cancer journal for clinicians.* Feb 3 2012.

What Organizations Are Involved in Radiation?

A variety of organizations are involved overseeing, regulating, or educating the public, health professionals, and policymakers about IR. The U.S. Nuclear Regulatory Commission (NRC) regulates nonmilitary industrial, medical, academic, and research use of IR in the United States.[10,11] The FDA through its Center for Devices and Radiological Health (CDRH) is responsible for enforcement of requirements for products that emit radiation as well as educating industry and consumers about radiation safety.[22] For example, the FDA provides educational materials related to X-ray imaging in children, but has specific regulatory responsibility for mammography facilities under the Mammography Quality Standards Act of 1992.[23]

The National Council on Radiation Protection and Measurements (NCRP) was chartered by the U.S. Congress in 1964. Their mission is "to support radiation protection by providing independent scientific analysis, information, and recommendations that represent the consensus of leading scientists."[12] Since 1928, another independent organization with membership from 30 countries, the International Commission on Radiological Protection (ICRP) has overseen the international system of radiological protection used for standard-setting and best practices.[24] United Nations Scientific Committee on the Effects of Atomic Radiation (UNSCEAR) was established in 1955 by the United Nations General Assembly.[13] UNSCEAR regularly issues reports about levels and health effects of IR exposure and is considered an international authority on these topics. UNSCEAR's work is used by other organizations such as the World Health Organization, United Nations, International Atomic Energy Agency, the ICRP, and others.[13]

Biological and Health Effects

Potential biological effects of IR on living cells include repair of injured cells with no damage, cell death, or incomplete or erroneous cell repair leading to cell changes.[20] Because of this, both short-term (acute) or longer-term (chronic) health risks are possible, depending on exposure dose and rate of exposure. At very high doses of exposure, *acute* radiation syndrome may occur. For example, workers during the 1986 Chernobyl nuclear power plant accident who were exposed in the range of 800 to 16,000 mSv in a short time period experienced acute radiation sickness, and more than 20% died within several months of their exposure.[20] Chronic health risks, which do not occur immediately but after a time period called the *latent* period, may include cancer, specifically leukemia, multiple myeloma, lung, breast, bladder, liver, esophagus, ovary, and stomach cancers.[20] The latent period from radiation exposure to the development of cancer may range from several years to decades.[13,19] Very young children may have higher risks from radiation exposure because they have many future years ahead in their lives, and they may be as much as four times more radiosensitive as adults.[19]

Errors in DNA repair, which cause changes in genetic material are related to later cancer development with the probability of cancer increasing with radiation dose.[19] Epidemiological evidence for radiation exposure and cancer comes predominantly from Japanese atomic bomb survivors and also from nuclear industry workers, and other environmentally and medically exposed populations.[19,25] A 2009 publication reported that the effects of the atomic bomb on leukemia deaths continues to be seen in survivors more than 50 years later.[26] A study of 400,000 nuclear industry workers in 15 countries showed a significant relationship between radiation exposure level and risk of cancer death, with increased risks of cancer from exposures between 5 and 150 mSv.[27]

Scientific evidence that supports elevated cancer risks with radiation doses higher than 100 mSv is well documented.[19] Health risks and how they are calculated are more controversial when exposures are lower (in the range of 10 to 100 mSv) and continue to be debated in exposure ranges less than 10 mSv.[19] Generally, the assumptions for these lower doses, extrapolated backwards from the evidence at the higher doses, is called a "linear no-threshold" (LNT) assumption, with cancer risks directly related to exposure at any level.[19] In recent literature, authors argue against[28] and for[29] the continued use of the LNT assumption, the most conservative and protective of public health. This issue continues to be discussed and debated in the scientific literature.[18,19,30–36]

The previous discussion, and controversy, is relevant because many medical radiological tests fall in the 10 mSv or less exposure category, and some single CT scans, depending on what part of the body is imaged, deliver doses of 10 mSv and can be higher in individuals with multiple studies.[19] Some authors argue that available data from epidemiological studies "directly suggest increased cancer risk in the 10 mSv to 100 mSv range, which is relevant to nuclear cardiac and many CT studies."[19] One commonly cited estimate, from the ICRP and NCRP, is a 5% excess risk of cancer death from a dose of 1,000 mSv.[19]

CT Scans—Benefits and Potential Risks

Many authors raise concerns about CT scans because of their increasing use and radiation exposure to patients.[3,9,14,23,27,37] According to the National Cancer Institute (NCI), CT scanning is a type of medical imaging that uses specialized X-ray equipment to create 2-D or 3-D images by taking multiple imaging "slices" of the part of the body being studied. CT scans may be used to diagnose such conditions as cancer, aneurysm, coronary artery disease, infection, or severe head injury, or to monitor the effectiveness of treatment.[14] The NCI also notes the "downside" of advances in imaging: CT scans and nuclear medicine tests expose patients to 50 to 500 times the IR dose from a routine chest X-ray.[9] And while CT scans, nuclear medicine studies, and interventional fluoroscopy studies comprise about 25% of medical imaging studies using IR, together, they contribute nearly 90% of the population exposure to IR from medical imaging[38] (see **Figure 19–2**).

As of 2007, more than 62 million CT scans are performed annually in the United States and at least 4 million are performed in children, a dramatic increase since the 1980s.[27] Fazel and colleagues studied cumulative

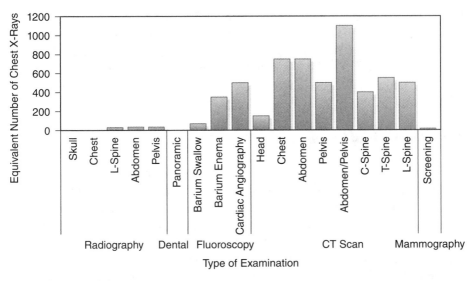

Figure 19–2 Medical imaging studies—Equivalent doses.

Data from Linet MS, Slovis TL, Miller DL, et al. Cancer risks associated with external radiation from diagnostic imaging procedures. *CA: a cancer journal for clinicians.* Feb 3 2012.

doses of radiation from medical imaging in 952,420 U.S. adults between the ages of 18 and 64, over a 3-year period.[39] They found nearly 70% of adults had at least one medical imaging procedure during the time of their study.[39] Moderate radiation doses (>3 to 20 mSv) were found in 193.8 individuals per 1,000 per year, and high (>20 to 50 mSv) or very high (>50 mSv) doses were noted in 18.6% or 1.9 individuals per 1,000 per year. Three-quarters of total radiation exposures were from CT and nuclear medical imaging, and the authors concluded that imaging tests were a substantial source of population radiation exposure.[39] Other authors concur, citing the growing use of CT scans and resultant population exposures (in ranges epidemiologically linked to cancer risk) as a potential public health issue.[27]

Miglioretti and colleagues studied CT use in children in seven health systems in the United States and estimated future cancer risks from radiation exposure.[40] Using cancer dose and risk models from the *Biological Effects of Ionizing Radiation* (BEIR) VII report,[41] they calculated lifetime attributable cancer risks. Overall, the authors predicted that nearly 5,000 additional cases of cancer would result from the 4 million CT cans of the head, abdomen/pelvis, chest, or spine done on an annual basis in the United States.[40] Berrington de Gonzalez and colleagues,[8] using the BEIR VII report,[41] estimated that about 2% of all cancers diagnosed in the United States (about 29,000 cancers) may be related to CT scans in the United States in 2007, an estimate similar to the 1.5–2% projected by Brenner and Hall.[27] The largest radiation doses were from CT scans of the abdomen and pelvis, chest, and head.[8]

Trends in Medical Imaging

According to the NCRP, increased radiation exposure from CT scanning, nuclear medicine tests, and fluoroscopy are major contributors to the near doubling of the U.S. population's exposure to IR over the past 20 years.[21,38] Using data from the National Hospital Ambulatory Medical Care Survey, Larson and colleagues found that emergency department (ED) visits in the United States that included a CT scan increased from 2.7 million to 16.2 million from 1995 to 2007.[42] This was accompanied by an increase from 2.8% to nearly 14% in the percentage of ED visits where patients received a CT scan.[42] CT use was higher in older patients, in urban settings, and most commonly prescribed for abdominal pain, chest pain, and headache.[42] In children, CT scan use increased from 0.33 to 1.65 million, from 1995 to 2008, most commonly for head injury, headache, and abdominal pain.[43] CT scans and nuclear medicine tests alone contribute to three-quarters of medical exposure to IR in the United States.[21]

These concerns are not limited to the United States. Researchers in Italy studied radiation exposure in 16,431 patients hospitalized for heart disease in a single hospital, during the time period 1970–2009.[44] The authors noted increasing radiation exposure over time in patients with heart disease, and exposures in patient with heart disease (37 mSv) were significantly higher than in patient without heart disease (13 mSv) when studied over the 5 most recent years.[44]

Using data from the NCRP and UNSCEAR, Mettler and colleagues reported on nuclear medicine use and other medical imaging studies in the United States and worldwide.[45] The United States performs a large number of medical imaging tests using IR, an estimated 377 million medical imaging tests and 18 million nuclear medicine tests in 2006. In addition, annual per capita radiation exposure from these tests has increased 600% in the United States since 1980 (from 0.5 mSv in 1980 to 3.0 mSv in 2006), whereas globally, medically related radiation exposure has doubled since about the mid-1990s, estimated at 0.6 mSV annually, slightly higher than the average U.S. exposure in 1980.[45]

Variation in Medical Imaging and Radiation Exposure

Variation in use of medical imaging and radiation exposure within the same medical imaging test, in different healthcare settings and in different geographic regions, has been reported. Smith-Bindman and colleagues estimated radiation doses from CT scans on 1,119 patients at four California hospitals.[46] They found that different types of CT studies resulted in very different radiation exposures for patients, with much higher doses seen in CT scans of the abdomen and pelvis than the head.[46] In addition, they found that radiation doses varied for each type of CT study, and doses also varied depending on which location the scan was performed. For each type of CT study, there was an average variation of thirteen times between the lowest and highest doses.[46]

In 2013, the first Dartmouth Atlas children's health report was released by the Dartmouth Institute, showing differences in rates of medical imaging in northern New England, depending on where children lived.[47] CT scans of the chest or abdomen (delivering the same radiation dose as about 200 chest X-rays) were performed much more often in children living in Bennington, VT (15.4 scans per 1,000 children) than in Brattleboro, VT (5.1 scans per 1,000 children).[47] Children living in Lewiston, ME and Manchester, NH had CT scans of the head 50% more frequently than children living near major academic medical centers in Vermont, Maine, and New Hampshire.[47] These findings raised questions about the variation in use of medical imaging, and related differences in radiation exposure, that may reflect geographic differences in medical practice rather than differences in rates of certain diseases.[47]

What Factors Contribute to Rising CT Use?

Hillman and Goldsmith write, "There is broad agreement that an unknown but substantial fraction of imaging examinations are unnecessary and do not positively contribute to patient care."[48] One study, using evidence-based criteria, reported that 26% of 286 outpatient CT scans ordered at one academic center by primary care physicians were not appropriate.[49] A variety of factors may contribute to increased use. Research assessing the impact of use of new imaging technologies on patient outcomes is lacking.[48] Fear of potential malpractice lawsuits is a contributor.[50] These lawsuits are more likely when a medical condition is not diagnosed, rather than from over use of medical imaging, creating a situation where fear of liability may influence imaging decisions.[48] One Massachusetts study reported that 28% of diagnostic imaging tests ordered were for this reason.[48] Subjective factors, such as the current culture of technology-intensive medical practice and its influence on clinical education of health professionals may also play a role. The Association of American Medical Colleges (2009) data shows that more than 80% of medical schools do not require radiology clerkships.[48]

Some authors contend that physician ownership in imaging facilities and "self-referral" contributes to increasing numbers of CT scans performed each year, as well as increasing health care costs.[48,50–54] Kilani and colleagues noted a 2.5-fold increase in imaging for healthcare providers who were "self-referrers" compared to those who were not, in a 2011 meta-analysis of nearly 77 million healthcare visits.[55] As of 2012, there are 235 physician-owned specialty hospitals, up from 50 a decade prior.[51] Numbers of independent diagnostic testing facilities (IDTFs) doubled in the period from 1996 to 2006, with 5,800 such facilities reported in 2006.[51] One study of magnetic resonance imaging (MRI) scans (a type of medical imaging test which is *not* a sources of IR exposure) found that more MRI scans were ordered (a 38% increase) when physicians were able to bill for these services.[56]

Many authors believe such arrangements create potential conflicts of interest for healthcare providers, and beginning in 1989, laws such as the "Stark Law," were passed to oversee this practice.[51] Subsequently, further growth of physician-owned facilities was prohibited by the Patient Protection and Affordable Care Act (ACA) in 2010.[51]

EVIDENCE BASE FOR PREVENTION AND PRACTICE

In 1986, Evans and McNeil reported that 1% of all cases of leukemia and less than 1% of all breast cancer cases could be attributed to diagnostic X-rays in a Maine population.[57] An accompanying editorial entitled "The Danger of X-Rays—Real or Apparent?" by John Boice wrote "Despite the uncertainties involved in estimating the effects of low-level radiation, most experts agree that even small amounts of radiation cannot be assumed to be entirely free of adverse consequences."[58] Both papers suggested then that avoiding unneeded tests, substituting tests that don't use IR when possible, training in radiology in medical schools, and lowering doses per exam by improving equipment, might all continue to ensure that the benefits of medical imaging outweigh potential risks.[57,58]

Decades later, population radiation exposures are increasing from medical sources, and controversy continues about assumptions made in determining cancer risks and the best ways to reduce them, while preserving the benefits of advances in medical technology. One author, writing about radiation exposure in children from CT scans, said "The simple answer is . . . it's complicated."[59]

Strategies to Reduce Patient Exposure to IR

One basic principle in reducing radiation exposure is that any exposure should be as low as reasonably achievable (ALARA).[15,36] There is also a call to reduce the number of CT scans by some experts,[9,27] suggesting that in about one-third of all CT scans, another test (not using IR) could be substituted or that the scan is not necessary. This translates to as many as 20 million adults and 1 million children receiving CT scans that are not medically needed.[27]

A variety of strategies are proposed, such as reducing doses to individual patients through machine settings and making sure that the dose to achieve a high-quality image is adjusted for patient size.[9,27] The NCI has a list of possible approaches to help reduce radiation exposure from medical imaging without compromising healthcare quality.[9] Another commonly discussed recommendation is to replace CT or other medical imaging techniques that use IR with other tests such as ultrasound or MRI whenever possible.[9,27]

In 2014, AuntMinnie.com, an Internet site for radiologists and other health professionals, reported on the dramatic reduction in CT-related radiation exposure at Ohio State University after they implemented scanning protocols.[60] The study, published in the *Journal of the American College of Radiology*, evaluated changes in radiation exposure from CT scans of the abdomen, head, sinus, and lumbar spine from 2008–2012 following the implementation of new protocols and technology improvements to reduce radiation doses to individual patients.[60,61]

Rayo and colleagues, in the Ohio State study, found a 37% decrease in the number of abdominal CT scans performed during the study period. In addition, they noted that the approaches adopted in their institution reduced radiation exposure by 30–52%, with an estimated reduction in radiation-related cancers of 63%.[61] Over the time period of the study, the percentage of patients receiving higher doses (a dose of 50 mSv or more each year) was reduced from 10% to 0.2%.[61] Generally, they found that the approaches they used to reduce individual patient doses—using protocols and improvements in technology (that are easily adoptable in other locations)—were associated with the greatest dose reductions.[61]

Strategies recently employed in healthcare settings to reduce radiation doses include computer programs to reduce inappropriate CT prescribing by health professionals and technology improvements during and after the scans themselves, to reduce patient doses without compromising image quality.[61,62] A primer on the technical aspects of CT scanning describes what information is needed for health professionals to help reduce patient doses during CT scanning.[63] New software developed by equipment manufacturers can help reduce doses while preserving image quality.[64] A systemic review of a technique called adaptive statistical iterative reduction (ASIR), a method used to improve image quality, reported dose reduction of 23–76%,[65] and one Massachusetts study demonstrated dose reductions of 24% in head CT scans in children.[66]

Reports from as early as 2009 have demonstrated population radiation dose reductions from systematically using currently available techniques.[67] A prospective, controlled (but not randomized) study in 15 Michigan hospitals in their Advanced Cardiovascular Imaging Consortium evaluated the experience of nearly 5,000 patients who underwent cardiac computed tomography angiography (CCTA) after "best-practices" were used to reduce doses to individual patients. The study authors found an average dose reduction of 53.3% after the intervention, without compromising quality of the images produced.[67]

Educating Health Professionals and Patients

Other suggested strategies include educating both patients and physicians about radiation doses, risks, and benefits of CT imaging.[9] A small study in one academic medical center evaluated adult patients in an ED who received a CT scan, asking how often patients received information about benefits and risks and physician knowledge.[68] Only 7% of patients said they were informed about risks and benefits of the CT scan. Only 9% of ED physicians believed CT scans resulted in increased cancer risks and neither patients nor physicians were able to compare radiation doses of chest X-rays and CT scans.[68]

A systematic review of physician knowledge about radiation doses and risks from CT scanning included 14 studies from six countries, including Turkey, England, Germany, Israel, Canada, and the U.S.[69] Despite the different designs and quality of the studies, the review found low to moderate physician knowledge.[69] Another study of patient involvement in decisions about CT scans found that 83% of the patients (246 of 296 participants) had a discussion with their physician. In addition, the decision to have a CT scan was a shared decision in 44% of cases, highlighting the important role of physician and patient conversations.[70]

The Alliance for Radiation Safety in Pediatric Imaging promotes the Image Gently campaign to educate health professionals and parents about ways to protect children from unnecessary radiation exposure.[71] The Image Wisely campaign promotes radiation safety for adults who undergo medical imaging.[72]

Tracking Patient Exposure to Medical Radiation

The NCI recommends individual patient radiation exposure be recorded and tracked, using such systems as the IAEA's proposed "Smart Card."[9] This approach, if used in electronic medical records, could allow medical imaging tests and related exposures to be available to patients and their healthcare providers, potentially avoiding repeating some imaging tests.[73] Such a practical approach was implemented in 2013, when a group of 22 hospitals and 185 clinics in Salt Lake City began using a system to measure and record patient cumulative radiation exposures from medical imaging tests.[74] This approach is also recommended by the FDA, which promotes maintaining medical imaging information in patients' records, as well as developing ways to help patients track their own medical imaging.[38] The National Institutes of Health (NIH) Clinical Center requires that radiation doses from medical imaging be recorded in patient electronic medical records.[14]

Federal Policy Initiatives

In 2010, the FDA began the Initiative to Reduce Unnecessary Radiation Exposure from Medical Imaging.[14,38] The FDA cited two overarching principles for radiation protection: *justification* for performing each test and *optimization* of the doses used.[38] Goals for use of medical imaging included safe use, increased patient awareness, and informed clinical decision making.[38] The FDA calls for manufacturers of medical imaging equipment to add additional safety features, such as design improvements and better training for individuals using the equipment. They recommend that the Centers for Medicare and Medicaid Services (CMS) include quality assurance practices into accreditation criteria for healthcare facilities.[38] In addition, the FDA endorses the development and use of diagnostic benchmarks (called "reference levels") through a national radiation dose registry. This approach could be used to monitor exposure trends over time and allow local comparisons to national levels.[38] The FDA also recommends that healthcare professionals continue to develop and disseminate criteria for appropriate use of CT, nuclear medicine tests, and fluoroscopy.[38]

The Joint Commission, an independent nonprofit organization that accredits and certifies more than 20,500 U.S. healthcare organizations and programs, announced changes in quality and safety standards for diagnostic medical imaging, effective July 1, 2014, with some requirements effective in 2015.[75] The requirements include minimum competency requirements for radiology technologists, annual checks of medical imaging equipment by a radiation physicist, imaging protocols for pediatric patients, data collection whenever radiation limits are exceeded, and documenting CT radiation doses in patient medical records.[75]

Health Professional Guidelines

The American College of Radiology (ACR) has developed evidence-based "appropriateness criteria" for healthcare providers.[76] These criteria are, in some healthcare institutions, increasingly integrated into computerized decision-support tools and then connected to the ordering of medical imaging tests.[50] The ACR has also developed the "Dose Index Registry" that allows healthcare facilities to compare their aggregated and anonymous CT doses to regional and national levels.[77] The American College of Cardiology (ACC) and the Royal College of Radiologists in the United Kingdom have also developed guidelines for health professionals.[15]

Choosing Wisely—Promoting Better Patient and Physician Decision Making

To promote better patient and physician conversations and reduce unnecessary healthcare spending, nine medical specialty societies joined the American Board of Internal Medicine (ABIM) Foundation and Consumer Reports to initiate the Choosing Wisely campaign in 2012.[78] In this initiative, each participating specialty society picked five tests or treatments they suspected were used too frequently.[50,78] The concept of Choosing Wisely is to support patient care that is evidence-based, does not repeat other tests or care, does not cause harm to patients, and is really needed.[79] Twenty-four of the 45 items on the initial list were related to diagnostic radiology and a final list included 18 medical imaging tests, highlighting consensus among physician specialty groups that some medical imaging tests are used too often.[50] At the same time the campaign was announced, a *New York Times* editorial asked "Do You Need That Test?" and called for more patient responsibility. The editors called the Consumer Reports and ABIM Choosing Wisely strategy "sound medicine and economics."[80]

How well are these strategies working? Although still early, some recent evidence supports an optimistic view. Between 2000 and 2007, of all physician services for Medicare patients, medical imaging studies grew the fastest.[50] The U.S. Government Accounting Office (GAO) reported to Congress in 2008 that physician spending for medical imaging services increased to $14 billion.[81] Healthcare spending for CT scans, MRIs, and nuclear medicine tests rose 17% each year from 2000 through 2006, and healthcare spending on medical imaging per Medicare patient varied geographically, from $62 in Vermont to $472 in Florida, in 2006.[81] However more recently, a 1.7% decrease in CT scans from 2009 to 2010 was observed in the Medicare population.[61] Longer follow-up, in this population and others, will determine if these approaches are working.

DISCUSSION QUESTIONS: TEMPLATE FOR DISCUSSION

1. Significance of this public health issue:
   a. Why is this health issue important?
   b. How many people does it impact?
   c. How serious is it?
   d. Is it preventable?
2. What is the evidence base for prevention?
3. What specific strategies should be used to achieve progress on this health issue?
   a. What evidence-based approach would you use?
   b. Where would you start if you are an individual citizen; public health professional; healthcare professional; or community, state, or federal policymaker?
4. Specific questions for this topic:
   a. Why is IR exposure from medical sources increasing?
   b. What are barriers to reducing potential risks while preserving medical benefits?

5. What is the controversy?
   a. Define the controversy.
   b. Is controversy a good or bad thing? (Does it help or hinder progress?)
6. *Why* is this health issue controversial?
   a. What specific factors are involved?
   b. Do economics, government, scientific uncertainty, or politics play a role?
   c. What is the role of the media?
7. How would you respond to the controversy?

PERSPECTIVES TO CONSIDER

Controversy over health risks at low levels of IR is ongoing and will likely continue in the near future.[19,27–29] In the meantime it makes sense, based on what is already known about exposure to IR at higher doses and observed trends in medical imaging, to take appropriate steps to reduce unnecessary risk to the public, a strategy endorsed by many experts, and professional and government organizations.[9,15,27,38] A variety of organizations are advocating for common-sense and practical ways to reduce radiation exposure in clinical medicine.[9] Notably, the Image Gently[71] effort and the Choosing Wisely[50] initiatives have growing support from professional societies. It seems clear that public and professional education are both needed to ensure high-quality, appropriate health care, while reducing risks to the health of individual patients and the public.

FOR ADDITIONAL STUDY

Linet MS, Slovis TL, Miller DL, et al. Cancer risks associated with external radiation from diagnostic imaging procedures. *CA: A cancer journal for clinicians.* Feb 3 2012.

REFERENCES

1. Neighmond P. FDA investigates radiation overdose at hospitals. *NPR.* 2009. http://www.npr.org/templates/story/story.php?storyId=121477802. Accessed August 5, 2014.
2. Chitale R. Doctors 'shocked' by radiation overexposure at Cedars-Sinai. *ABC News.* 2009. http://abcnews.go.com/Health/CancerPreventionAndTreatment/doctors-shocked-radiation-exposure/story?id=8818377. Accessed August 5, 2014.
3. Smith-Bindman R. Is computed tomography safe? *N Engl J Med.* 2010;363(1):1–4.

4. Federico F. Benefits of eliminating overuse in medical imaging *Institute for Healthcare Improvement Safety First Blog.* 2014. http://www.ihi.org/communities/blogs/_layouts/ihi/community/blog/itemview.aspx?List=0f316db6-7f8a-430f-a63a-ed7602d1366a&ID=23. Accessed August 5, 2014.

5. Butterfield S. How many are too many for CT scans? *ACP Internist.* 2011. http://www.acpinternist.org/archives/2011/02/CT.htm. Accessed August 5, 2014.

6. Brody JE. Medical radiation soars, with risks often overlooked. *The New York Times.* 2012. http://well.blogs.nytimes.com/2012/08/20/medical-radiation-soars-with-risks-often-overlooked/. Accessed August 5, 2014.

7. Redberg RF, Smith-Bindman R. We are giving ourselves cancer. *The New York Times.* 2014. http://www.nytimes.com/2014/01/31/opinion/we-are-giving-ourselves-cancer.html. Accessed August 5, 2014.

8. Berrington de Gonzalez A, Mahesh M, Kim KP, et al. Projected cancer risks from computed tomographic scans performed in the United States in 2007. *Arch Intern Med.* 2009;169(22):2071–2077.

9. NCI. The downside of diagnostic imaging. 2010. http://www.cancer.gov/cancertopics/research/downside-of-diagnostic-imaging/print. Accessed November 4, 2014.

10. US NRC. Ionizing radiation. 2014. http://www.nrc.gov/reading-rm/basic-ref/glossary/ionizing-radiation.html. Accessed August 5, 2014.

11. US NRC. Frequently asked questions (FAQ) about radiation protection. 2014. http://www.nrc.gov/about-nrc/radiation/related-info/faq.html. Accessed August 5, 2014.

12. NCRP. National Council on Radiation Protection and Measurements. 2014. http://www.ncrponline.org/Index.html. Accessed August 5, 2014.

13. UNSCEAR. United Nations Scientific Committee on the Effects of Atomic Radiation. 2014. http://www.unscear.org/. Accessed August 5, 2014.

14. NCI. Computed tomography (CT) scans and cancer. 2014. http://www.cancer.gov/cancertopics/factsheet/detection/CT. Accessed August 5, 2014.

15. Linet MS, Slovis TL, Miller DL, et al. Cancer risks associated with external radiation from diagnostic imaging procedures. *CA.* February 3, 2012. http://www.ncbi.nlm.nih.gov/pmc/articles/PMC3548988/. Accessed August 5, 2014.

16. US EPA. Sources of radiation exposure. 2013. http://www.epa.gov/radiation/sources/index.html. Accessed August 5, 2014.

17. US EPA. RadTown USA: Basic tnformation. 2012. http://www.epa.gov/radtown/basic.html. Accessed August 5, 2014.

18. Stabin MG. Doses from medical radiation sources. 2014. http://hps.org/hpspublications/articles/dosesfrommedicalradiation.html. Accessed November 4, 2014.

19. Lin EC. Radiation risk from medical imaging. *Mayo Clinic Proc.* 2010;85(12):1142–1146; quiz 1146.

20. US NRC. Fact sheet on biological effects of radiation. 2011. http://www.nrc.gov/reading-rm/doc-collections/fact-sheets/bio-effects-radiation.html. Accessed August 5, 2014.

21. NCRP. NCRP Report No. 160, Ionizing radiation exposure of the population of the United States. 2006. http://www.ncrponline.org/Publications/Press_Releases/160press.html. Accessed August 5, 2014.

22. FDA. Radiation safety. 2014. http://www.fda.gov/Radiation-EmittingProducts/RadiationSafety/default.htm. Accessed August 5, 2014.

23. FDA. Radiation-emitting products. 2014. http://www.fda.gov/Radiation-EmittingProducts/default.htm. Accessed August 5, 2014.
24. ICRP. International commission on radiological protection. 2014. http://www.icrp.org/index.asp. Accessed August 5, 2014.
25. Little MP. Cancer and non-cancer effects in Japanese atomic bomb survivors. *J Radiol Protect.* 2009;29(2A):A43–59.
26. Richardson D, Sugiyama H, Nishi N, et al. Ionizing radiation and leukemia mortality among Japanese atomic bomb survivors, 1950–2000. *Rad Res.* 2009;172(3):368–382.
27. Brenner DJ, Hall EJ. Computed tomography—an increasing source of radiation exposure. *N Engl J Med.* 2007;357(22):2277–2284.
28. Tubiana M, Feinendegen LE, Yang C, Kaminski JM. The linear no-threshold relationship is inconsistent with radiation biologic and experimental data. *Radiology.* 2009;251(1):13–22.
29. Little MP, Wakeford R, Tawn EJ, Bouffler SD, Berrington de Gonzalez A. Risks associated with low doses and low dose rates of ionizing radiation: Why linearity may be (almost) the best we can do. *Radiology.* 2009;251(1):6–12.
30. Mothersill C, Seymour C. Implications for human and environmental health of low doses of ionising radiation. *J Environ Rad.* 2014;133:5–9.
31. Strzelczyk JJ, Damilakis J, Marx MV, Macura KJ. Facts and controversies about radiation exposure, part 1: Controlling unnecessary radiation exposures. *J Am Col Radiol.* 2006;3(12):924–931.
32. Strzelczyk JJ, Damilakis J, Marx MV, Macura KJ. Facts and controversies about radiation exposure, part 2: Low-level exposures and cancer risk. *J Am Col Radiol.* 2007;4(1):32–39.
33. Morgan WF, Bair WJ. Issues in low dose radiation biology: The controversy continues. A perspective. *Rad Resh.* 2013;179(5):501–510.
34. Storrs C. How much do CT scans increase the risk of cancer? *Scientific American.* 2013. http://www.scientificamerican.com/article/how-much-ct-scans-increase-risk-cancer/. Accessed August 5, 2014.
35. Kendall GM, Little MP, Wakeford R, et al. A record-based case-control study of natural background radiation and the incidence of childhood leukaemia and other cancers in Great Britain during 1980–2006. *Leukemia.* 2013;27(1):3–9.
36. Costello JE, Cecava ND, Tucker JE, Bau JL. CT radiation dose: Current controversies and dose reduction strategies. *Am J Roentgenol.* 2013;201(6):1283-1290.
37. Redberg RF. Cancer risks and radiation exposure from computed tomographic scans: How can we be sure that the benefits outweigh the risks? *Arch Intern Med.* 2009;169(22):2049–2050.
38. FDA. White Paper: Initiative to reduce unnecessary radiation exposure from medical imaging. 2010. http://www.fda.gov/Radiation-emittingProducts/RadiationSafety/RadiationDoseReduction/default.htm. Accessed August 5, 2014.
39. Fazel R, Krumholz HM, Wang Y, et al. Exposure to low-dose ionizing radiation from medical imaging procedures. *N Engl J Med.* 2009;361(9):849–857.
40. Miglioretti DL, Johnson E, Williams A, et al. The use of computed tomography in pediatrics and the associated radiation exposure and estimated cancer risk. *JAMA Pediatrics.* 2013;167(8):700–707.
41. *Health Risks from Exposure to Low Levels of Ionizing Radiation: BEIR VII Phase 2.* Washington, DC: The National Academies Press; 2006.

42. Larson DB, Johnson LW, Schnell BM, Salisbury SR, Forman HP. National trends in CT use in the emergency department: 1995–2007. *Radiology*. 2011;258(1):164–173.

43. Larson DB, Johnson LW, Schnell BM, Goske MJ, Salisbury SR, Forman HP. Rising use of CT in child visits to the emergency department in the United States, 1995–2008. *Radiology*. 2011;259(3):793–801.

44. Carpeggiani C, Landi P, Michelassi C, Marraccini P, Picano E. Trends of increasing medical radiation exposure in a population hospitalized for cardiovascular disease (1970–2009). *PLoS One*. 2012;7(11):e50168.

45. Mettler FA, Jr., Bhargavan M, Faulkner K, et al. Radiologic and nuclear medicine studies in the United States and worldwide: frequency, radiation dose, and comparison with other radiation sources: 1950–2007. *Radiology*. 2009;253(2):520–531.

46. Smith-Bindman R, Lipson J, Marcus R, et al. Radiation dose associated with common computed tomography examinations and the associated lifetime attributable risk of cancer. *Arch Intern Med*. 2009;169(22):2078–2086.

47. Where children live affects care, exposing some to unnecessary treatment, imaging and medication. [press release]. 2013. http://tdi.dartmouth.edu/press/press-releases/where-children-live-affects-their-health-care-exposing-some-to-unnecessary-. Accessed August 5, 2014.

48. Hillman BJ, Goldsmith JC. The uncritical use of high-tech medical imaging. *N Engl J Med*. 2010;363(1):4–6.

49. Lehnert BE, Bree RL. Analysis of appropriateness of outpatient CT and MRI referred from primary care clinics at an academic medical center: How critical is the need for improved decision support? *J Am Col Radiol*. 2010;7(3):192–197.

50. Rao VM, Levin DC. The overuse of diagnostic imaging and the Choosing Wisely initiative. *Ann Intern Med*. 2012;157(8):574–576.

51. Center for Healthcare Research and Transformation (CHRT). Physician ownership in hospitals and outpatient facilities: CHRT Policy Paper 2013. http://www.chrt.org/public-policy/policy-papers/physician-ownership-in-hospitals-and-outpatient-facilities/. Accessed August 5, 2014.

52. Casalino LP, et al. Physician self-referral and physician-owned specialty facilities 2008. http://www.rwjf.org/content/dam/farm/reports/issue_briefs/2008/rwjf28861/subassets/rwjf28861_1. Accessed August 5, 2014.

53. Hillman BJ, Goldsmith J. Imaging: The self-referral boom and the ongoing search for effective policies to contain it. *Health Aff (Millwood)*. 2010;29(12):2231–2236.

54. Pear R. Doctors who profit from radiation prescribe it more often, study finds. *The New York Times*. 2013. http://www.nytimes.com/2013/08/19/us/doctors-who-profit-from-radiation-prescribe-it-more-often-study-finds.html?_r=0. Accessed August 5, 2014.

55. Kilani RK, Paxton BE, Stinnett SS, Barnhart HX, Bindal V, Lungren MP. Self-referral in medical imaging: A meta-analysis of the literature. *J Am Col Radiol*. 2011;8(7):469–476.

56. Baker LC. Acquisition of MRI equipment by doctors drives up imaging use and spending. *Health Aff (Millwood)*. 2010;29(12):2252–2259.

57. Evans JS, Wennberg JE, McNeil BJ. The influence of diagnostic radiography on the incidence of breast cancer and leukemia. *N Engl J Med*. 1986;315(13):810–815.

58. Boice JD. The danger of X-rays —real or apparent? *N Engl J Med*. 1986;315(13):828–830.

59. Frush DP. Radiation, CT, and children: The simple answer is ... it's complicated. *Radiology*. 2009;252(1):4–6.

60. Casey B. Ohio hospital slashes CT radiation dose—and cancer risk. *AuntMinnie. com.* 2014. http://www.auntminnie.com/index.aspx?sec=ser&sub=def&pag=dis&Ite mID=107954. Accessed August 5, 2014.

61. Rayo MF, Patterson ES, Liston BW, White S, Kowalczyk N. Determining the rate of change in exposure to ionizing radiation from CT scans: A database analysis from one hospital. *J Am Col Radiol.* 2014;11(7):703–708.

62. Wang SS. Dialing back on radiation in CT scans to lower risk. *The Wall Street Journal Online.* 2012. http://online.wsj.com/news/articles/SB1000142405270230341040457 7468950681647544. Accessed August 5, 2014.

63. Maldjian PD, Goldman AR. Reducing radiation dose in body CT: A primer on dose metrics and key CT technical parameters. *Am J Roentgenol.* 2013;200(4): 741–747.

64. Linebaugh K. New efforts look to cut radiation from CT scans. *The Wall Street Journal Online.* 2013. http://online.wsj.com/news/articles/SB100014241278873246624045783 32592947022334. Accessed August 5, 2014.

65. Willemink MJ, Leiner T, de Jong PA, et al. Iterative reconstruction techniques for computed tomography part 2: Initial results in dose reduction and image quality. *Eur J Radiol.* 2013;23(6):1632–1642.

66. Iterative reconstruction techniques reduce pediatric head CT dose. *Diagn Imaging.* 2014. http://www.diagnosticimaging.com/pediatric-imaging/iterative-reconstruction-techniques-reduce-pediatric-head-ct-dose. Accessed August 5, 2014.

67. Raff GL, Chinnaiyan KM, Share DA, et al. Radiation dose from cardiac computed tomography before and after implementation of radiation dose-reduction techniques. *JAMA.* 2009;301(22):2340–2348.

68. Lee CI, Haims AH, Monico EP, Brink JA, Forman HP. Diagnostic CT scans: Assessment of patient, physician, and radiologist awareness of radiation dose and possible risks. *Radiology.* 2004;231(2):393–398.

69. Krille L, Hammer GP, Merzenich H, Zeeb H. Systematic review on physician's knowledge about radiation doses and radiation risks of computed tomography. *Eur J Radiol.* 2010;76(1):36–41.

70. Caoili EM, Cohan RH, Ellis JH, Dillman J, Schipper MJ, Francis IR. Medical decision making regarding computed tomographic radiation dose and associated risk: The patient's perspective. *Arch Intern Med.* 2009;169(11):1069–1071.

71. Image Gently: The Alliance for Radiation Safety in Pediatric Imaging. 2014. http://www.imagegently.org/Home.aspx. Accessed August 5, 2014.

72. Image Wisely: Radiation safety in adult medical imaging. 2014. http://www.imagewisely.org/. Accessed August 5, 2014.

73. IAEA.org. IAEA calls for enhanced radiation protection of patients. 2014. http://www.iaea.org/newscenter/pressreleases/iaea-calls-enhanced-radiation-protection-patients. Accessed August 5, 2014.

74. Landro L. New tracking of a patient's radiation exposure. *The Wall Street Journal Online.* 2012. http://online.wsj.com/news/articles/SB100014241278873247670045784 8849413973896412. Accessed August 5, 2014.

75. The Joint Commission. Accreditation and certfication: New and revised diagnostic imaging standards effective July 1, 2014. 2014. http://www.jointcommission.org/issues/article.aspx?Article=3gWOB9f%2BbQs0mm5VSuT6O9ehvaSIz%2FLl7aMI8E2NJIU%3D. Accessed August 5, 2014.

76. ACR. American College of Radiology (ACR) appropriateness criteria. 2014. http://www.acr.org/Quality-Safety/Appropriateness-Criteria. Accessed August 8, 2014.
77. ACR. Dose index registry. 2014. http://www.acr.org/Quality-Safety/National-Radiology-Data-Registry/Dose-Index-Registry. Accessed August 5, 2014.
78. Cassel CK, Guest JA. Choosing wisely: Helping physicians and patients make smart decisions about their care. *JAMA*. 2012;307(17):1801–1802.
79. Choosing Wisely: An initiative of the ABIM foundation. 2014. http://www.choosingwisely.org/about-us/. Accessed June 4, 2014.
80. Editorial. Do you need that test? *The New York Times*. 2012. http://www.nytimes.com/2012/04/09/opinion/do-you-really-need-that-medical-test.html?_r=0. Accessed August 5, 2014.
81. GAO. Medicare Part B imaging services: Rapid spending growth and shift to physician offices indicate need for CMS to consider additional management practices. 2008. http://www.gao.gov/new.items/d08452.pdf. Accessed August 5, 2014.

CHAPTER 20

Physical Activity—
Is Sitting Death?

LEARNING OBJECTIVES

- Describe the data and trends in physical activity and inactivity in the United States and globally.
- Identify health risks associated with physical inactivity generally and sitting specifically.
- Discuss the cumulative health impact of physical inactivity in the United States and globally.
- Describe the health benefits of physical activity for children, adolescents, and adults.
- Identify barriers to physical activity in children, adolescents, and adults, and in different geographic areas and populations.
- Propose evidence-based practices that are effective in promoting and increasing physical activity in individuals and populations.

THE CONTROVERSY

"Don't just sit there. It may be killing you,"[1] warns a *USA Today* report about an epidemic of sedentary behavior in the United States termed the "sitting disease."[1] A Mayo Clinic expert reports that 34 chronic conditions, such as type 2 diabetes, heart disease, and stroke, are related to regular and prolonged sitting.[1] Most people in the United States sit for at least 8 hours per day, with more time spent sitting associated with increased risk of death from all causes, in a variety of scientific studies.[1-4] In addition, contrary to public perception, the relationship between sitting time and death risk is *independent* of the level of overall physical activity,[3,4] suggesting that even if people follow guidelines for daily physical activity, too much sitting is still a health risk.[2] The *Harvard Women's Health Watch* joins the chorus, warning of risks from too much computer use, couch-sitting, and TV watching.[5] Citing results of a 2014 study of 92,234 women followed for 12 years,[6] the study showed a relationship between time inactive and risk of death, no matter what age, race, or ethnicity; weight; or level of physical activity.[6]

The benefits of physical activity are well known, reducing risks from many chronic diseases, and helping people maintain a healthy weight.[7] The Centers for Disease Control and Prevention (CDC) notes that fewer than 50% of adults in the United States are following the currently recommendations for 150 minutes of moderate physical activity each week; this percentage is higher in older individuals and women.[7] In 2011, about 20% of U.S. adults met the 2008 recommendations for aerobic exercise and muscle strengthening activities,[8] and fewer than 30% of high school students are active for at least one hour per day.[9] One *Lancet* study estimates that more than 5.3 million of the 57 million deaths globally in 2008 were related to physical inactivity.[10,11] Furthermore, the World Health Organization (WHO) reports that globally nearly one-third (31%) of adults are not active enough.[12]

There are many reasons why adults say they can't exercise—too busy, too old, or hating the monotony,[13] but these factors may be modifiable obstacles for many people. Experts give many types of encouragement and practical advice about ways to get up and move more often, even for people who are older or who have disabilities.[1] Standing and treadmill desks are finding their way into workplace settings, and reminders to get up and walk around every hour are recommended by researchers in the field.[5] A systematic review even suggests that financial incentives, even modest ones, may increase exercise participation in adults, at least in the short term.[14] And to make it even easier, new phone apps can create these incentives: one website and iPhone application pays you if you keep your activity commitment and charges you if you don't.[15,16] Not so fast, argue some observers, calling a recent discussion of financial incentives for workers in the United Kingdom a "radical government strategy," while others simply call it "desperation."[17]

BACKGROUND AND SCOPE OF THE PUBLIC HEALTH AND HEALTH POLICY ISSUE

Health Benefits of Physical Activity

The CDC website has information about health benefits, data and statistics, and strategies to increase physical activity in individuals and populations.[18] Health benefits of regular physical activity include maintaining a healthy weight, improved mental acuity, reduced risk of depression, reduced age-related bone density loss, and reduced risks for chronic conditions, including cardiovascular disease, type 2 diabetes, and colon and breast cancers.[18]

In addition, regular physical activity reduces risks for premature death.[18] Moderate-intensity physical activity, such as walking, for a minimum of 150 minutes per week, can reduce risks for premature death. More active minutes per week are even better: individuals active for 7 hours per week have a 40% reduction in risk for premature death.[18] Exercise lengthens life and helps older individuals maintain optimal function.[19] Being more active improves the ability of the body to use insulin and regulate glucose and is recommended to help prevent type 2 diabetes.[20]

Physical activity, in structured programs, may prevent mobility disability in high-risk older individuals.[21] Evidence also supports these same health benefits in people with disabilities. CDC reports that of the 21 million adults in the United States with disabilities, nearly 50% have no aerobic physical activity, even though most are able to participate in some activity and would be much more likely to be active if it were recommended by their health professional.[22]

Epidemiology of Sedentary Behavior

The 2008 Physical Activity Guidelines for Americans (PAG) for children, adults, and older adults provide goals for all ages.[23] For example, the guidelines recommend 60 minutes or more of daily physical activity for children and adolescents and weekly recommendations for moderate or vigorous-intensity physical activity and muscle-strengthening activities for all adults and older adults.[23]

Only 48% of adults in the United States are achieving the recommended levels of physical activity, and less than 30% of adolescents are achieving daily physical activity goals.[9] Specifically among U.S. students in grades 9 through 12, in 2010, just over half (51%) met target for muscle-strengthening activity, and only 15.3% met the aerobic physical activity objective; only 12.2% met targets for both.[24] In 2011, 20.6% of adults overall met targets for both aerobic and muscle-strengthening physical activity, higher (30.7%) in younger (aged 18–24 years) adults.[8] Adults with higher education (27.4%) were more likely to be physically active and engage in muscle-strengthening activities.[8] The percentage of adults meeting guidelines for both aerobic and muscle-strengthening activities was higher in men (23.4%) than women (17.9%); fewer Hispanic adults (18.4%) than non-Hispanic black adults (21.2%) and non-Hispanic white adults (20.7%) met these targets.[8]

Detailed information about differences in physical activity levels in different states is gathered from the Behavioral Risk Factor Surveillance System (BRFSS), which highlights geographic variation in activity levels across the United States.[9] Physical *inactivity* levels are highest in southern states and parts of the Midwest in the United States (see **Figure 20–1**).[9]

Globally, the WHO reports that 31% of the world's adults are not active enough, with percentages varying across continents (see **Figure 20–2**).[12]

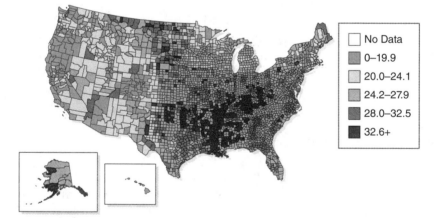

Figure 20–1 2010 age-adjusted estimates of the percentage of adults who are physically inactive.

Reproduced from Centers for Disease Control and Prevention. Physical Activity: Facts about Physical Activity. Available at http://www.cdc.gov/physicalactivity/data/facts.html

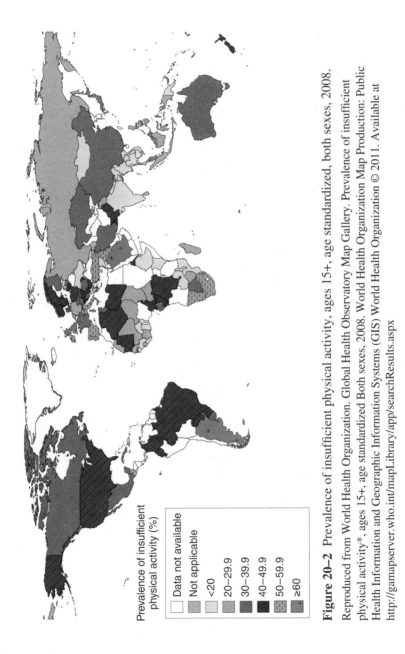

Figure 20–2 Prevalence of insufficient physical activity, ages 15+, age standardized, both sexes, 2008.

Reproduced from World Health Organization. Global Health Observatory Map Gallery. Prevalence of insufficient physical activity*, ages 15+, age standardized Both sexes, 2008. World Health Organization Map Production: Public Health Information and Geographic Information Systems (GIS) World Health Organization © 2011. Available at http://gamapserver.who.int/mapLibrary/app/searchResults.aspx

Lee and colleagues calculated that physical inactivity was responsible for about 9% of premature deaths (5.3 million of a total of 57 million) globally, in 2008.[10] They estimated that between 6% and 10% of chronic conditions, such as heart disease, breast and colon cancer, and type 2 diabetes, were related to physical inactivity.[10]

How Do Weight and Fitness Levels Compare as Health Risks?

Both obesity and cardiorespiratory fitness (CRF) have been reported to have independent effects on risk of death in the published literature.[25] For example, McGee and colleagues reported a meta-analysis of 26 studies evaluating the relationship between body mass index (BMI) and death.[26] Using well-established BMI categories from the National Institutes of Health and WHO, the authors studied 388,622 individuals overall, with gender, racial and ethnic diversity, and international representation. Taking into account the effects of age and smoking, the investigators found that obese individuals (BMI of 30 or higher) had a significantly higher risk of death, death from coronary heart disease (CHD), and cardiovascular disease (CVD), and a slightly increased risk of death from cancer.[26]

Kodama and colleagues studied the effect of CRF on death from all causes and from cardiovascular disease in an analysis of 33 published studies.[27] They found that individuals with low CRF (compared to those with high CRF) had a significantly higher risk of death from all causes (RR = 1.70) and also for combined cardiovascular diseases (RR = 1.56).[27] A retrospective study of women in Japan began with 510 students in 1943 followed successfully (98%) for 64 years.[28] Results showed that physical fitness during adolescence was associated with a reduced risk of death years later, both before age 50 and after age 70.[28]

Several studies try to tease apart the relationship between being overweight and fitness levels in risk for premature death. Pedersen's literature review concludes there is an independent association between physical fitness and deaths from all causes unrelated to BMI levels, and observed health benefits are greater with greater levels of physical fitness.[29] Fogelholm published a systematic review of 36 studies, comparing normal-weight but physically inactive individuals to obese but physically active individuals.[30] He found that obese but fit individuals had lower risks for death from all causes and also from cardiovascular disease than unfit individuals of normal weight. However, even fit individuals who were obese had higher risks for type 2 diabetes.[30]

A 2014 meta-analysis of 10 articles, by Barry and colleagues, empha-sized the effect of both CRF and BMI on risk of death.[25] The authors established five categories of combinations of fit and unfit (for CRF), and normal weight, overweight, and obese (based on BMI) and compared them to normal weight-fit individuals. They found that fitness was the driving factor for mortality risk rather than weight; unfit individuals had double the risk of death, no matter what weight category they were in. In addition, normal weight-fit, overweight-fit and obese-fit individuals all had similar risks of death.[25]

Why Too Much Sitting Is a Health Risk

A variety of studies illustrate associations between the amount of sedentary time and subsequent death; some of these relationships are independent of overall levels of moderate to vigorous physical activity (MVPA).[3,4,6,31–34] Researchers hypothesize that prolonged sitting may result in metabolic changes conducive to elevated risks for diabetes, cardiovascular diseases, and other chronic conditions.[35] Some researchers term the metabolic changes seen with prolonged sitting as the "inactivity physiology."[36]

Many studies investigating relationships between sitting and health out-comes differ in their methods, and whether or not self-reported information or objective measures of activity were used, such as using accelerometers.[37] A 2010 study used accelerometer data from nearly 2,000 individuals from the National Health and Nutrition Examination Survey (NHANES), and followed them for 2.8 years.[32] Those individuals with more sedentary time also had a statistically significant increased risk of death, after con-trolling for overall levels of MVPA, social, and demographic factors.[32] A cross-sectional study of NHANES data investigated possible associa-tions between MVPA, television viewing, and sedentary time on obesity.[38] MVPA showed the strongest inverse relationship to obesity, and differences as small as 5 to 10 minutes of physical activity were related to substantial differences in obesity risk.[38]

Matthews and colleagues studied 240,819 adults aged 50–71years for 8.5 years, using self-reported information.[33] Sedentary behavior was signifi-cantly associated with increased risk for death, after adjusting for a variety of factors, including MVPA. Increased sitting time was associated with increased risk of death from all causes.[33] More television viewing time was significantly associated with both cardiovascular deaths and deaths from all causes, even if these individuals also exercised frequently.[33] Katzmarzyk and colleagues prospectively studied 17,013 Canadians aged 18–90 years, finding a significant association with sitting time and risk of death from all causes and also from cardiovascular disease.[31] Importantly, these elevated risks were independent of overall physical activity levels. In this study, the risk of death increased as time spent sitting increased.[31]

A study of 222,497 Australian adults by van der Ploeg and colleagues, using self-reported information, found significant associations between sitting and deaths from all causes, in individuals sitting 8 or more hours per day.[3] Highest risks were observed in people sitting 11 hours or more per day, and all elevated risks independent of levels of overall physical activity.[3] Patel and colleagues reported increased risk of deaths with more time spent sitting in a prospective American Cancer Society study of 53,440 men and 69,776 women who were followed for 14 years.[4] In this study, sitting 6 or more hours per day compared to sitting less than 3 hours per day resulted in an increased risk of death (especially from cardiovascular disease) in both men and women, which was independent of level of physical activity.[4]

A 2013 study from the Women's Health Initiative (WHI) by Chomistek and colleagues examined associations of sitting and physical activity on the subsequent risk of cardiovascular disease.[34] In this study of more than 71,000 women ages 50 to 79 years, more daily sitting was an independent risk factor for developing cardiovascular disease. Risk for cardiovascular disease was significantly increased for women sitting 10 or more hours per day compared to those sitting 5 or fewer hours per day, and was highest in the women who were physically inactive and sat 10 or more hours per day.[34]

A 2014 study of older women by Seguin and colleagues, also from the WHI, evaluated the relationship of time spent being sedentary and deaths from all causes, as well as deaths from CVD, CHD, and cancer.[6] This study of 92,234 women lasted for 12 years. In their analysis, the investigators took into account the effects of age, race/ethnicity, BMI, overall physical activity, and existing chronic diseases, to try and determine the independent effect of time spent sedentary on risk for death.[6] The total amount of daily sedentary time was divided into four categories, from the least sedentary (4 or less hours per day) to the most sedentary (11 or more hours per day). Women who reported the most time spent sedentary had significantly increased risks of death from all causes, CHD, and cancer, and risks were higher with increasing levels of sedentary time.[6] What was especially important from this large and diverse study of older women was that the association of time spent sedentary and risk of death was independent of the level of physical activity or the presence of chronic conditions.[6]

EVIDENCE BASE FOR PREVENTION AND PRACTICE

Many authors suggest we can improve longevity by being more active and sitting less.[10,39,40] And in the United States, it is well-documented that as the weekly number of minutes of physical activity increases, whether at moderate or more intense levels, risk of premature death declines[41] (see **Figure 20–3**).

Lee and colleagues projected substantial global increases in life expectancy if physical activity was increased, averaging about 0.68 years, but ranging from 0.41 years to 0.95 years in different geographic regions[10] (see **Figure 20–4**).

In the United States, a life-table analysis evaluating the relationships between television viewing, sitting, and life expectancy, estimated that life expectancy in the United States could be increased by 2 years if sitting time decreased to less than 3 hours per day.[40] Further, life expectancy could be increased by 1.38 years if television viewing was reduced to under 2 hours per day.[40] However, this may be challenging in practice, as a 2014 report that described the epidemiology of sitting in nearly 6,000 U.S. adults, found that average self-reported sitting in men was 4.75 hours per day and 4.68 hours per day in women.[39] In the United States, hours sitting varied by age, by whether individuals were normal weight or overweight, by ethnicity, and by education level, but not between men and women.[39]

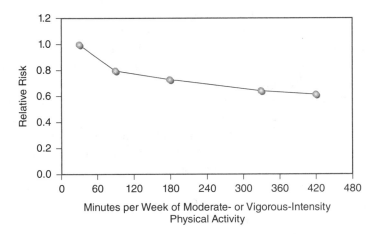

Figure 20–3 The risk of dying prematurely declines as people become physically active.

Reproduced from Health.gov: Office of Disease Prevention and Health Promotion. Available at http://www.health.gov/paguidelines/guidelines/chapter2.aspx

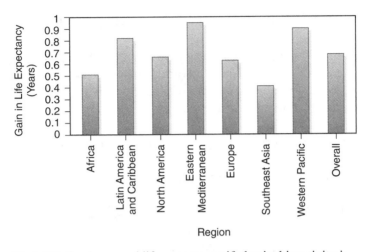

Figure 20–4 Median increased life expectancy if physical inactivity is eliminated, by WHO region, 2012.

Data from Lee IM, Shiroma EJ, Lobelo F, Puska P, Blair SN, Katzmarzyk PT. Effect of physical inactivity on major non-communicable diseases worldwide: an analysis of burden of disease and life expectancy. *The Lancet.* 2012;380(9838):219–229.

The U.S. Preventive Services Task Force and Community Preventive Services Task Force

The U.S. Preventive Services Task Force (USPSTF), an independent panel of experts in preventive and evidence-based medicine, reviews scientific evidence and publishes recommendations in a wide-range of clinical prevention areas.[42] For example, they make recommendations in areas of cancer screening, infectious diseases, mental health, and counseling in many areas, including behavioral risk factors for chronic conditions. Their focus is on clinical prevention and those services, tests, or interventions that might be used in a healthcare setting.[42] In 2014, they recommended intensive behavioral counseling in primary care settings for overweight or obese adults to reduce risks for CVD. These recommendations include both diet and physical activity—health behaviors related to CVD risk.[43,44]

Analogous to the USPSTF focus on individual patients, the Community Preventive Services Task Force (CPSTF) publishes "The Community Guide: What Works to Promote Health" to guide community-based prevention.[45] The CPSTF uses a systematic review process to review the scientific evidence for interventions that are effective in population-based settings.[45] In the area of physical activity, systematic reviews were conducted of three areas: behavioral and social approaches, campaigns and informational approaches, and environmental and policy approaches.[46] In the first area, the CPSTF recommends health behavior change programs for individuals (such as goal-setting and reinforcing positive behavior changes), community programs providing social support (such as creating groups for social support), and improved school-based physical education (such as using more active games).[46] Well-publicized, comprehensive, community-wide campaigns to increase physical activity are also recommended. In the area of environmental and policy approaches, based on a systematic review of the scientific evidence, several strategies were recommended.[46] Urban design and land-use changes that improve access to schools, recreation areas, stores, and improve "walkability" in communities (by improving safety, physical appearance, and availability of sidewalks) were all recommended.[46] Creating additional places to be active, such as walking and bicycle trails, and improving access to places to exercise were also recommended.[46] Evaluation of these approaches shows that such interventions are both effective and cost-effective, and represent practical public health approaches to increase physical activity.[47] Other systematic reviews are also available from the Cochrane database.[48]

Physical Activity: Role of the Built Environment

The potential positive role of environmental changes that make it easier to be physically active is being actively promoted; for example, CDC's emphasis on healthy community design.[49] Locating children's parks closer to their homes can result in increased use.[50] The Active Living Research initiative from the Robert Wood Johnson Foundation has contributed to increasing the scientific evidence, including environmental and policy strategies to increase physical activity in order to prevent obesity.[51,52]

One review emphasizes the critical role of "ecological models" in approaches to increase physical activity, recognizing the need for change at the level of the individual, social environment, built environment, and policies.[53] Physical activity can be characterized into categories: leisure-time physical activity, activity at school or work, activity related to transportation, and activity during household responsibilities, all outside of the realm of health care.[53] In children, adolescents, and adults, the availability of conveniently located recreation (i.e., places to be active) including walking and biking trails and parks increases physical activity.[54] Whether or not these locations are clean and well-designed may increase how often they are used.[53] How communities are designed and configured is also important. Whether or not there are sidewalks, protection from traffic, and whether schools, stores, and parks are located in walking distance, all may impact activity levels.[53]

Many national organizations have published recommendations for promoting the built environment and policies to increase physical activity, such as the American Academy of Pediatrics, American Heart Association, CDC, Institute of Medicine, and the White House Task Force on Childhood Obesity.[53] CDC recommends evidence-based strategies for individuals, worksites, and communities, for people of all ages[18] and their Healthy Community Design Initiative focuses on the built environment and health.[49] Many of their recommended areas are consistent with recommendations from the Community Guide[45] and emphasize the importance of making it easier for people to be active by modifying the surrounding physical environment.[49] Such strategies are especially important in communities with a high percentage of racial and ethnic minority populations and in communities where more families with less education or lower incomes are living. These neighborhoods are far less likely to have places available for outdoor or other recreation; traffic safety concerns and crime are also more common.[53,55,56]

Examples of successful community-based environment interventions to reduce obesity and/or improve physical fitness have been reported from Somerville, MA in the Shape Up Somerville intervention,[57] Healthy Living Cambridge Kids, in Cambridge, MA[58] and an intervention to increase biking, walking, and use of public transportation in Jackson, MI called Project U-Turn.[59]

Standing More and Sitting Less

Excessive sitting during the day, whether for prolonged periods at worksites, or even in schools, has resulted in new thinking about ways to reduce sedentary behavior. A feasibility study of adding standing desks to elementary schools in New Zealand found that both children and teachers supported their use, and using standing desks in classrooms resulted in more movement and standing.[60] A worksite intervention called Stand Up Australia used an approach that engaged workplace management, changed the physical environment (by adding adjustable height work stations), and coached individual employees; initial pilot testing supported workplace feasibility.[61] A controlled trial in adults (aged 20 to 65) engaged in desk occupations in three separate parts of the University of Queensland, Brisbane, Australia, found that the intervention successfully reduced workplace sitting.[62]

DISCUSSION QUESTIONS: TEMPLATE FOR DISCUSSION

1. Significance of this public health issue:
   a. Why is this health issue important?
   b. How many people does it impact?
   c. How serious is it?
   d. Is it preventable?
2. What is the evidence-base for prevention?
3. What specific strategies should be used to achieve progress on this health issue?
   a. What evidence-based approach would you use?
   b. Where would you start if you are an individual citizen; public health professional; healthcare professional; community, state, or federal policymaker?
4. Specific questions for this topic:
   a. What are the barriers to being physical active?
   b. How aware is the general public about the evidence for sedentary behavior (prolonged sitting) as an independent health risk?
   c. How can the importance of more physical activity as well as less sitting be communicated?
5. What is the controversy?
   a. Define the controversy.
   b. Is controversy a good or bad thing? (Does it help or hinder progress?)
6. *Why* is this health issue controversial?
   a. What specific factors are involved?
   b. Do economics, government, scientific uncertainty, or politics play a role?
   c. What is the role of the media?
7. How would you respond to the controversy?

PERSPECTIVES TO CONSIDER

The evidence for health risks from physical inactivity is compelling. Internationally, experts estimate that physical *inactivity* contributed to an estimated 5.3 million deaths in 2008.[10] Physical inactivity is far too common across diverse populations and geographic areas. The WHO estimates nearly one-third of adults globally are inactive,[12] and in the United States, less than one-half of all adults and one-third of adolescents are active enough.[9]

Importantly, the evidence for health benefits from physical activity in increasing longevity, reducing risks of deaths from chronic conditions, maintaining a healthy weight, and many other benefits is extensive.[18] Living a longer life is just one of a long list of health benefits.[10,40]

The relationships between obesity and physical activity as risk factors for premature death are complex, but important. Several investigators have found an independent role for fitness level and risk of premature death, no matter whether people were normal weight or obese,[25,29,30] reinforcing the life-saving potential of current physical activity recommendations, even though they are challenging to implement in practice.

Many studies, in different and diverse populations, have also tried to answer the question of whether sitting time, separate from total physical activity levels, is an independent risk for premature death. Some authors have found that not only is sitting an independent risk, but more sitting time was associated with higher risks in some studies.[3,4,6,31–34]

Literature about the health benefits of physical activity in normal weight, overweight, and obese individuals has important implications for public health and clinical practice. In addition, fitness aside, whether or not the general public is even aware that sitting for many hours on a daily basis is a health risk in its own right (independent of how active they are) is not known. This too, has implications for health care and public health practice, as stronger advice to individuals and entire populations must include specific messages about physical activity, fitness, and *less* sitting—important messages in comprehensive recommendations, educational initiatives, and advice to patients.

Available research has increased dramatically in areas of environmental and policy strategies to make entire communities places where it is easier to be active, but many barriers remain.[51,52] Many national and professional organizations are now emphasizing the important role of environmental and policy approaches in promoting physical activity at the community and population level,[53] complementing individual approaches.[44] One important point made in a review of the built environment[53] is that these approaches are largely out of the purview of healthcare professionals, but impact public health in a substantial way. Both public health and healthcare professionals have a critical role in advocating for such evidence-based approaches, promoting physical activity and improving the health of patients and populations.

For Additional Study

Gremeaux V, Gayda M, Lepers R, Sosner P, Juneau M, Nigam A. Exercise and longevity. *Maturitas.* 2012;73(4):312–317.

Baker PR, Francis DP, Soares J, Weightman AL, Foster C. Community wide interventions for increasing physical activity. *The Cochrane Database of Systematic Reviews.* 2011;(4):CD008366.

References

1. Hellmich N. Retirees: Sitting disease may be killing you. *USA Today.* 2014. http://www.usatoday.com/story/money/personalfinance/2014/07/19/retirement-sitting-disease/12750061/. Accessed August 14, 2014.
2. Woodham C. Are you sitting youself to death? *US News and World Report.* 2012. http://health.usnews.com/health-news/articles/2012/05/02/are-you-sitting-yourself-to-death. Accessed August 14, 2014.
3. van der Ploeg HP, Chey T, Korda RJ, Banks E, Bauman A. Sitting time and all-cause mortality risk in 222,497 Australian adults. *Arch Intern Med.* 2012;172(6):494–500.
4. Patel AV, Bernstein L, Deka A, et al. Leisure time spent sitting in relation to total mortality in a prospective cohort of US adults. *Am J Epidemiol.* 2010;172(4):419–429.
5. Watson S. Too much sitting linked to an early death. *Harvard Women's Health Watch* 2014. http://www.health.harvard.edu/blog/too-much-sitting-linked-to-an-early-death-201401297004. Accessed August 14, 2014.
6. Seguin R, Buchner DM, Liu J, et al. Sedentary behavior and mortality in older women: The women's health initiative. *Am J Prev Med.* 2014;46(2):122–135.
7. CDC. More people walk to better health. *CDC Vital Signs.* 2012. http://www.cdc.gov/vitalsigns/walking/index.html. Accessed August 14, 2014.
8. Adult participation in aerobic and muscle-strengthening physical activities—United States, 2011. *MMWR.* 2013;62(17):326–330.
9. CDC. Physical activity: Facts about physical activity. 2014. http://www.cdc.gov/physicalactivity/data/facts.html. Accessed August 14, 2014.
10. Lee IM, Shiroma EJ, Lobelo F, Puska P, Blair SN, Katzmarzyk PT. Effect of physical inactivity on major non-communicable diseases worldwide: An analysis of burden of disease and life expectancy. *Lancet.* 2012;380(9838):219–229.
11. Jaslow R. Inactivity tied to 5.3 million deaths worldwide, similar to smoking. *CBS News.* 2012. http://www.cbsnews.com/news/inactivity-tied-to-53-million-deaths-worldwide-similar-to-smoking/. Accessed August 14, 2014.
12. WHO. Global Health Observatory: Prevalence of insufficient physical activity. 2014. http://www.who.int/gho/ncd/risk_factors/physical_activity/en/. Accessed August 14, 2014.
13. Hobson K. 10 excuses for not exercising, and why they won't fly. *U.S. News.* 2009. http://health.usnews.com/health-news/diet-fitness/fitness/slideshows/fitness-excuses/2. Accessed August 5, 2014.
14. Mitchell MS, Goodman JM, Alter DA, et al. Financial incentives for exercise adherence in adults: Systematic review and meta-analysis. *Am J Prev Med.* 2013;45(5):658–667.

15. Kristof K. How to get paid to exercise *CBS News*. 2012. http://www.cbsnews.com/news/how-to-get-paid-to-exercise/. Accessed August 14, 2014.

16. Almendrala A. Does getting paid to exercise work? This app says yes. *The Huffington Post*. 2014. http://www.huffingtonpost.com/2014/05/08/paid-to-exercise_n_5283708.html. Accessed August 14, 2014.

17. Smith R. Obesity crisis: Get paid to lost weight. *The Telegraph*. 2008. http://www.telegraph.co.uk/news/uknews/1576430/Obesity-crisis-get-paid-to-lose-weight.html. Accessed August 14, 2014.

18. CDC. Physical activity. 2014. http://www.cdc.gov/physicalactivity/index.html. Accessed August 14, 2014.

19. Gremeaux V, Gayda M, Lepers R, Sosner P, Juneau M, Nigam A. Exercise and longevity. *Maturitas*. 2012;73(4):312–317.

20. HSPH. Simple steps to preventing diabetes. *The Nutrition Source*. 2014. http://www.hsph.harvard.edu/nutritionsource/preventing-diabetes-full-story/. Accessed August 14, 2014.

21. Pahor M, Guralnik JM, Ambrosius WT, et al. Effect of structured physical activity on prevention of major mobility disability in older adults: The LIFE study randomized clinical trial. *JAMA*. 2014;311(23):2387–2396.

22. CDC. Adults with disabilities. *CDC Vital Signs*. 2014. http://www.cdc.gov/vitalsigns/disabilities/. Accessed August 14, 2014.

23. CDC. Physical activity: How much physical activity do you need? 2011. http://www.cdc.gov/physicalactivity/everyone/guidelines/index.html. Accessed August 14, 2014.

24. Physical activity levels of high school students—United States, 2010. *MMWR*. 2011;60(23):773–777.

25. Barry VW, Baruth M, Beets MW, Durstine JL, Liu J, Blair SN. Fitness vs. fatness on all-cause mortality: A meta-analysis. *Prog Cardiovasc Dis*. 2014;56(4):382–390.

26. McGee DL, Diverse Populations, Collaboration. Body mass index and mortality: A meta-analysis based on person-level data from twenty-six observational studies. *Ann Epidemiol*. 2005;15(2):87–97.

27. Kodama S, Saito K, Tanaka S, et al. Cardiorespiratory fitness as a quantitative predictor of all-cause mortality and cardiovascular events in healthy men and women: A meta-analysis. *JAMA*. 2009;301(19):2024–2035.

28. Sato M, Kodama S, Sugawara A, Saito K, Sone H. Physical fitness during adolescence and adult mortality. *Epidemiology*. 2009;20(3):463–464.

29. Pedersen BK. Body mass index-independent effect of fitness and physical activity for all-cause mortality. *Scand J Med Sci Sports*. 2007;17(3):196–204.

30. Fogelholm M. Physical activity, fitness and fatness: Relations to mortality, morbidity and disease risk factors. A systematic review. *Obesity Rev*. 2010;11(3):202–221.

31. Katzmarzyk PT, Church TS, Craig CL, Bouchard C. Sitting time and mortality from all causes, cardiovascular disease, and cancer. *Med Sci Sports Exercise*. 2009;41(5):998–1005.

32. Koster A, Caserotti P, Patel KV, et al. Association of sedentary time with mortality independent of moderate to vigorous physical activity. *PLoS One*. 2012;7(6):e37696.

33. Matthews CE, George SM, Moore SC, et al. Amount of time spent in sedentary behaviors and cause-specific mortality in US adults. *Am J Clin Nutr*. 2012;95(2):437–445.

34. Chomistek AK, Manson JE, Stefanick ML, et al. Relationship of sedentary behavior and physical activity to incident cardiovascular disease. *J Am Col Cardiol*. 2013;61(23):2346–2354.

35. HSPH. Staying active. *The Nutrition Source.* 2014. http://www.hsph.harvard.edu/nutritionsource/staying-active/. Accessed August 14, 2014.

36. Raynor HA, Bond DS, Freedson PS, Sisson SB. Sedentary behaviors, weight, and health and disease risks. *J Obesity.* 2012;2012:852743. http://www.ncbi.nlm.nih.gov/pmc/articles/PMC3236513/. Accessed August 5, 2014.

37. Kavanagh JJ, Menz HB. Accelerometry: A technique for quantifying movement patterns during walking. *Gait & Post.* 2008;28(1):1–15.

38. Maher CA, Mire E, Harrington DM, Staiano AE, Katzmarzyk PT. The independent and combined associations of physical activity and sedentary behavior with obesity in adults: NHANES 2003–2006. *Obesity.* 2013;21(12):E730–E737.

39. Harrington DM, Barreira TV, Staiano AE, Katzmarzyk PT. The descriptive epidemiology of sitting among US adults, NHANES 2009–2010. *J Sci Med Sport/Sports Med Australia.* 2014;17(4):371–375.

40. Katzmarzyk PT, Lee IM. Sedentary behaviour and life expectancy in the USA: A cause-deleted life table analysis. *BMJ Open.* 2012;2(4):e000828. http://www.ncbi.nlm.nih.gov/pmc/articles/PMC3400064/. Accessed August 5, 2014.

41. DHHS. Physical activity guidelines: chapter 2: Physical activity has many health benefits. 2008. http://www.health.gov/paguidelines/guidelines/chapter2.aspx. Accessed August 26, 2014.

42. USPSTF. U.S. Preventive Services Task Force. 2014. http://www.uspreventiveservicestaskforce.org/. Accessed January 31, 2014.

43. Campbell J, Li A. USPSTF recommends behavioral counseling to reduce cardiovascular disease *2 minute medicine.* 2014. http://www.2minutemedicine.com/uspstf-recommends-behavioral-counseling-to-reduce-cardiovascular-disease/. Accessed August 14, 2014.

44. LeFevre ML, USPSTF. Behavioral counseling to promote a healthful diet and physical activity for cardiovascular disease prevention in adults with cardiovascular risk factors: U.S. Preventive Services Task Force recommendation statement. *Ann Intern Med.* 2014;161(8):587–593.

45. The Community Guide: What works to promote health. 2014. http://www.thecommunityguide.org/index.html. Accessed January 31, 2014.

46. The Community Guide: Increasing physical activity. *The Community Guide: What works to promote health.* 2013. http://www.thecommunityguide.org/pa/index.html. Accessed August 14, 2014.

47. Roux L, Pratt M, Tengs TO, et al. Cost effectiveness of community-based physical activity interventions. *Am J Prev Med.* 2008;35(6):578–588.

48. Baker PR, Francis DP, Soares J, Weightman AL, Foster C. Community wide interventions for increasing physical activity. *Cochrane Database Syst Rev.* 2011(4): CD008366.

49. CDC. Designing and building healthy places. 2014. http://www.cdc.gov/healthyplaces/. Accessed August 14, 2014.

50. Dunton GF, Almanza E, Jerrett M, Wolch J, Pentz MA. Neighborhood park use by children: Use of accelerometry and global positioning systems. *Am J Prev Med.* 2014;46(2):136–142.

51. Sallis JF, Cutter CL, Lou D, et al. Active living research: Creating and using evidence to support childhood obesity prevention. *Am J Prev Med.* 2014;46(2):195–207.

52. Barker DC, Gutman MA. Evaluation of active living research: Ten years of progress in building a new field. *Am J Prev Med.* 2014;46(2):208–215.

53. Sallis JF, Floyd MF, Rodriguez DA, Saelens BE. Role of built environments in physical activity, obesity, and cardiovascular disease. *Circulation.* 2012;125(5):729–737.

54. Ding D, Sallis JF, Kerr J, Lee S, Rosenberg DE. Neighborhood environment and physical activity among youth a review. *Am J Prev Med.* 2011;41(4):442–455.

55. Sallis JF, Slymen DJ, Conway TL, et al. Income disparities in perceived neighborhood built and social environment attributes. *Health & Place.* 2011;17(6):1274–1283.

56. Gordon-Larsen P, Nelson MC, Page P, Popkin BM. Inequality in the built environment underlies key health disparities in physical activity and obesity. *Pediatrics.* 2006;117(2):417–424.

57. Economos CD, Hyatt RR, Goldberg JP, et al. A community intervention reduces BMI z-score in children: Shape Up Somerville first year results. *Obesity.* 2007;15(5): 1325–1336.

58. Chomitz VR, McGowan RJ, Wendel JM, et al. Healthy living Cambridge kids: A community-based participatory effort to promote healthy weight and fitness. *Obesity.* 2010;18(Suppl 1):S45–S53.

59. TenBrink DS, McMunn R, Panken S. Project U-Turn: Increasing active transportation in Jackson, Michigan. *Am J Prev Med.* 2009;37(6 Suppl 2):S329–S335.

60. Hinckson EA, Aminian S, Ikeda E, et al. Acceptability of standing workstations in elementary schools: A pilot study. *Preven Med.* 2013;56(1):82–85.

61. Neuhaus M, Healy GN, Fjeldsoe BS, et al. Iterative development of Stand Up Australia: A multi-component intervention to reduce workplace sitting. *Int J Behav Nutr Phys Act.* 2014;11(1):21.

62. Neuhaus M, Healy GN, Dunstan DW, Owen N, Eakin EG. Workplace sitting and height-adjustable workstations: A randomized controlled trial. *Am J Prev Med.* 2014; 46(1):30–40.

Index

Note: Page numbers followed by *f* and *t* indicate material in figures and tables respectively.